Instructional Course Lectures

Volume XL 1991

American Academy
of Orthopaedic Surgeons

Instructional Course Lectures

Volume XL 1991

Edited by
Hugh S. Tullos, MD
Head, Division of Orthopaedic Surgery
Baylor College of Medicine
Houston, Texas

With 219 illustrations

American Academy
of Orthopaedic Surgeons

American Academy of Orthopaedic Surgeons

Instructional Course Lectures
Volume XL

Director of Communications and Publications: Mark W. Wieting
Assistant Director, Publications: Marilyn L. Fox, PhD
Senior Editor: Wendy O. Schmidt
Medical Editor: Bruce A. Davis
Editorial Assistant: Monica M. Trocker

Design: James Buddenbaum Design, Wilmette, Illinois
Typesetting: Impressions, Inc., Madison, Wisconsin
Printing: Mack Printing Company, Easton, Pennsylvania
Binding: Zonne Bookbinders, Chicago, Illinois
Stock: Acid-free Somerset

International Standard Book Number 0-89203-043-7

Library of Congress Catalog Card Number 43-17054

Contributors

Steven P. Arnoczky, DVM, Director, Laboratory for Comparative Orthopaedic Research, The Hospital for Special Surgery, New York, New York

Robert L. Buly, MD, MS, Fellow in Hip Surgery, Maurice E. Müller Foundation, Bern, Switzerland

E. Brantley Burns, MD, Orthopaedic Surgeon, Knoxville, Tennessee

John J. Callaghan, MD, Associate Professor, Department of Orthopaedics, University of Iowa Hospital and Clinics, Iowa City, Iowa

John C. Chae, MD, Research Assistant, Dartmouth Biomedical Engineering Center, Hanover, New Hampshire

John P. Collier, DE, Director, Thayer School of Engineering, Dartmouth College, Hanover, New Hampshire

Dennis K. Collis, MD, Clinical Instructor, Department of Orthopaedics, University of Oregon Health Sciences Center, Portland, Oregon

Ralph W. Coonrad, MD, Associate Clinical Professor, Duke University, Durham, North Carolina

Daniel E. Cooper, MD, Clinical Instructor, Department of Orthopaedics, University of Texas Health Science Center, Dallas, Texas

Les A. Dauphinais, Research Assistant, Dartmouth Biomedical Engineering Center, Hanover, New Hampshire

Jeffrey P. Davies, MS, Research and Design Engineer, Orthopaedic Biomechanics Laboratory, Massachusetts General Hospital, Boston, Massachusetts

Luciano S. Dias, MD, Associate Professor, Department of Orthopaedic Surgery, Northwestern University Medical School, Chicago, Illinois

Anthony M. DiGioia III, MD, Senior Resident, Department of Orthopaedic Surgery, University of Pittsburgh, Pittsburgh, Pennsylvania

James C. Drennan, MD, Professor, Department of Orthopaedics, University of New Mexico School of Medicine, Albuquerque, New Mexico

Charles A. Engh, MD, Clinical Assistant Professor of Orthopaedic Surgery, Georgetown University, Washington, DC

Harry E. Figgie III, MD, Assistant Professor of Orthopaedics and of Biomechanics, Case Western Reserve University School of Medicine, Cleveland, Ohio

Mark P. Figgie, MD, Instructor in Surgery, Cornell University Medical College, New York, New York

M. A. R. Freeman, MD, FRCS, Senior Consultant Orthopaedic Surgeon, The London Hospital Medical College, London, England

Andrew H. Glassman, MD, Chief, Department of Orthopaedic Surgery, The National Hospital for Orthopaedics and Rehabilitation, Arlington, Virginia

Victor M. Goldberg, MD, Professor and Chairman, Department of Orthopaedics, Case Western Reserve University, Cleveland, Ohio

Scott R. Grewe, MD, Sports Medicine Director, Portland Orthopedic Clinic, P.C., Portland, Oregon

William H. Harris, MD, Chief, Hip and Implant Service, Massachusetts General Hospital, Boston, Massachusetts

Thomas Huddleston, MD, Fellow, Joint Replacement Service, University of Pittsburgh, Pittsburgh, Pennsylvania

Michael H. Huo, MD, Department of Orthopaedic Surgery, Georgetown University Medical Center, Washington, DC

Allan E. Inglis, MD, Professor of Clinical Surgery, Professor of Anatomy in Cell Biology and Anatomy, Cornell University Medical College, The Hospital for Special Surgery, New York, New York

Murali Jasty, MD, Assistant Clinical Professor in Orthopaedics, Harvard Medical School, Boston, Massachusetts

Robert E. Jensen, MS, Research Assistant, Dartmouth Biomedical Engineering Center, Hanover, New Hampshire

Frank W. Jobe, MD, Clinical Professor, Department of Orthopaedics, University of Southern California School of Medicine, Los Angeles, California

Jesse B. Jupiter, MD, Assistant Professor of Orthopaedic Surgery, Harvard Medical School, Boston, Massachusetts

Matthew J. Kraay, MD, University Hospitals of Cleveland, Case Western Reserve School of Medicine, Cleveland, Ohio

Ronald S. Kvitne, MD, Assistant Clinical Professor, Department of Orthopaedics, University of Southern California, Los Angeles, California

Glenn C. Landon, MD, Assistant Professor, Division of Orthopaedic Surgery, Baylor College of Medicine, Houston, Texas

Richard E. Lindseth, MD, Professor and Vice Chairman, Department of Orthopaedic Surgery, Indiana University School of Medicine, Indianapolis, Indiana

Michael B. Mayor, MD, Assistant Professor Clinical Surgery, Director of Orthopaedic Research, Dartmouth-Hitchcock Medical Center, Hanover, New Hampshire

John R. Moreland, MD, Assistant Clinical Professor of Orthopedics, UCLA School of Medicine, Los Angeles, California

Bernard F. Morrey, MD, Chairman, Department of Orthopedics, Mayo Clinic, Rochester, Minnesota

Philip C. Noble, MS, Research Associate Professor, Division of Orthopaedic Surgery, Baylor College of Medicine, Houston, Texas

Frank R. Noyes, MD, Clinical Professor, Department of Orthopaedic Surgery, University of Cincinnati, Cincinnati, Ohio

Lonnie E. Paulos, MD, Associate Clinical Professor, University of Utah School of Medicine, Salt Lake City, Utah

Harry E. Rubash, MD, Assistant Professor of Orthopaedic Surgery, University of Pittsburgh, Pittsburgh, Pennsylvania

Eduardo A. Salvati, MD, Professor of Clinical Surgery (Orthopaedics), The Hospital for Special Surgery and New York Hospital, New York, New York

Sonya Shortkroff, MS, Research Associate, The Brigham and Women's Hospital, Boston, Massachusetts

Clement B. Sledge, MD, John B. Buckminster Brown Professor, Orthopaedic Surgery, Harvard Medical School, Boston, Massachusetts

Myron Spector, PhD, Director of Orthopedic Research, The Brigham and Women's Hospital, Harvard Medical School, Boston, Massachusetts

Helene P. Surprenant, Research Assistant, Dartmouth Biomedical Engineering Center, Hanover, New Hampshire

Victor A. Surprenant, BA, Research Assistant, Dartmouth Biomedical Engineering Center, Hanover, New Hampshire

Robert E. Tennant, MD, Orthopaedic Surgeon, St. Vincent's Hospital, Portland, Oregon

Thomas S. Thornhill, MD, Associate Professor of Orthopedic Surgery, The Brigham and Women's Hospital, Harvard Medical School, Boston, Massachusetts

Hugh S. Tullos, MD, Head, Division of Orthopaedic Surgery, Baylor College of Medicine, Houston, Texas

Jon J. P. Warner, MD, Assistant Professor of Orthopaedic Surgery, Center for Sports Medicine and Rehabilitation, University of Pittsburgh, Pittsburgh, Pennsylvania

Russell F. Warren, MD, Professor of Orthopaedic Surgery, Cornell University Medical College, New York, New York

Andrew J. Weiland, MD, Surgeon-in-Chief, The Hospital for Special Surgery, Cornell University Medical Center, New York, New York

Kaye E. Wilkins, MD, Clinical Professor of Orthopaedics and Pediatrics, University of Texas Health Science Center at San Antonio, San Antonio, Texas

Edward M. Wojtys, MD, Assistant Professor, Department of Surgery, University of Michigan, Ann Arbor, Michigan

Phillip E. Wright II, MD, Associate Professor of Orthopaedic Surgery, University of Tennessee, Memphis, Tennessee

Preface

This 40th volume of the *Instructional Course Lectures* series reflects the continuing commitment of the American Academy of Orthopaedic Surgeons to postgraduate education. As in the preceding volumes, the lectures selected for publication were chosen to provide in-depth coverage in areas that have not been included in recent volumes and those that would contribute best to the continuity of this volume. This selection process ensures that many fine manuscripts remain for publication in succeeding volumes.

This volume also includes a cumulative index to volumes 26 through 40 of the *Instructional Course Lectures*. The index lists the names of all contributors to those volumes and serves as a detailed guide to all topics covered in those 15 volumes. An index for this series has not been published since 1977, when it appeared as a separate volume. The Academy's Committee on Publications, in response to comments from recent purchasers of the *Lectures*, decided to provide the index to readers as a service and to include it with volume 40.

As chairman in 1990 of the Instructional Course Committee, I am indebted to Newton C. McCollough III, MD, past president of the American Academy of Orthopaedic Surgeons, for the opportunity to participate in the Instructional Course Committee.

Finally, the primary credit for this volume should be directed to the Academy members who participated in the 1990 Instructional Course Lectures in New Orleans, and who then provided the manuscripts for this volume; to the membership, who endorse the lectures; and to the Academy's publications staff, who do the editorial and production work. In particular, I would like to thank Bruce A. Davis, medical editor, who served as project manager and principal editor of the copy; Monica M. Trocker, editorial assistant, who coordinated the permissions and manuscript processing and review; Wendy O. Schmidt, senior editor, who reviewed copy and layout and indexed this volume as well as the 15 volumes in the cumulative index; and Lee Lambos, secretary, who assisted with word processing. Marilyn L. Fox, PhD, assistant director, publications, assisted in the overall development and production process, and Mark W. Wieting, director, communications and publications, provided general oversight of the entire project.

Hugh S. Tullos, MD
Houston, Texas
Chairman
Committee on Instructional Courses

Joseph S. Barr, Jr, MD
Boston, Massachusetts

Robert E. Eilert, MD
Denver, Colorado

Walter B. Greene, MD
Chapel Hill, North Carolina

James D. Heckman, MD
San Antonio, Texas

Contents

The Elbow

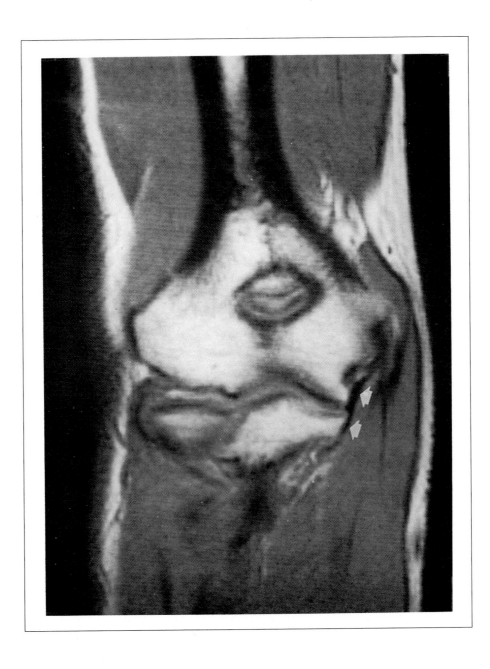

Fractures of the Medial Epicondyle in Children

Kaye E. Wilkins, MD

Most concern regarding elbow injuries in children focuses on the most common injury, the supracondylar fracture, which can produce either a compartment syndrome or the cosmetically unattractive cubitus varus deformity. The literature also describes intra-articular fractures of the lateral condylar physis and/or epiphysis, which if improperly treated can produce a significant functional disability. Little attention, however, is given to fractures of the medial epicondyle, because these injuries involve only a small bony prominence that is not part of the articular surface and does not contribute significantly to the growth of the distal humerus. It is important, however, to have a clear picture of the overall contribution of this epicondyle to elbow function. This knowledge allows the treating surgeon to determine a proper plan of management when a medial epicondyle fracture occurs, either as an isolated fracture or as part of a more extensive elbow injury.

Anatomic Considerations

The medial epicondyle is a true apophysis and serves as the origin of the pronator teres and common flexors of the wrist. In infants it is a part of the common distal humeral epiphysis (Fig. 1). As the child's distal humerus grows, the medial epicondyle becomes an isolated apophysis separated from the distal epiphysis by a metaphyseal bridge (Fig. 2). This metaphyseal bridge serves as the origin of the ulnar collateral ligaments. The medial capsule of the elbow joint is lateral to this collateral ligament origin. Thus, an isolated injury to this apophysis is both extra-articular and extracapsular.

One aspect of the anatomy of the medial epicondyle not often appreciated is that it is on the posterior aspect of the distal humerus. This is important when it is used as a landmark for percutaneous fixation of supracondylar fractures. It is also important to recognize this fact when interpreting radiographs of the distal humerus in young children. Because it is posterior, the edge of the medial humeral metaphysis overlies this epicondylar ossification center. This can produce a double density, which can be misinterpreted as a fracture through the apophysis (Fig. 3).

In small children, this apophysis is unossified. Ossification begins at 4 to 6 years of age. The medial epicondyle is the final ossification center to join the distal humerus, fusing with it at approximately 15 years of age.[1,2] This delayed fusion accounts for the increased

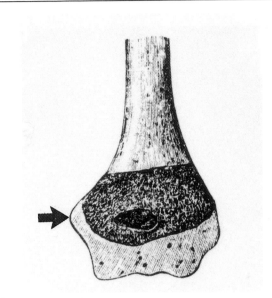

Fig. 1 In the very young child, the medial epicondyle (arrow) is included with the common distal humeral epiphysis.

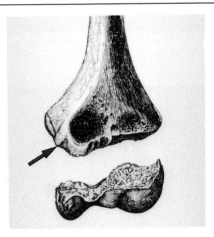

Fig. 2 In older children, there is a bridge of metaphyseal bone (arrow) between the distal humeral epiphysis and the medial epicondyle. (From Poland J: *A Practical Treatise on Traumatic Separation of the Epiphyses.* London, Smith-Elder, 1889.)

incidence of medial epicondylar fractures in adolescents.

The key to elbow stability—the ulnar collateral ligament—is composed of three bands: anterior, posterior, and oblique. The anterior band is composed of an anterior portion, which is taut in extension, and a pos-

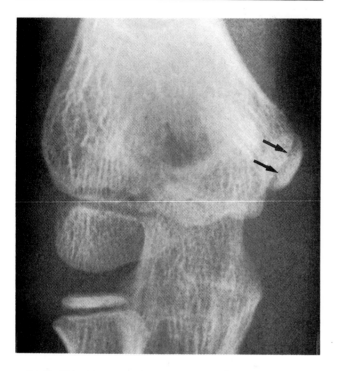

Fig. 3 The posterior location of the medial epicondyle allows it to be overlapped by the metaphyseal margin. This can create a double density (arrows) that may be misinterpreted as a fracture line (pseudofracture).

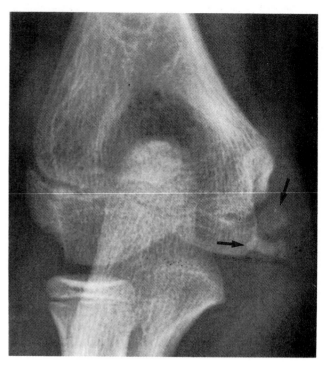

Fig. 4 Fragmentation of the medial epicondyle (arrows) caused by a direct blow.

terior portion, which, along with the posterior band, is taut in flexion. Thus, the anterior portion of the anterior band is the major stabilizing force when the elbow is in extension and is more vulnerable to injury.[3] In flexion, both the posterior portion of the anterior band and the posterior band provide stability. The third band of the ulnar collateral ligament, the oblique band, attaches only to the olecranon process of the ulna and thus does not contribute to elbow stability.

Incidence

In the overall incidence of fractures in the elbow region, fractures involving the medial epicondyle constitute 14.1% of the fractures involving only the distal humerus and 11.5% of all fractures that occur on both sides of the elbow joint.[4] Medial epicondyle fractures are most commonly associated with dislocation of the elbow. Information regarding the overall incidence of this injury is included in the extensive review of elbow injuries by Marion and associates.[5] In their series, 34.8% of the medial epicondyle fractures were associated with pure uncomplicated elbow dislocations. Another 14% involved complicated elbow dislocations, in which the fragment was incarcerated in the joint. Thus, the overall incidence with all elbow dislocations was 56.8%. Because of its high association with elbow dis-

locations, the medial epicondyle fracture often occurs during the second decade. Peak ages are 9 to 12 years.[4]

Mechanism of Injury

This injury can occur as the result of one of three mechanisms: direct blow, pure avulsion, or in association with an elbow dislocation.

Direct Blow

This is probably the rarest mechanism for this injury. There has been only one case report, by Watson-Jones,[6] in which this mechanism was definitely proven. I have had one case in which a direct blow produced comminution of the epicondylar fragment with very little displacement (Fig. 4).

Pure Avulsion

This is probably the second most common mechanism of injury. The individual falls on the outstretched hand, forcing it into dorsiflexion. This, plus the normal valgus angulation of the elbow, places a tension force on the flexor muscles. The weakest area—the epicondylar apophysis—fails first. This fracture can be associated with other ipsilateral injuries, such as greenstick fracture of the olecranon or fracture of the radial neck. Avulsion injuries can also occur from the extreme muscle forces that develop with throwing in adolescent baseball pitchers (Fig. 5).

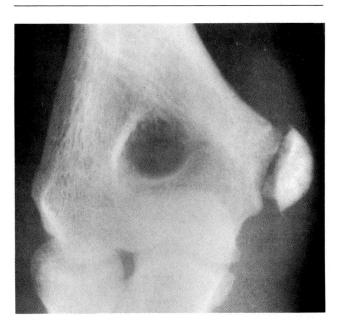

Fig. 5 Avulsion of the medial epicondyle sustained in the act of pitching by a 15-year-old athlete.

Association With Elbow Dislocation

This is the most common mechanism. This is a true avulsion injury, but it is complicated by the associated elbow dislocation. In many cases, the elbow dislocation reduces spontaneously. With these injuries, there is a risk that the fragment will become incarcerated within the joint. In addition, there is usually injury to the lateral collateral ligaments.[1,7] There can also be greater loss of elbow motion with these injuries because of the trauma to the capsule and collateral ligaments.

Classification

In Outline 1, I have combined the classifications of others[5,7–9] to create a more comprehensive classification that can serve as a basis for treatment. Fracture patterns are determined by the clinical findings, the history, and the radiographic findings.

Treatment

Most medial epicondyle fractures can be managed without surgery. The decision to use surgical intervention is not based on the amount of displacement alone. Other factors must be considered in determining the appropriate treatment. These factors will be discussed as we review the treatment of the various types of this fracture.

Acute Injuries With Minimal or No Displacement

There is usually very little argument for surgical management of these injuries. Such injuries are usually im-

Outline 1
Medial epicondyle fracture classification

Acute injuries
  Undisplaced
  Minimally displaced
  Significantly displaced
    Elbow not dislocated
    Elbow dislocated
  Entrapment of fragment in joint
    Elbow not dislocated
    Elbow dislocated
  Fractures through the epicondylar apophysis
    Without displacement
    With displacement
Chronic tension stress injuries
  (Little League elbow syndrome)

mobilized for a brief period of time with a temporary splint, and motion is initiated early. The major long-term problem with these injuries is elbow stiffness. Motion, under controlled conditions, should be begun after three or four days. The splint is removed early to allow active motion. Once the swelling and tenderness have decreased significantly, the splint can be removed and replaced by a simple sling. Passive motion or physical therapy is usually not indicated unless it is designed to strengthen the forearm flexor and extensor muscles and the muscles about the shoulder in older athletes.

Acute Injuries With Significant Displacement

There are articles in the literature supporting both surgical and nonsurgical treatment. The best argument for nonsurgical management is found in the review by Josefsson and Danielsson,[10] who examined 56 patients treated without surgery. At an average of 35 years after injury, 31 had developed pseudarthrosis, but the function and range of motion were good in all cases. In Oklahoma, where the practice was to surgically repair all fractures displaced more than 2 mm, Hines and associates[11] found that the majority of their patients had a good range of motion and stability with no neurologic symptoms.

Clinical judgment, however, plays an important role in deciding whether or not to operate. In athletes, who need a stable elbow, Woods and Tullos[3] found that minor degrees of valgus instability can produce disability during high-performance activities. They used a simple gravity stress test to determine if the elbow was unstable and required surgical intervention (Fig. 6). Any significant displacement of the fragment with gravity alone was taken as an indication that it should be stabilized surgically. I believe that the activity of the patient is more important than the extent of displacement as an indication for surgical intervention. If the injury is to the dominant extremity in an athlete who throws baseballs or footballs, in which a significant valgus stress is applied to the extremity, there is no question that the fragment must be replaced anatomically by an open

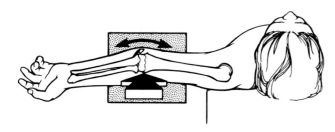

Fig. 6 The gravity stress test: The position of the elbow and the radiographs for performing the valgus stress examination. The elbow must be flexed about 15 degrees. (Redrawn with permission from Schwab GH, Bennet JB, Woods GW, et al: Biomechanics of elbow instability: The role of the medial collateral ligament. *Clin Orthop* 1980;146:42–52.)

reduction. The same is true for either extremity in a gymnast or wrestler. An injury, however, to the non-dominant extremity in an individual who leads a sedentary life can probably be best treated nonsurgically even though the epicondyle is significantly displaced.

After closed treatment, motion should be initiated early, with immobilization being kept to a minimum whatever the degree of displacement (Fig. 7). Two other factors must be kept in mind in determining whether surgery can be avoided. First, it must be established that the fragment is not incarcerated in the joint. If the fragment is at the level of the joint, it is probably safest to assume that it is in the joint until proven otherwise. This can usually be determined by the freedom of motion of the elbow, especially if a dislocation has been reduced. If there is free smooth motion, the fragment is probably not incarcerated in the joint. If it is difficult to obtain any motion whatsoever, then other methods, such as an arthrogram, can be used to locate accurately the position of the fragment. Second, the function of the ulnar nerve must be carefully assessed. Minor paresthesias or small sensory deficits usually subside rapidly. If, however, there is motor dysfunction, the fracture must be explored surgically to be sure that the ulnar nerve is not impinging on the fracture site or the joint itself.

If the epicondyle requires surgical stabilization, fixation should be sufficient to allow early active motion. Fortunately, the fragment is usually large enough to be stabilized with a small cancellous screw in which interfragmentary compression can be applied (Fig. 8). Stabilization allows the patient to begin motion as soon as the incision is adequately healed. Kirschner wires or small Steinmann pins should be avoided because often more than one must be used to stabilize the fragment. Even if they are cut off under the skin, they

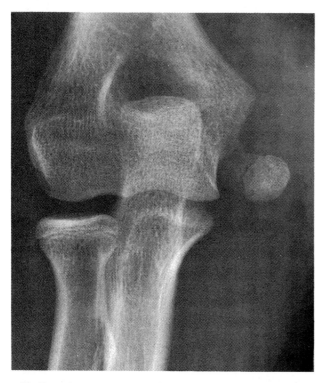 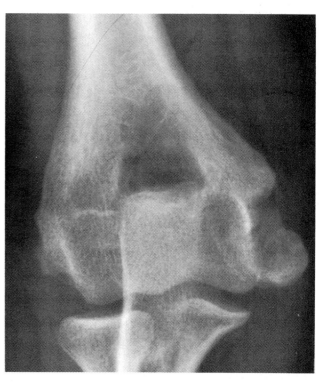

Fig. 7 Left, The position of the medial epicondyle after reduction of a dislocated elbow in the nondominant extremity of a 13-year-old girl. **Right,** The position of the fragment 18 months after injury. This patient had a full range of motion and was completely asymptomatic.

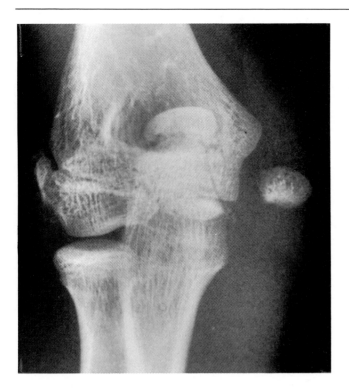 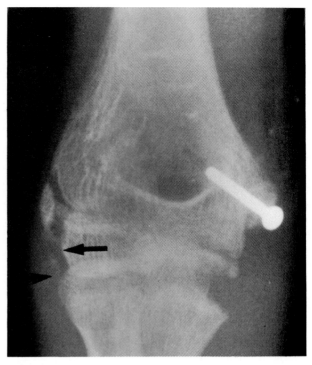

Fig. 8 **Left**, The displacement of the medial epicondyle in a 12-year-old female gymnast who sustained an acute injury to her dominant upper extremity. **Right**, Four weeks after the injury, there is evidence of calcification of the lateral collateral ligaments (arrows), indicating that there was probably a partial dislocation of the elbow as part of this injury. The medial epicondyle was secured with a single screw.

protrude far enough to cause irritation and inhibit active motion.

Early Incarceration in the Joint

Early incarceration of the fracture fragment into the joint is almost always associated with elbow dislocation. Often the fragment appears to be incarcerated in the joint when the elbow is dislocated, only to become extruded from the joint when the elbow is reduced. If, however, after a reduction, the fragment is at the level of the joint, if there is lack of smooth motion, or if the joint space appears widened, then the fragment must be considered to be incarcerated in the joint (Fig. 9).

Once it has been determined that the fragment is incarcerated in the joint, the question arises as to whether it can be extracted adequately from the joint without surgery. In 1934, Roberts[12] reported successful manipulation without surgery in four cases. Fibrous union was attained with good functional results. His technique was to place a valgus stress on the elbow while supinating the forearm and dorsiflexing the wrist and fingers, thus using the forearm flexor muscles to aid in extracting the fragment. The same year Fairbank and Buxton[13] confirmed during surgical exploration that this technique would extract the fragment if performed early. This technique was subsequently adopted by many other authors.[9,14-16] After 24 hours, the ability to

extract the fragment by this manipulative technique decreases.[14,16]

Patrick[17] recommended using faradic electrical stimulation of the flexor muscles to facilitate the extraction process.

Even though Schmier[16] found that cases in which the fragment could be extracted by closed methods had better results than those that required open extraction, I believe that all of these need to be explored surgically without manipulation. In my experience, fragments that are incarcerated in the joint often have the ulnar nerve entwined within the fragment as well. Manipulation risks further injury to the ulnar nerve. After the fragment is extracted from the joint, it is stabilized with a screw, if possible, to allow early motion.

Late Incarceration in the Joint

Originally the chance of regaining elbow function in cases in which the incarceration was discovered late (four to six weeks after injury) was considered slim even if the fragment was removed surgically. Patrick[17] found that by the fourth week the fragment had become fused to the articular surface of the coronoid process. Forcible removal of the fragment after this period was found to produce a raw defect in the articular surface of the coronoid process. This defect subsequently scarified the opposing trochlear articular surface. In ad-

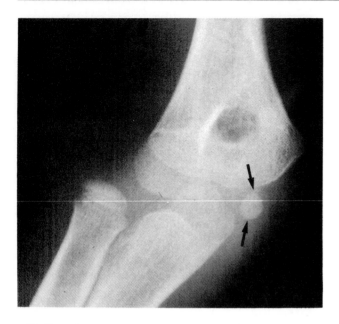 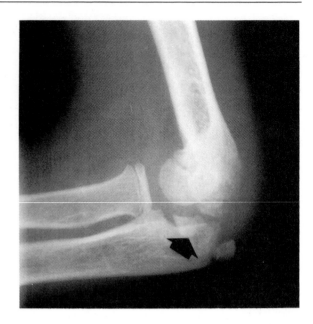

Fig. 9 **Left,** Posterior lateral elbow dislocation with a displaced medial epicondyle (arrows). **Right,** After reduction, the medial epicondyle remained entrapped within the elbow joint (arrow).

dition, the long-term presence of the fragment in the joint subluxates the joint, stretching the capsule and ligaments. If the fragment is removed after these ligaments and capsules have undergone secondary changes, elbow stability may be lost. Blount[18] recommended against treating fractures with the fragment incarcerated in the joint if more than six weeks had passed since the original injury.

This pessimism has been reversed by a more recent review of late removal. Fowles and associates,[19] working in Tunisia, found that if the elbow was carefully explored and the fragment removed, children could regain at least 80% of their normal elbow motion without significant pain. In their six cases the function was satisfactory and there were no neurologic sequelae when the fragment was removed late.

Fractures Through the Apophysis These fractures are usually partial avulsion or injuries caused by a direct blow. Even displaced fractures can usually be managed without surgery and with early motion.

Chronic Tension Stress Injuries

In chronic tension stress injuries (Little League elbow), the history is usually quite characteristic. It is found in young baseball pitchers who are throwing an excessive number of pitches or who are just starting to throw curve pitches.[20] Clinically, this syndrome is manifested by a decrease in elbow extension. Medial epicondylar pain is accentuated by a valgus stress to the elbow in extension. Local tenderness and swelling over the medial epicondyle are usually significant.

On radiographs, the density of the bone of the distal humerus is increased because of the chronic stress. The physeal line is irregular and widened (Fig. 10). If the stress has continued for a long time, there may be hy-

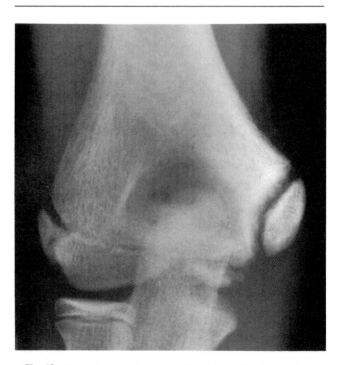

Fig. 10 Chronic stress fracture: Widening of the physeal line of the medial epicondyle in a 13-year-old baseball pitcher who was pitching excessively.

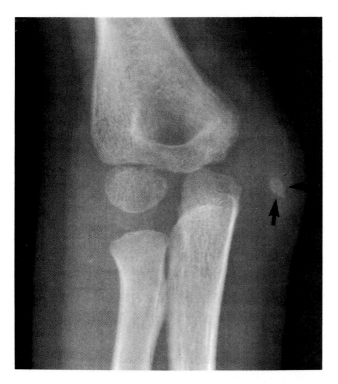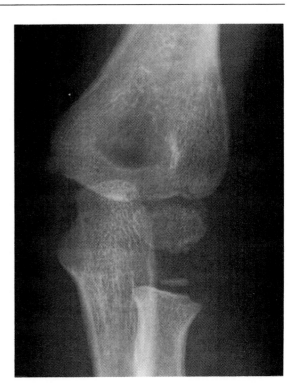

Fig. 11 **Left,** Injury film of a fracture of the medial condyle misinterpreted as a medial epicondyle fracture. The unossified trochlear surface is not visualized. The presence of a markedly displaced medial epicondyle fragment in a very young child should alert one that this is more than a medial epicondyle fracture. **Right,** Normal side (for comparison).

pertrophy of the distal humerus with acceleration of bone growth. The bone age of the elbow is greater than the patient's chronological age.

These individuals must stop pitching altogether until their symptoms have subsided and they have regained their full range of motion. During this period, they should continue specific exercises designed to strengthen all the muscles about the elbow and shoulder. Because the number of pitches thrown is a major factor producing this syndrome, a reduction in pitching time after they resume play is certainly indicated.

Differentiation From Medial Condyle Fractures

In younger individuals in whom trochlear ossification has not developed, a fracture of the medial condyle can be confused with a fracture of the medial epicondyle (Fig. 11). The following clues can help differentiate these two injuries.

First, any significant effusion within the elbow joint (for example, positive fat-pad signs) raises the possibility that the injury is intra-articular. Isolated medial epicondyle injuries are extra-articular and rarely produce a significant elbow effusion.[21] Second, in fractures of the medial epicondyle there is often a metaphyseal flake of bone associated with the epicondylar fragment.

Finally, one must always be suspicious of the occurrence of medial epicondyle fractures in young children. Elbow dislocation, which is usually associated with this injury, is uncommon before the age of 8 or 9 years. Thus, if there is any significant displacement of the medial epicondyle it must be assumed that the medial condyle is involved, and it must be proven beyond a doubt that the articular surface is not involved. This usually can be done with an arthrogram. Magnetic resonance imaging may also be helpful in localizing the intra-articular component of the medial condylar fracture.

Summary

In conclusion, medial epicondyle fractures must be taken seriously. Good results can be obtained by both surgical and nonsurgical methods. For individuals who require a stable elbow for high-performance activities, surgical stabilization probably is superior. Whether surgical or not, the method chosen should allow for early active elbow motion to avoid residual stiffness. Incarcerated fragments must be removed surgically. Even if there is a delay in diagnosing the incarceration, surgery can provide a good result. Chronic tension stress injuries, such as are seen in skeletally immature baseball pitchers, require complete rest coupled with an aggressive muscle-strengthening program and a reduction in pitching activity. Finally, in the very young child, these injuries must be differentiated from medial condyle fractures, which can produce significant disability.

References

1. Brodeur AE, Silberstein MJ, Graviss ER: *Radiology of the Pediatric Elbow*. Boston, GK Hall Medical Publishers, 1981.

2. Silberstein MJ, Brodeur AE, Graviss ER, et al: Some vagaries of the medial epicondyle. *J Bone Joint Surg* 1981;63A:524–528.

3. Woods GW, Tullos HS: Elbow instability and medial epicondyle fractures. *Am J Sports Med* 1977;5:23–30.

4. Wilkins KE: Fractures and dislocations of the elbow regions, in Rockwood CA Jr, Wilkins KE, King RE (eds): *Fractures in Children*. Philadelphia, 1984, vol 3, pp 363–575.

5. Marion J, LaGrange J, Faysse R, et al: Les fractures de l'éxtremité inférieure del' humerus chez l'enfant [Fractures of the lower extremity of the humerus in children]. *Rev Chir Orthop* 1962;48:490.

6. Watson-Jones R: Primary nerve lesions in injuries of the elbow and wrist. *J Bone Joint Surg* 1930;12:121–140.

7. Bede WB, Lefebure AR, Rosman MA: Fractures of the medial humeral epicondyle in children. *Can J Surg* 1975;18:137–142.

8. Smith FM: *Surgery of the Elbow*, ed 2. Philadelphia, WB Saunders, 1972.

9. Watson-Jones R: *Fractures and Joint Injuries*, ed 3. Baltimore, Williams & Wilkins, 1943.

10. Josefsson PO, Danielsson LG: Epicondylar elbow fracture in children: 35-year follow-up of 56 unreduced cases. *Acta Orthop Scand* 1986;57:313–315.

11. Hines RF, Herndon WA, Evans JP: Operative treatment of medial epicondyle fractures in children. *Clin Orthop* 1987;223:170–174.

12. Roberts NW: Displacement of the internal epicondyle into the elbow-joint: 4 cases successfully treated by manipulation. *Lancet* 1934;2:78–79.

13. Fairbank HAT, Buxton JD: Displacement of the internal epicondyle into the elbow-joint, letter. *Lancet* 1934;2:218.

14. Blount WP: *Fractures in Children*. Baltimore, Williams & Wilkins, 1955.

15. Brewster AH, Karp M: Fractures in the region of the elbow in children: An end-result study. *Surg Gynecol Obstet* 1940;71:643–649.

16. Schmier AA: Internal epicondylar epiphysis and elbow injuries. *Surg Gynecol Obstet* 1945;80:416–421.

17. Patrick J: Fracture of the medial epicondyle with displacement into the elbow joint. *J Bone Joint Surg* 1946;28:143–147.

18. Blount WP: Unusual fractures in children, in Banks SW, Larmon WA, Virgin HW Jr, et al (eds): American Academy of Orthopaedic Surgeons *Instructional Course Lectures, XI*. Ann Arbor, JW Edwards, 1954, pp 57–71.

19. Fowles JV, Kassab MT, Moula T: Untreated intra-articular entrapment of the medial humeral epicondyle. *J Bone Joint Surg* 1984;66B:562–565.

20. Brogdon BG, Crow NE: Little leaguer's elbow. *Am J Roentgenol* 1960;83:671–675.

21. Harrison RB, Keats TE, Frankel CJ, et al: Radiographic clues to fractures of the unossified medial humeral condyle in young children. *Skeletal Radiol* 1984;11:209–212.

Anatomy and Kinematics of the Elbow

Bernard F. Morrey, MD

Effective treatment of pathologic conditions of the elbow requires a clear understanding of the interrelationship of its anatomy and biomechanics. The applied anatomy of the elbow as it relates to the biomechanics of the joint has been previously described,[1] but since that time further progress has been made toward understanding and applying an expanding knowledge of the anatomy and biomechanics of the elbow joint.

The Articular Surface

Several aspects of the articular surfaces of the elbow joint are worth noting. While the precise orientation of these articular relationships has been previously described, additional relationships are worthy of mention.

Humeral Articulation

The articular surface of the capitellum is anterior to the lateral supracondylar bony column.

Application In applying an internal fixation device over the posterolateral column, bending the plate makes it possible to place an additional one or two screws in the distal fragment. This is particularly helpful in treating low transverse fractures (Figs. 1 and 2). Because the narrowness of the supracondylar column medially and the posterior extension of the trochlear articular surface, combined with the presence of the ulnar nerve, limit plate application in this plane, the most effective fixation of the medial column is a medially oriented plate placed at a 90-degree angle to the lateral fixation.

Ulnar Articulation

The hyaline cartilage on the articular surface of the greater sigmoid fossa is not continuous. Because the midportion of the articular surface is composed of fi-

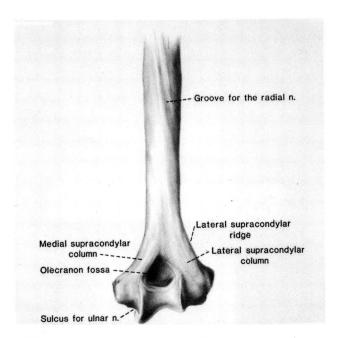

Fig. 1 Posterior and distal aspect of the lateral column of the distal humerus is flat and void of cartilage (arrow). (Reproduced with permission from the Mayo Foundation.)

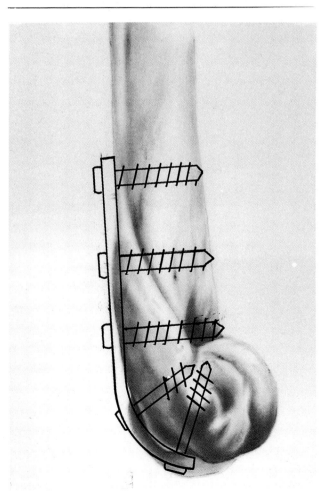

Fig. 2 Plate fixation of the lateral column extends distally, providing additional fixation points for fractures.

brofatty tissue,[2] there is no strong subchondral bone in the midportion of the greater sigmoid fossa (Fig. 3).

Application This anatomic aspect of the ulnar articulation means that fractures of the olecranon are not anatomically reproduced by the opposing articular surface. Instead, the opposing surface tends to narrow the anterior and posterior dimensions of the greater sigmoid fossa, which can cause impingement and degenerative arthritis. Olecranon fractures are best managed by aligning the cortex, thus restoring the proper anteroposterior dimension even if there has been comminution and loss of bone and articular surface in the midportion of the greater sigmoid fossa. In addition, this anatomic characteristic may be employed to design the transolecranon osteotomy to expose the elbow if this is the exposure of preference. By so doing, violation of the hyaline cartilage can be avoided. Finally, by recognizing this anatomic feature arthroscopically, it is possible to avoid mistaking a deficiency of the articular cartilage for a pathologic entity, which could lead to debriding or abrading the normal anatomic structure.

The Radius

The articular margin of the radial head consists of approximately 280 degrees of articular cartilage and approximately 80 degrees of nonchondral margin. The articulation of the radial head in the lesser sigmoid fossa allows approximately 160 to 170 degrees of fore-

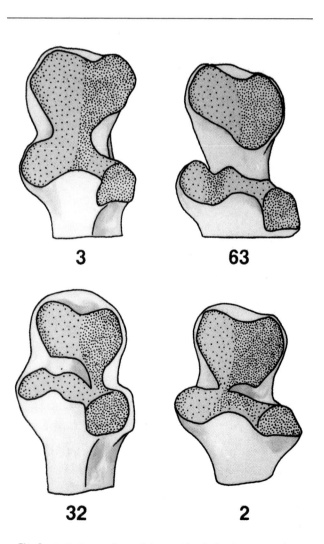

Fig. 3 Articular surface of the proximal ulna is not continuous with hyaline cartilage but is void of articular surface in its midpoint as is shown by the relative percents of the distribution patterns. (Adapted with permission from Tillman BH: *Contribution to the Function Morphology of Articular Surfaces.* Stuttgart, George Thieme, 1978.)

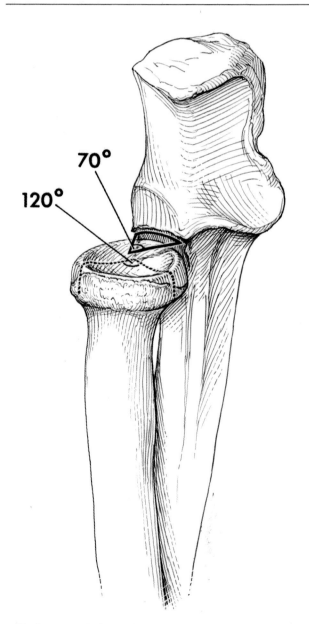

Fig. 4 The lack of strong subchondral bone around one third of the radial articular margin accounts, in part, for the shear fractures that occur through this segment. Similarly, this fragment can be accurately reduced and fixed without the fixation impinging in the lesser sigmoid fossa. (Reproduced with permission from the Mayo Foundation.)

arm rotation, made possible by the 15-degree angulation of the radial neck away from the radial tuberosity.

Application The unique orientation of the radial neck, as well as the lack of strong subchondral bone covering the anterolateral aspect of the radial head, accounts for the frequent slice or shear fractures that occur in the anterolateral segment (Fig. 4). When a fracture occurs in this area, the fracture fragment may be fixed by countersinking small screws through the fracture fragment. Because this portion does not articulate with the lesser sigmoid fossa, there is little risk of articular impingement.

Ulnohumeral Articular Orientation

The 30-degree anterior rotation of the distal humerus, coupled with the posterior rotation of the open-

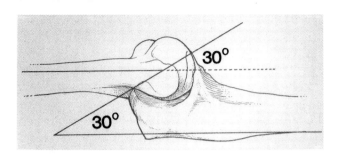

Fig. 5 The posterior orientation of the opening angle of the greater sigmoid fossa matches the anterior rotation of the distal humerus, providing stability to the elbow when it is fully extended. (Reproduced with permission from the Mayo Foundation.)

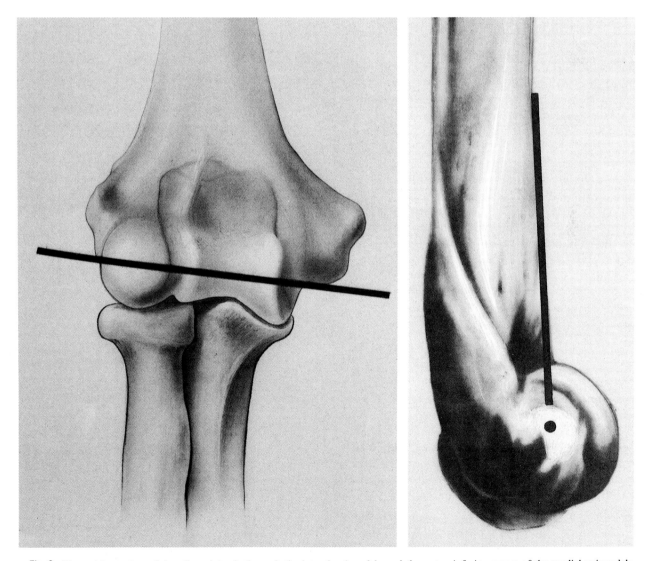

Fig. 6 The axial rotation of the elbow joint is through the lateral epicondyle and the anteroinferior aspect of the medial epicondyle (**left**) and at the center of the lateral epicondyle colinear with the anterior humeral cortex on the lateral projection (**right**). (Reproduced with permission from the Mayo Foundation.)

ing of the greater sigmoid fossa, allows the elbow to pass through an arc of 150 degrees of flexion and extension and still remain stable in full extension (Fig. 5). This relationship, particularly as it relates to the ulnar articulation, has not been emphasized in the past.

Application The posterior opening angle of the ulna is particularly helpful when assessing olecranon and coronoid fractures. A loss of coronoid substance, estimated by recognizing this angular relationship, can be useful in designing reconstructive procedures to avoid instability.

Elbow Motion Axis of Rotation

Identification of the axis of rotation of the flexion and extension arc is a most important and clinically relevant biomechanical and anatomic consideration. The axis lies in the middle of the lateral epicondyle, which is the center of the projection of the capitellum (Fig. 6).[3] It passes through the center of the capitellum and the trochlea and lies at the anteroinferior aspect of the medial epicondyle on the anteroposterior plane (Fig. 6).[4]

Application Restoration of the axis of rotation is important in elbow reconstructive surgery, because even a slight alteration in the location of the axis of rotation by a prosthetic implant can affect the postoperative flexion strength of the elbow joint.[5] It has been observed that even if the entire distal humerus is lost because of tumor or a fracture, the axis of rotation can be reestablished by using certain prosthetic designs, thus avoiding the need for custom implants.

In my practice, one other important application of this information has been in treating the stiff elbow. By applying a distraction device employing the axis of rotation about which the ulna may be allowed to move with uniform separation, improved flexion and extension have been observed after an elbow capsular release.[4]

Elbow Joint Capacity

Although the anterior capsule of the elbow is thin and filamentous, it does provide significant varus-valgus elbow stability when the elbow is in full extension.[6] A recent study found the capacity of the elbow joint to be approximately 25 ml.[7] It has also been documented that the maximum capacity with the capsule fully distended occurs with the elbow in approximately 80 degrees of flexion. Finally, the resistance of the elbow joint to rupture from distention was observed to be relatively low, averaging about 85 mm H_2O.

Application This information helps explain why patients hold their elbows in 80 to 90 degrees of flexion after an injury resulting in a hemarthrosis. This angle is also the most common position in which the elbow becomes ankylosed or stiff.[4] Further, awareness of the normal capacity of the elbow is worthwhile when per-

forming arthroscopy. Any marked variation from normal capacity suggests a scarred capsular structure, if the volume is less than normal, or a redundant or unstable joint, if the capacity is significantly increased.

Finally, the low rupture pressure of the elbow joint should cause the arthroscopist some concern if a mechanical device is used to distend the joint during an arthroscopic procedure.

The Collateral Ligaments

The details of the anatomy of the collateral ligament structures have been provided in the past.[1,8] The functional significance of the lateral ulnar collateral ligament has been clarified by recent investigations conducted by O'Driscoll and associates (Fig. 7).[9] The origin of this structure has been confirmed to be at the midportion of the lateral epicondyle, and the insertion is at the tubercle of the crista musculi supinatoris. The release of this ligament, even with an intact radial collateral ligament, allows the elbow to subluxate in an inferior rotatory type of mechanism. Release of the radial collateral ligament with an intact ulnar collateral ligament does not allow this instability pattern.

Application Recognition of the existence and function of the lateral ulnar collateral ligament explains the recently described pivot shift phenomenon of the elbow joint.[9] This ligament, which has been shown to function as a lateral guy wire, complements the anterior ulnar collateral ligament. It provides stability to the ulno-

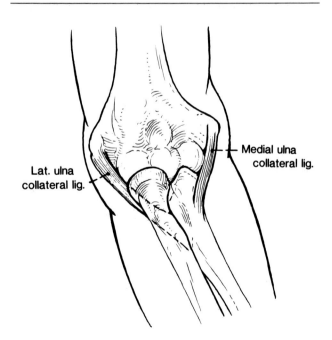

Fig. 7 The presence of a lateral ulnar collateral ligament anatomically matches the anterior medial ulnar collateral ligament. These structures provide varus-valgus stability to the ulnohumeral joint independent of the presence of a radial head.

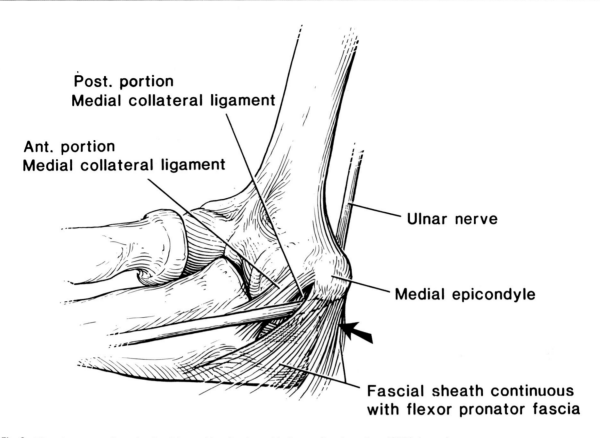

**Post. portion
Medial collateral ligament**

**Ant. portion
Medial collateral ligament**

Ulnar nerve

Medial epicondyle

**Fascial sheath continuous
with flexor pronator fascia**

Fig. 8 The ulnar nerve is maintained in position by the cubital tunnel retinaculum (CTR) (arrow).

humeral joint independent of the radial collateral ligament or the presence of the radial head. Furthermore, the origin of the lateral ulnar collateral ligament at the axis of rotation allows proper reconstruction of the lateral complex that effectively eliminates recurrent subluxation or dislocation of the joint. This procedure has been performed ten times in my clinical practice and in no case has the problem recurred. Anatomic restoration of the origin of the medial collateral ligament is an essential feature of the procedure described by Jobe and associates.[10]

The Cubital Tunnel

Although the ulnar nerve is frequently explored and decompressed, the detailed anatomy of the "roof" of the cubital tunnel has not been previously provided. This area has been carefully dissected in my laboratory and a discrete structure originating from the medial epicondyle and inserting on the ulna has been defined.[11] This structure, termed the cubital tunnel retinaculum, is independent of the brachial fascia as well as the superficial forearm fascia (Fig. 8). It functions as the major constraint of the ulnar nerve as it passes behind the medial epicondyle. Of particular significance was the observation that, when the elbow is

flexed, the cubital tunnel retinaculum becomes taut and flattens the space through which the ulnar nerve passes to reach the flexor carpi ulnaris. When the elbow is extended, the cubital tunnel retinaculum becomes lax, providing ample room for the nerve.

Application Knowledge of the detailed anatomy of the cubital tunnel retinaculum helps explain the phenomenon of ulnar nerve impingement and irritation that is observed when the elbow is fully flexed. Furthermore, a more detailed appreciation of this structure allows an accurate understanding of the dissection of this region.

Finally, it has been observed in the dissections in my laboratory that approximately 10% of individuals do not possess a discrete cubital tunnel retinaculum. It was also observed that in these individuals the ulnar nerve is lax and rides over the medial epicondyle with flexion and extension. Thus, the essential cause of congenital subluxation of the ulnar nerve appears to be the absence of the cubital tunnel retinaculum.

Summary

Despite the fact that the anatomy of the elbow has been generally well described and clearly recognized for many years, additional features have been further elucidated in recent times. These features have direct application in many of the surgical reconstructive procedures performed at the elbow.

References

1. Morrey BF: Applied anatomy and biomechanics of the elbow joint, in Anderson LD (ed): American Academy of Orthopaedic Surgeons *Instructional Course Lectures, XXXV*. St. Louis, CV Mosby, 1986, pp 59–68.
2. Tillman BH: *Contribution to the Function Morphology of Articular Surfaces*. Stuttgart, George Thieme, 1978.
3. London JT: Kinematics of the elbow. *J Bone Joint Surg* 1981; 63A:529–535.
4. Morrey BF: Post-traumatic contracture of the elbow: Operative treatment, including distraction arthroplasty. *J Bone Joint Surg* 1990;72A:601–618.
5. Morrey BF: Joint replacement of the elbow, in Morrey BF (ed): *The Elbow and Its Disorders*. Philadelphia, WB Saunders, 1985.
6. Morrey BF, An KN: Articular and ligamentous contributions to the stability of the elbow joint. *Am J Sports Med* 1983;11:315–319.
7. O'Driscoll SW, Morrey BF, An KN: The capsular capacity of the elbow joint. *J Arthrosc*, in press.
8. Morrey BF, An KN: Functional anatomy of the ligaments of the elbow. *Clin Orthop* 1985;201:84–90.
9. O'Driscoll SW, Bell DF, Morrey BF: Posterolateral rotatory instability of the elbow: Clinical and radiographic features. *J Bone Joint Surg*, in press.
10. Jobe FW, Stark H, Lombardo SJ: Reconstruction of the ulnar collateral ligament in athletes. *J Bone Joint Surg* 1986;68A:1158–1163.
11. O'Driscoll SW, Hori A, Carmichael S, et al: The cubital tunnel retinaculum. *J Bone Joint Surg*, in press.

Elbow Instability in the Athlete

Frank W. Jobe, MD

Ronald S. Kvitne, MD

Introduction

Overhand or throwing athletes are at risk for developing a variety of elbow problems.[1-3] The incidence of injury appears to be directly related to the duration of exposure and to the intensity of their athletic participation.[4] Although sudden traumatic injuries are quite common, most symptomatic pathologic syndromes result from chronic excessive repetitive stress.[5-11] In order to treat those injuries that are unique to the throwing athlete, it is important to have a thorough understanding of the pertinent regional anatomy, the biomechanics of throwing, and the relationship of elbow motion and stability.

Background

Anatomy

Laboratory investigations have shown that elbow stability is partly a function of its bony configuration (50%). The remaining 50% is a function of the anterior joint capsule, the ulnar (medial) collateral ligament, and the radial (lateral) collateral ligament.[7,9]

The ulnar collateral ligament complex (Fig. 1) consists of anterior and posterior bundles and an oblique band (transverse ligament). The anterior bundle, which inserts on the medial aspect of the coronoid process of the ulna, is functionally the most important factor in resisting valgus stress at the elbow. Its humeral origin is eccentrically located with respect to the axis of elbow flexion and extension, thus providing stability throughout a full range of motion. The thinner posterior bundle is much weaker and provides stability primarily beyond 90 degrees of elbow flexion. The oblique band does not cross the joint but exists as a thickening of the caudal-most portion of the joint capsule to expand the greater sigmoid notch.

The radial collateral ligament complex is less consistent and not as well understood as the ulnar collateral ligament complex. The radial collateral ligament "proper" originates from the lateral epicondyle and inserts onto the annular ligament (Fig. 2). A posterior bundle, present in approximately 90% of the population,[7] crosses the radiocapitellar joint, superficial to the annular ligament, and inserts onto the crista musculi supinatoris. This portion of the radial ligament complex is functionally more important in providing stability to resist varus stress, especially in patients who have undergone a previous radial head resection.

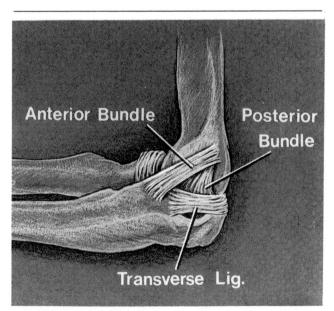

Fig. 1 Ulnar collateral ligament complex. Anterior and posterior bundles and transverse ligament.

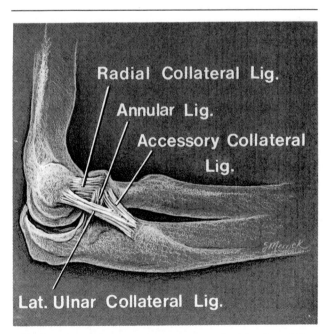

Fig. 2 Radial collateral ligament complex. Radial collateral ligament and lateral ulnar collateral ligament.

Fig. 3 Throwing motion. Wind-up, early cocking, late cocking, acceleration, and follow-through. (Reproduced with permission from Glousman R, Jobe F, Tibone J, et al: Dynamic electromyographic analysis of the throwing shoulder with glenohumeral instability. *J Bone Joint Surg* 1988;70A:221.)

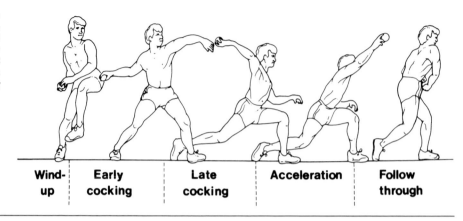

Wind-up | Early cocking | Late cocking | Acceleration | Follow through

Fig. 4 Stability testing. Valgus stress testing of ulnar collateral ligament for instability. (Reproduced with permission from Jobe FW, Kvitne RS: Shoulder and elbow injuries among professional baseball players. *Jpn J Sports Sci* 1990;9(7):429–442.)

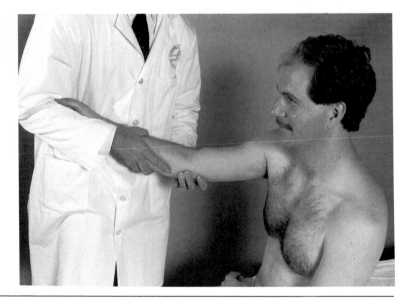

Biomechanics of Throwing

The throwing motion has been divided into five stages (Fig. 3). Stage I, which begins with the wind-up or preparation phase, ends when the ball leaves the nondominant gloved hand. Stage II, or early cocking, begins as the ball is released from the gloved hand, as the shoulder abducts and externally rotates, and terminates with contact of the forward foot on the ground. Stage III is termed late cocking, as the dominant shoulder continues to achieve maximal external rotation. Stage IV, or acceleration phase, starts with internal rotation of the humerus and ends with ball release. Stage V consists of the follow-through or deceleration phase, during which the energy from the throwing motion is dissipated, and ends when all motion is complete.

During the late cocking and acceleration phases of overhand or throwing activities, tremendous valgus forces are generated about the medial aspect of the

elbow. Initially, these stresses are transmitted to the medial flexor-pronator musculature and the ulnar collateral ligament. With proper mechanics, conditioning, and warm-up, most athletes can tolerate these forces. However, poor mechanics, conditioning, or flexibility, or fatigue can have a cumulative effect that leads to muscle strain and allows further stress to be transmitted to the ulnar collateral ligament. If these additional stresses are applied at a rate that is greater than the rate of tissue repair, progressive microscopic damage can occur. This progressive damage appears initially as edema and inflammation within the ulnar collateral ligament, with resultant pain, tenderness, and swelling about the medial aspect of the elbow joint. With further stress, dissociation of the ligament fibers occurs, progressing to calcification and, later, ossification. The resultant scar tissue within the ligament then serves as a stress riser. Over time, the ulnar collateral ligament can

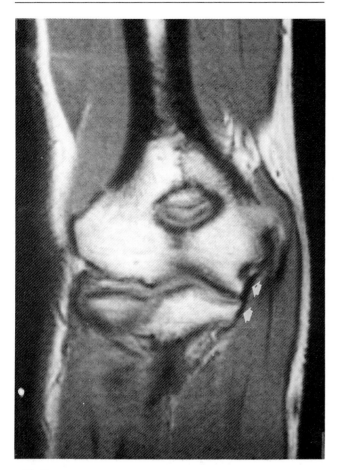

Fig. 5 Magnetic resonance imaging of elbow shows a normal ulnar collateral ligament.

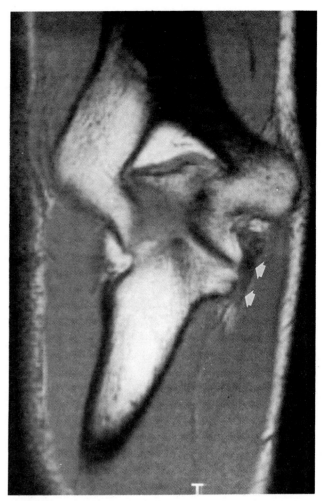

Fig. 6 Magnetic resonance imaging of elbow shows complete disruption of ulnar collateral ligament.

become attenuated and, therefore, functionless. The ligament can, on occasion, become avulsed from its ulnar insertion or, less commonly, can rupture in its midsubstance or even, rarely, become detached from the medial epicondyle. Any of these conditions can cause the athlete's performance to suffer, as the elbow joint loses its primary soft-tissue stabilizer and the basic biomechanics of the elbow joint becomes altered.

Diagnosis

The diagnosis of elbow instability is based on the athlete's history, on the physical findings, and on radiographic evaluation. Patients often have a history of repetitive overhand or throwing activities. Localized pain about the medial aspect of the elbow during the late cocking or acceleration phases of their particular sport will help pinpoint the problem area. Tenderness to palpation over the ulnar collateral ligament complex can be present or absent, depending on the amount of inflammation at the time of examination. Ulnar nerve symptoms are present in a significant number of pa-

tients with chronic elbow instability. These symptoms are caused by extensive inflammation about the ulnar collateral ligament, which secondarily irritates the ulnar nerve as it passes through the cubital tunnel.

Testing for elbow instability is best performed with the athlete in the seated position with the patient's hand and wrist held securely between the examiner's elbow and trunk. By grasping the patient's elbow and proximal forearm and simultaneously palpating the ulnar collateral ligament with the long finger, varus and valgus stress testing can be carried out (Fig. 4). While stressing the collateral ligament for a determination of end-point laxity, it is important to flex the elbow beyond 25 degrees to unlock the olecranon from its fossa.

Radiographs taken during stability testing and compared with those of the contralateral elbow can often document excessive laxity of the elbow even when the clinical findings are equivocal. Gravity valgus stress testing can also be used to assess the degree of elbow instability, especially in the apprehensive patient.[9,11]

Recently we have used magnetic resonance imaging

Fig. 7 Incision through common flexor-pronator origin.

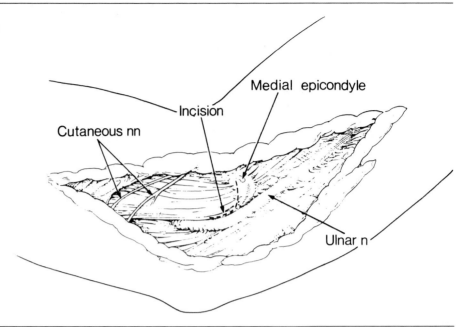

Fig. 8 Exposure of ulnar collateral ligament.

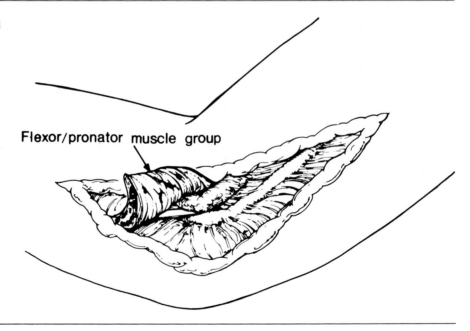

as an investigational tool in evaluating the collateral ligaments. Our preliminary results indicate that magnetic resonance imaging is sometimes helpful in assessing the elbow for ligament abnormalities (Figs. 5 and 6). Although not diagnostic, standard radiographs can provide useful information in identifying (1) ossification within the ulnar collateral ligament, (2) heterotopic bone formation at the tip of the olecranon or in the fossa, (3) marginal osteophytes about either the radiocapitellar joint or the ulnohumeral articulation, (4) loose bodies, or (5) osteochondritic lesions within the elbow joint. Although arthrography can be useful in cases of acute ulnar collateral ligament rupture, it often gives false-negative findings in cases of chronic ulnar collateral ligament laxity or instability.

Nonsurgical Treatment

Once the diagnosis has been established, a specific treatment program can be initiated. Because most elbow injuries in overhand athletes result from chronic,

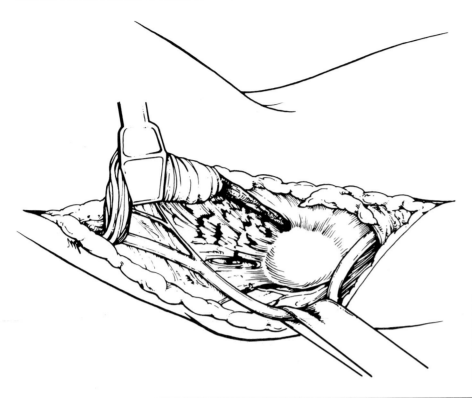

Fig. 9 Mobilization of ulnar nerve. (Reproduced with permission from Jobe FW, Kvitne RS: Ulnar neuritis and ulnar collateral ligament instabilities in overarm throwers, in Torg JS, Welsh RP, Shephard RJ (eds): *Current Therapy in Sports Medicine - 2.* Philadelphia, BC Decker, 1990, p 423.)

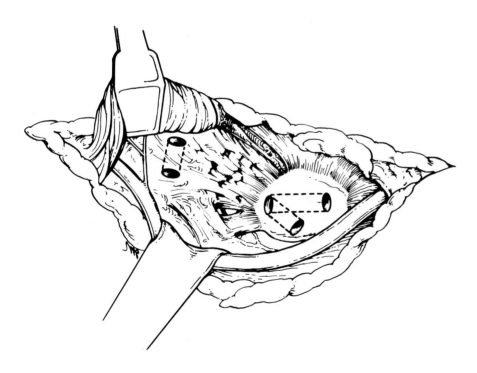

Fig. 10 Convergent drill holes creating tunnels for graft in medial epicondyle and proximal ulna. (Reproduced with permission from Jobe FW, Kvitne RS: Ulnar neuritis and ulnar collateral ligament instabilities in overarm throwers, in Torg JS, Welsh RP, Shephard RJ (eds): *Current Therapy in Sports Medicine - 2.* Philadelphia, BC Decker, 1990, p 423.)

repetitive microtrauma, an initial period of rest (no throwing) is recommended. Oral nonsteroidal anti-inflammatory medication is begun. Local injections of cortisone, however, are not generally recommended, because further attenuation of the ligament can occur.

A supervised muscle stretching and strengthening

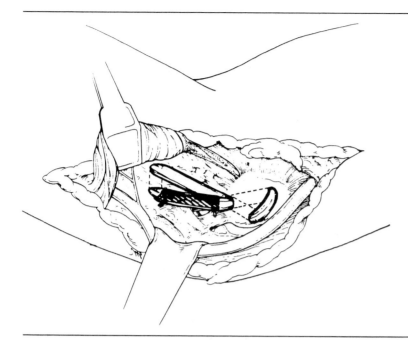

Fig. 11 Graft passed through tunnels with an isometric figure-of-8 configuration. (Reproduced with permission from Jobe FW, Kvitne RS: Ulnar neuritis and ulnar collateral ligament instabilities in overarm throwers, in Torg JS, Welsh RP, Shephard RJ (eds): *Current Therapy in Sports Medicine - 2*. Philadelphia, BC Decker, 1990, p 424.)

program for all the muscles about the elbow is extremely important to restore the necessary muscle tone and endurance needed to provide dynamic support to the elbow. This can be accomplished isometrically, isotonically, or isokinetically.

Various kinds of physical therapy can also be used, including contrast baths, phonophoresis or iontophoresis, or electrical stimulation. These measures can help diminish swelling and promote more rapid healing.

Surgical intervention is necessary for athletes with an acute complete disruption of the ulnar collateral ligament or for patients with chronic pain and instability who show little improvement after at least six months of conservative treatment. The goal of surgery is to reestablish valgus stability in the presence of acute or chronic symptomatic laxity.

Surgical Management of Ulnar Collateral Ligament Ruptures

Surgical Technique

Under tourniquet control, an incision is made over the medial epicondyle and is extended 2 to 3 fingerbreadths, both proximally and distally. Care is taken to protect the ulnar nerve and the branches of the medial antebrachial cutaneous nerve as dissection is carried down to the deep muscle fascia.

The ulnar collateral ligament is then exposed by incising the common flexor-pronator bundle at its origin on the medial epicondyle (Fig. 7). A fringe of its tendinous origin is left behind on the epicondyle to facilitate its reattachment at the end of the procedure. As the flexor-pronator bundle is elevated and reflected

distally (Fig. 8), a thin "carpet" of muscle tissue is left behind overlying the ulnar collateral ligament and joint capsule to serve as a bed onto which the ulnar nerve will be transposed.

Examination of the ulnar collateral ligament may reveal soft-tissue calcification and degeneration, attenuation, or complete disruption of the ligament. A longitudinal incision made through the ligament allows inspection of the underlying joint. Synovitis, osteochondral loose bodies, osteophytes, or degenerative changes may be identified and treated at this time. Impingement symptoms involving the posterior compartment (noted preoperatively) may be addressed at this time by inspection and debridement of the olecranon and olecranon fossa.

Next, the ulnar nerve is mobilized proximally to the level of the arcade of Struthers. A small portion of the medial intermuscular septum is also removed proximally to prevent impingement of the ulnar nerve as it is transposed anteriorly. Distal mobilization of the nerve involves carefully splitting the intermuscular septum between the ulnar and humeral heads of the flexor carpi ulnaris 2.5 cm beyond the medial epicondyle. The ulnar nerve can now be retracted out of harm's way, using a 6.4-mm Penrose drain (Fig. 9).

Convergent 3.2-mm drill holes are then made in the medial epicondyle and proximal ulna, creating bone tunnels through which the graft will be passed (Fig. 10). The drill holes placed in the proximal ulna are oriented vertically, are spaced approximately 1 cm apart, and are located at the level of the tubercle of the coronoid process. The holes within the medial epicondyle are placed within the cubital tunnel posterior, and are drilled in such a fashion as to create a single exit hole anteriorly. Tunnels drilled in this manner allow isometric placement of the tendon graft.

At this point, attention is turned to harvesting a suitable tendon for graft. The palmaris longus tendon can be obtained from either upper extremity without sacrificing strength, power, or endurance. However, it is essential to document the presence of the tendon preoperatively. Alternative autogenous graft sources include the plantaris tendon or a 3- to 5-mm medial strip of Achilles tendon.

The palmaris longus tendon is harvested by first creating a 2-cm transverse skin incision in the distal flexor crease at the wrist. The median nerve and its palmar cutaneous branch are protected as the tendon is isolated at its insertion into the palmar fascia. A second transverse skin incision is made 7.5 to 10 cm proximal to the wrist, exposing the proximal palmaris longus musculotendinous junction. The tendon is transected distally and brought out through the proximal incision with the tension applied distally to the tendon. It is divided at its musculotendinous junction, providing a free autogenous graft approximately 15 cm in length. These incisions are then irrigated and closed routinely.

A single No. 1 nonabsorbable braided suture is placed in one end of the free tendon graft, and a flexible suture passer is used to thread the tendon through the bone tunnels, creating a figure-of-8 configuration. With the elbow held in neutral varus-valgus position and 45 degrees of elbow flexion, the graft is pulled taut and sutured to itself with additional sutures (Fig. 11). The elbow is then brought through a full passive range of motion to verify the isometricity and stability of the reconstruction. For additional support, the graft is also sutured to any remnants of the underlying ulnar collateral ligament.

Anterior transposition of the ulnar nerve is carried out by positioning the nerve anterior to the medial epicondyle and submuscularly beneath the flexor-pronator bundle. A portion of the intermuscular septum and muscle fibers of the flexor-pronator group is also resected to prevent impingement on the nerve as it is reattached to the medial epicondyle.

The tourniquet is then released, hemostasis is achieved with electrocautery, and the wound is closed in routine fashion. A long arm posterior plaster splint is used to immobilize the elbow in 90 degrees of flexion and neutral rotation. The wrist and hand are left free. A postoperative brace or orthosis is not necessary because the elbow is inherently stable.

Postoperative Care and Rehabilitation

Postoperative rehabilitation begins immediately, with the patient gently squeezing a soft sponge or rubber ball on the day of surgery. The splint is removed two weeks later, and active elbow and shoulder range-of-motion exercises are begun. Within four weeks of surgery, isometric, isotonic, and progressive resistive strengthening exercises are instituted, concentrating on elbow flexion, extension, pronation, and supination. Rotator cuff muscle stretching and strengthening exercises are also used at this time to avoid the development of a stiff shoulder. At four months after surgery, elbow range of motion and strength have usually returned sufficiently to allow the athlete to begin a short toss-long toss throwing program. The development of pain or swelling about the surgical site demands at least two weeks of rest (no throwing), with a gradual resumption of activities as symptoms permit. By seven months, pitching from the mound can begin at 75% of normal speed. As the strength, power, and endurance of the elbow and shoulder muscles improve over the next few months, performance will become maximized as the athlete returns to a preinjury competitive level of sports activity. This usually occurs by 12 to 18 months after surgery.

References

1. Indelicato PA, Jobe FW, Kerlan RK, et al: Correctable elbow lesions in professional baseball players: A review of 25 cases. *Am J Sports Med* 1979;7:72–75.
2. Tullos HS, Erwin WD, Woods GW, et al: Unusual lesions of the pitching arm. *Clin Orthop* 1972;88:169–182.
3. DeHaven KE, Evarts CM: Throwing injuries of the elbow in athletes. *Orthop Clin North Am* 1973;4:801–808.
4. Albright JA, Jokl P, Shaw R, et al: Clinical study of baseball pitchers: Correlation of injury to the throwing arm with method of delivery. *Am J Sports Med* 1978;6:15–21.
5. Jobe FW, Stark H, Lombardo SJ: Reconstruction of the ulnar collateral ligament in athletes. *J Bone Joint Surg* 1986;68A:1158–1163.
6. Miller JE: Javelin thrower's elbow. *J Bone Joint Surg* 1960;42B:788–792.
7. Morrey BF, An KN: Articular and ligamentous contributions to the stability of the elbow joint. *Am J Sports Med* 1983;11:315–319.
8. Norwood LA, Shook JA, Andrews JR: Acute medial elbow ruptures. *Am J Sports Med* 1981;9:16–19.
9. Schwab GH, Bennett JB, Woods GW, et al: Biomechanics of elbow instability: The role of the medial collateral ligament. *Clin Orthop* 1980;146:42–52.
10. Barnes DA, Tullos HS: An analysis of 100 symptomatic baseball players. *Am J Sports Med* 1978;6:62–67.
11. Woods GW, Tullos HS: Elbow instability and medial epicondyle fractures. *Am J Sports Med* 1977;5:23–30.

Tendonopathies at the Elbow

Ralph W. Coonrad, MD

Tendon injuries about the elbow are essentially problems of the middle-aged and of week-end sports participants. They are rarely seen in adolescents or young athletes. For the purpose of classification, tendon injuries consist of lateral epicondylitis, medial epicondylitis, and avulsion, or rupture, of the biceps or triceps. The terms epicondylitis and rupture, although they are commonly applied to these entities, do not necessarily describe accurately the actual injury involved.[1-5] Tendonopathies are essentially avulsion injuries occurring at either the muscle origin or its insertion. They are usually partial, but can be complete, and can be either microscopic or macroscopic. These injuries can be symptomatic at any stage of disruption and can progress from microscopic to macroscopic.

The most consistent predisposing factors to these conditions are age and preexisting degenerative changes. The peak incidence is in the fourth and fifth decades. They are, therefore, similar in etiology and pathology to degenerative rotator cuff tears at the shoulder, avulsion of the quadriceps tendon or patellar tendon at the knee,[6] and avulsion or tearing of the heel cord at the os calcis. The significant and contrasting difference in this group of tendonopathies is the greater incidence of partial or microscopic avulsion injuries in tennis elbow occurring at the muscle origin, contrasted with the greater frequency of complete lesions involving the biceps or triceps at the muscle insertion.[7]

Lateral Tennis Elbow

Etiology

Runge[8] first described the clinical entity known as lateral epicondylitis in 1873, and Major[9] the symptoms associated with lawn tennis in 1883. Macroscopic tears found at surgery as an explanation for the distinct clinical findings were reported in the 1970s by Coonrad and Hooper,[10] as well as by Nirschl and Pettrone,[11] Froimson,[12] and others. The condition has a peak age incidence in the early 40s and a variable, but nearly equal, sex incidence. It is far more common in nonathletes. Lateral epicondylitis has been reported to be resistant to conservative measures in 4% to 10% of cases, and the time from onset of symptoms until consideration of surgery, when necessary, usually has been more than 12 months. By avoiding steroid therapy and

using the conservative measures described by Nirschl[3] and others, which are discussed below, my experience has been that fewer patients have required surgery in recent years. The primary site of abnormality demonstrated at surgery has been the extensor carpi radialis brevis origin. Occasionally, the extensor communis or extensor carpi radialis longus origin is involved. Lateral tennis elbow is significantly more common than the similar entity on the medial side of the elbow. Although it can occur with the repetitive use associated with some vocations, it is far more likely to occur with sudden force-overload injuries in sports.[13]

The first controlled histologic study of this entity, reported by Regan and associates[5] in 1990, clearly demonstrated a lack of any inflammatory component in surgical specimens. However, vascular and fibroblastic proliferation had previously been reported by Goldie,[2] Nirschl,[3] and others,[10] along with hyaline degeneration and the added feature of calcium deposition in cases in which steroids had been administered. The lack of inflammatory response observed in the study of Regan and associates[5] led these authors to suggest, as an explanation for the clinical course of tennis elbow, that initial avulsion of tendon origin or insertion results in an incomplete healing response characterized by vascular and fibrous proliferation in an area of poor vascularity at middle age.

Diagnosis

The diagnosis is made by finding consistent point tenderness at the conjoined tendon origin, usually precisely localized to the extensor brevis portion. Anatomically, this area is partially, or completely, covered by the adjacent extensor carpi radialis longus and extensor communis. The area of point tenderness lies just above and 1 to 2 mm distal to the midpoint of the lateral epicondyle. Grasping or pinching with the wrist in extension (the "coffee-cup" test), usually reproduces pain precisely at the point of tenderness. Clinical findings[14-16] may include effusion of the elbow joint, which usually does not occur until six to nine months after symptom onset. I attribute this effusion to muscle dysfunction, caused by pain similar to that associated with inadequate quadriceps function at the knee. Effusion on this basis is more likely to occur at the elbow or the knee in athletes, or in any patient who puts stress on a joint with poor muscle stability.

The only real concern in differential diagnosis is the

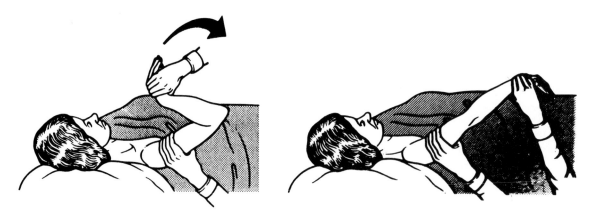

Fig. 1 Manipulative management of lateral tennis elbow under general anesthesia. (Reproduced with permission from Wadsworth TG (ed): *The Elbow*. Edinburgh, Churchill Livingstone, 1982, p 285.)

radial tunnel syndrome,[17-19] a compression neuropathy involving the deep branch of the radial nerve. This syndrome is characteristically associated with tenderness 3.8 cm, or more, distal to the lateral epicondyle and usually directly over the radial tunnel. Compression of the nerve can occur at four different levels in the radial tunnel: (1) from a fibrous band anterior to the radial head at the entrance of the radial tunnel, (2) from the recurrent branch of the radial artery just below this point, (3) from the distal tendinous margin of the extensor carpi radialis brevis, or (4) from the margin of the supinator at the arcade of Frohse. Pain experienced at the elbow when the long finger is extended against resistance—a common but inconsistent finding with the radial tunnel syndrome—is not ordinarily associated with tennis elbow.[20] A diagnostic nerve block of the deep branch of the radial nerve in the radial tunnel differentiates radial tunnel syndrome from typical tennis elbow (J.A. Nunley, personal communication, October 1989). Electrodiagnostic studies of the radial nerve in radial tunnel compression syndrome can be helpful if polyphasic potentials are present; however, conduction velocities are usually normal.[19] Nirschl[3] reported normal electromyographic findings in 20 unselected patients with classic tennis elbow findings.

Treatment

In the majority of patients tennis elbow responds to conservative measures. In recent years, however, it has been common practice to inject a painful tennis elbow on the initial office visit or early in the course of symptoms without a trial of other effective measures. Few reported surgical series for the treatment of tennis elbow list any patients who have not had steroid injections. Yet, experience and experimental data[21-23] have shown that repeated administration of local steroids can atrophy skin and subcutaneous fat and can gradually destroy tendon, sometimes making a chronic

problem of a tennis elbow that might otherwise have subsided even without treatment. Although one or two local injections of steroid may relieve the symptoms and be relatively harmless, in my opinion repeated steroid therapy may constitute a more frequent cause of chronic tennis elbow than is commonly appreciated. Many patients, advised of the possible side effects of local steroid use, are willing to forgo the immediate relief of injectable steroid for other conservative, but just as effective, methods of relieving the aggravating, but seldom incapacitating, symptoms of tennis elbow.

A conservative approach calls for an initial period of rest and avoidance of chronic abuse or overuse. This period, which can be as long as six to 12 weeks in athletes or strenuously active individuals, is followed by a graduated resistive exercise program tailored to the individual patient. Initially, a patient should learn to grasp and pinch only in supination. An exercise program should be carefully and precisely adjusted so that the pain threshold is never reached. Grip strength and both flexion and extension strength at the elbow can be monitored at a level that does not produce pain. Endurance exercises can be added gradually. I find isotonic exercises, using weights in the hand or pulled by hand through an arc of wrist motion, along with isometric exercises without any arc of motion, to be effective. The program should include strengthening exercises for the entire upper extremity, including the shoulder, elbow, wrist, and hand. If pain recurs during exercise, the level of resistance or the frequency should be reduced.

The patient with a history of overuse in industrial compensation or similar situations requires a special and often more detailed approach. Initially, a Minnesota Multiphasic Personality Inventory evaluation or psychologic consultation may help to measure the level of the patient's motivation, cooperation, and effectiveness for rehabilitative effort. The level of discomfort

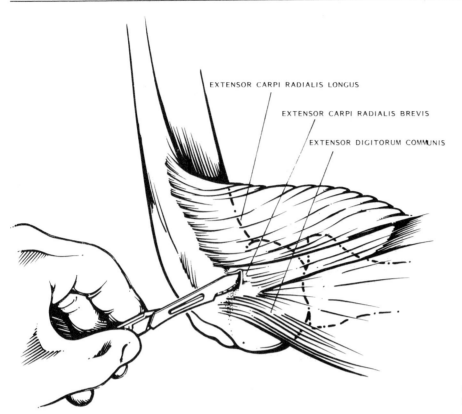

EXTENSOR CARPI RADIALIS LONGUS

EXTENSOR CARPI RADIALIS BREVIS

EXTENSOR DIGITORUM COMMUNIS

Fig. 2 Elevation of the brevis portion of the conjoined tendon at the midportion of the lateral epicondyle.

Fig. 3 Fimbriated tendon and scar tissue at the brevis origin.

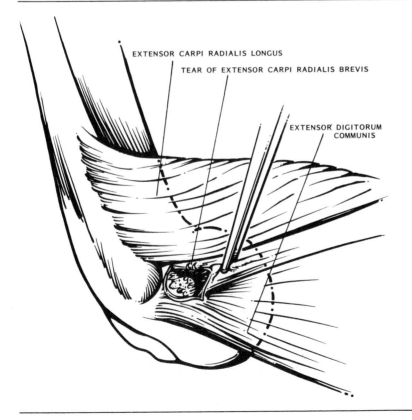

EXTENSOR CARPI RADIALIS LONGUS

TEAR OF EXTENSOR CARPI RADIALIS BREVIS

EXTENSOR DIGITORUM COMMUNIS

with tennis elbow is generally not severe enough to be incapacitating, and alternative techniques of accomplishing a repetitive task can usually be formulated. Instilling confidence in a patient and stimulating a desire to succeed with conservative measures can be as important as the manner in which an exercise program is initiated and carried out.

Early in the course of symptoms, anti-inflammatory drugs can be helpful in some patients. The use of a Froimson band[12] or air splint in overuse situations can help to avoid or delay surgery.

With more resistant problems that fail to respond to an exercise program, it may be necessary to consider surgery. Patients who have had symptoms for a number of months or a year often have a mild flexion contracture of a few degrees or pain with attempted full elbow extension. In these patients, complete relief of symptoms can sometimes be achieved, and surgery avoided, by forcibly extending the elbow, as described by Mills[24] and later by Wadsworth,[25] under general anesthesia (Fig. 1). With the wrist and fingers flexed, the forearm fully pronated, and the elbow extended, the elbow is suddenly and forcibly taken into full extension, or slight hyperextension; this is followed by firm thumb-pressure massage exerted over the extensor origin at the point of maximum tenderness, pressuring the brevis origin heavily. An audible snap may sometimes be felt at the time of manipulation. The results of this procedure are frequently dramatic in long-standing cases, and it can eliminate the need for surgery.

When surgery is considered necessary because of incapacitation and failure of conservative measures over a reasonable period of time, and if directed at the demonstrated abnormality, it is successful about 95% of the time with few complications. Many surgical procedures have been described for tennis elbow.[26–29] These can be classified under four general types: (1) intra-articular, for which no pathologic justification has been demonstrated[30]; (2) complete tenotomy of the extensor origin, which always leaves significant weakness for varying periods of time[31]; (3) distal lengthening of the extensor carpi radialis brevis tendon, which was described by Garden[32] and Carroll and Jorgensen[33] but for which there are few subsequent reports of satisfactory results; and (4) excision of avulsed portion of the extensor brevis tendon, or scar tissue replacement, and direct repair to bone.[3,32,34,35]

The fourth procedure—excision of avulsed tendon ends or scar tissue replacement with direct repair—has been previously reported to produce satisfactory results over a period of 15 years by Coonrad,[34] Froimson,[36] Nirschl and Pettrone,[3,11] and others. Because the procedure has been well described by these authors, it will not be given in detail here. However, it consists essentially of identifying, prior to surgery, the characteristic point of maximum tenderness at the brevis origin. Then, under magnification, a curvilinear incision is made that completely exposes the lateral epicondyle. The superficial fascia is incised and the common extensor tendon origin elevated sharply from the bone in the direction of the elbow joint, starting at its midpoint. Normal-appearing Sharpey's fibers of the tendon are elevated with a small scalpel tip (Fig. 2) until a defect, fimbriated tendon ends, or discolored scar tissue can be identified (Fig. 3). The abnormal tendon is excised and normal tendon reattached firmly to the triceps margin and periosteum from which the common tendon was elevated. Surgery is followed by five days in a bulky, well-padded, long arm cast, graduated resistive exercise at five to six weeks, and sports or other strenuous activity after six months.

Results

A follow-up of 379 elbows with typical findings of tennis elbow during a ten-year period from 1978 to 1988 revealed successful results in 341 elbows treated

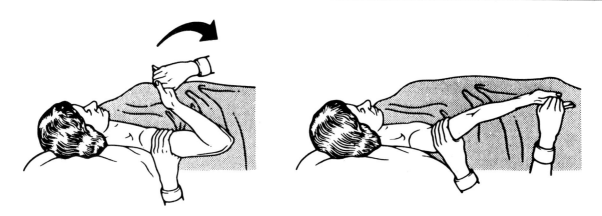

Fig. 4 Manipulative management of medial tennis elbow with the patient anesthetized. (Reproduced with permission from Wadsworth TG (ed): *The Elbow*. Edinburgh, Churchill Livingstone, 1982, p 285.)

conservatively. Of these, 71 were treated without steroids and 270 with local steroid injection. During this period, 38 elbows were treated surgically. A chart review revealed that three of the surgically treated patients had transient pain for six to nine months, and one had a suspected wound infection with a negative culture. All returned to their former activities, occupations, and sports, but none was a professional athlete and none underwent a repeat surgical procedure.

The results of surgical treatment by Nirschl (R.P. Nirschl, personal communication, April 1990) and Froimson (A.I. Froimson, personal communication, April 1990) in separate series, using essentially the procedure described above, were as follows.

Results reported in 1986 by Nirschl, after one to 15 years of follow-up, showed that relief was complete in 85% of the 325 elbows and partial in 12%; 3% were failures. A sample of patients was found by Cybex testing to have strength maintained after one year.

Results for 120 elbows reported in 1987 by Froimson, after one to three years of follow-up, revealed no failures, although one patient had transient pain for nine months. This group, 36 men and 84 women, included 76 patients who played either tennis or golf.

Medial Tennis Elbow

Medial tennis elbow is 5% as common as lateral tennis elbow, with which it is often associated. Medial tennis elbow is caused by avulsion that may be macroscopic or microscopic at the pronator teres or flexor carpi radialis origin from the medial epicondyle.

The diagnosis is made by finding localized tenderness at the site of avulsion and a history of pain with resistive pronation or flexion. It must be differentiated from ulnar nerve neuropathy and medial collateral ligament instability. Nirschl[3] reported ulnar nerve findings of neuropraxia in 60% of patients with medial epicondylar origin symptoms, and in only 15% of those with both medial and lateral epicondylar involvement. In my experience, associated ulnar neuropathy is much less common, involving only a few sports- and work-related injuries. Complete medial collateral ligament instability can often be demonstrated with valgus gravity stress testing, as described by Schwab and associates[37] for displaced medial epicondylar fracture. This is carried out with the patient supine, the shoulder placed in full external rotation, and the elbow passively extended over a fulcrum. Gravity weight of the forearm and a little

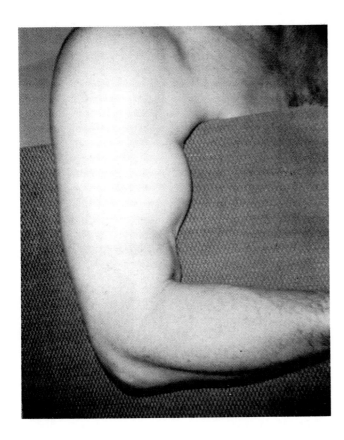
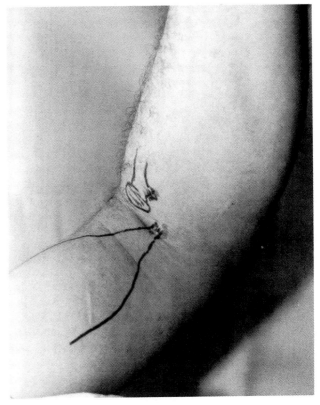

Fig. 5 Distal biceps avulsion in a 59-year-old man.

passive pressure produces valgus stress for radiographic documentation. Incomplete medial collateral ligament instability is better confirmed by testing under axillary, regional intravenous Bier block, or general anesthesia.

Treatment is the same for medial and for lateral tennis elbow. Conservative treatment is usually successful when a real effort is made with an exercise rehabilitation program after an initial rest period. The use of an air splint or Froimson band can also be helpful. Surgery should be considered as a last resort. Here again, steroid use should be avoided early, or until surgery is a consideration. If steroid is used, care should be taken to avoid direct infiltration of the steroid into the anterior oblique portion of the medial collateral ligament. If a mild flexion contracture is present, manipulation of the elbow under general anesthesia, as described by Mills[24] and Wadsworth,[25] may produce sustained relief and avoid a surgical procedure. The elbow is suddenly extended while held in full extension, with the forearm in full supination and the wrist dorsiflexed (Fig. 4).

Distal Biceps Avulsion

Distal biceps tendon avulsion or disruption is relatively uncommon (only 152 cases, all men, were reported in the world literature by 1956).[38] The mechanism of injury is usually from a sudden force overload with the elbow near mid-flexion.[39-41] Degenerative changes in the tendon predispose to disruption.[39] The incidence peaks in the sixth decade of life, with 80% of reported cases involving the dominant arm.[42]

The diagnosis is made by a characteristic history of sudden pain in the antecubital fossa, ecchymosis and swelling at the site, and marked weakness of elbow flexion. In addition, examination reveals a bulge in the distal arm on contraction of the biceps muscle (Fig. 5). Partial avulsions with only tenderness near the insertion are not uncommon,[43] sometimes with delayed rupture. As pain subsides, and if repair is not carried out for a complete disruption, testable strength gradually increases. Radiographs may show degenerative irregularity at the bicipital tuberosity.

Although Hovelius and Josefsson[44] reported that nonsurgical treatment gave satisfactory results in up to 50% of their cases, Morrey[38] demonstrated, in clinical studies, a loss of about 40% of both flexion and supination strength without surgical repair. In his experience, immediate repairs resulted in near normal testable function. Delayed repair or transfer into the brachialis improved supination and pronation, but was associated with residual flexion weakness.

The technique of repair is somewhat controversial.[35] Transfer of the torn tendon to the brachialis for reinforcement carries less risk of injury to the radial nerve but results in the loss of functional strength. Direct

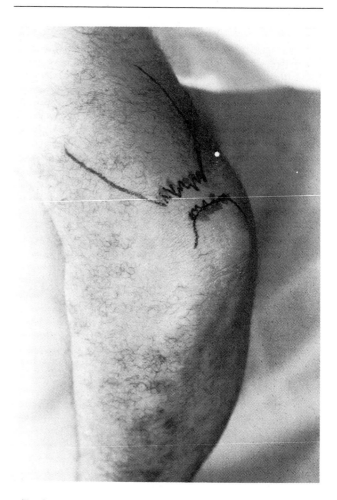

Fig. 6 Triceps rupture from a direct blow injury sustained by a 49-year-old man.

reattachment to the tubercle of the radius by a two-incision exposure,[40] later recommended as the procedure of choice by Morrey,[38] is the safest technique, but can result in ectopic bone formation.

My preferred method of treatment for the active patient, within 48 hours of injury, is direct reattachment of the tendon to the radial tubercle using multiple drill holes in bone. The Henry exposure is used with a transverse incision over the antecubital fossa. Extending this proximally on the lateral side and distally on the medial side gives sufficient exposure to identify the radial and median nerves and their proximal branches.

In the active patient, seen more than 48 hours and less than two weeks after the injury, my approach of choice would be the two-incision exposure of Boyd and Anderson[45] and repair as described by Morrey.[38] For patients who require late reconstruction, indications for surgery should be carefully evaluated, weighing heavily the lesser degree of improvement that should be expected beyond what transfer into the brachialis might contribute.

Distal Triceps Avulsion

Complete avulsion of the triceps from its insertion is considered the least common of all tendon disruptions in the body. A total of only 30 cases was reported between 1868 and 1985.[38] Partial tears are also uncommon.[22] The most common mechanisms of injury have been described as either a decelerating counterforce during active extension of the elbow or a direct blow.[41,46,47] Disruption also probably occurs more commonly than reported as a complication after surgical repair, in exposure for total elbow arthroplasty where the triceps is tenotomized.

The history of sudden total loss of extension at the elbow and a palpable defect (Fig. 6) leave little doubt as to the diagnosis. Radiographs may show small bone fragments with the avulsed tendon if the disruption occurs with trauma.[48] Other causes of avulsion include systemic disorders such as lupus erythematosus, Marfan's syndrome, and renal osteodystrophy.[38]

Treatment for either a late or recent injury is carried out by direct repair[7,43] through drill holes in the olecranon, with fascial reinforcement if necessary, as described by Bennett.[47] Reported results have generally been satisfactory, with a mild flexion contracture being the most frequently reported complication.[24]

References

1. Cyriax JH: The pathology and treatment of tennis elbow. *J Bone Joint Surg* 1936;18:921–940.
2. Goldie I: Epicondylitis lateralis humeri (epicondylalgia or tennis elbow): A pathogenetical study. *Acta Chir Scand* 1964;339(suppl):1–119.
3. Nirschl RP: Muscle and tendon trauma: Tennis elbow, in Morrey BF (ed): *The Elbow and Its Disorders.* Philadelphia, WB Saunders, 1985, pp 481–496.
4. Sarkar K, Uhthoff HK: Ultrastructure of the common extensor tendon in tennis elbow. *Virchows Arch* 1980;386:317–330.
5. Regan W, Wold L, Coonrad RW, Morrey BF: Microscopic histopathology of lateral epicondylitis. Presented at the 57th Annual Meeting of the American Academy of Orthopaedic Surgeons, New Orleans, Feb 8–13, 1990.
6. Colosimo AJ, Bassett FH: Jumper's knee: Diagnosis and treatment. *Orthop Rev* 1990;19:139.
7. McMaster PE: Tendon and muscle ruptures: Clinical and experimental studies on the causes and location of subcutaneous ruptures. *J Bone Joint Surg* 1933;15:705–722.
8. Runge F: Zur Genese und Behandlung des Schreibekrampfes. *Berl Klin Wochenschr* 1873;10:245–248.
9. Major HP: Lawn-tennis elbow, letter. *Br Med J* 1883;2:557.
10. Coonrad RW, Hooper WR: Tennis elbow: Its course, natural history, conservative and surgical management. *J Bone Joint Surg* 1973;55A:1177–1182.
11. Nirschl RP, Pettrone FA: Tennis elbow: The surgical treatment of lateral epicondylitis. *J Bone Joint Surg* 1979;61A:832–839.
12. Froimson AI: Treatment of tennis elbow with forearm support band. *J Bone Joint Surg* 1971;53A:183–184.
13. Nirschl RP: Tennis elbow. *Orthop Clin North Am* 1973;4:787–800.
14. Osgood RB: Radiohumeral bursitis, epicondylitis, epicondylalgia (tennis elbow). *Arch Surg* 1922;4:420–433.
15. Stack JK: Acute and chronic bursitis in the region of the elbow joint. *Surg Clin North Am* 1949;29:155–162.
16. Spencer GE Jr, Herndon CH: Surgical treatment of epicondylitis. *J Bone Joint Surg* 1953;35A:421–424.
17. Roles NC, Maudsley RH: Radial tunnel syndrome: Resistant tennis elbow as a nerve entrapment. *J Bone Joint Surg* 1972;54B:499–508.
18. Spinner M, Linscheid RL: Nerve entrapment syndromes, in Morrey BF (ed): *The Elbow and Its Disorders.* Philadelphia, WB Saunders, 1985, pp 691–712.
19. Eversmann WW Jr: Entrapment and compression neuropathies, in Green DP (ed): *Operative Hand Surgery.* New York, Churchill Livingstone, 1982, vol 2, pp 957–1009.
20. Werner CO: Lateral elbow pain and posterior interosseous nerve entrapment. *Acta Orthop Scand* 1979;174(suppl):1–62.
21. Balasubramaniam P, Prathap K: The effect of injection of hydrocortisone into rabbit calcaneal tendons. *J Bone Joint Surg* 1972;54B:729–734.
22. Tarsney FF: Rupture and avulsion of the triceps. *Clin Orthop* 1972;83:177–183.
23. Unverferth LJ, Olix ML: The effect of local steroid injections on tendon. *J Sports Med* 1973;1(4):31–37.
24. Mills GP: Treatment of tennis elbow. *Br Med J* 1928;1:12.
25. Wadsworth TG (ed): *The Elbow.* Edinburgh, Churchill Livingstone, 1982.
26. Kaplan EB: Treatment of tennis elbow (epicondylitis) by denervation. *J Bone Joint Surg* 1959;41A:147–151.
27. Kaplan EB: The etiology and treatment of epicondylitis. *Bull Hosp Joint Dis* 1968;29:77–83.
28. Bosworth DM: Surgical treatment of tennis elbow: A follow-up study. *J Bone Joint Surg* 1965;47A:1533–1536.
29. Boyd HB, McLeod AC Jr: Tennis elbow. *J Bone Joint Surg* 1973;55A:1183–1187.
30. Bosworth DM: The role of the orbicular ligament in tennis elbow. *J Bone Joint Surg* 1955;37A:527–533.
31. Michele AA, Krueger FJ: Lateral epicondylitis of the elbow treated by fasciotomy. *Surgery* 1956;39:277–284.
32. Garden RS: Tennis elbow. *J Bone Joint Surg* 1961;43B:100–106.
33. Carroll RE, Jorgensen EC: Evaluation of the Garden procedure for lateral epicondylitis. *Clin Orthop* 1968;60:201–204.
34. Coonrad RW: Tennis elbow, in Anderson LD (ed): American Academy of Orthopaedic Surgeons *Instructional Course Lectures,* XXXV. St. Louis, CV Mosby, 1986, pp 94–101.
35. Norman WH: Repair of avulsion of insertion of biceps brachii tendon. *Clin Orthop* 1985;193:189–194.
36. Froimson AI: Tenosynovitis and tennis elbow, in Green DP (ed): *Operative Hand Surgery.* New York, Churchill Livingstone, 1982, vol 2, pp 1507–1521.
37. Schwab GH, Bennett JB, Woods GW, et al: Biomechanics of elbow instability: The role of the medial collateral ligament. *Clin Orthop* 1980;146:42–52.
38. Morrey BF: Tendon injuries about the elbow, in Morrey BF (ed): *The Elbow and Its Disorders.* Philadelphia, WB Saunders, 1985, pp 452–463.
39. Davis WM, Yassine Z: An etiological factor in tear of the distal tendon of the biceps brachii: Report of two cases. *J Bone Joint Surg* 1956;38A:1366–1368.
40. Dobbie RP: Avulsion of the lower biceps brachii tendon: Analysis of 51 previously unreported cases. *Am J Surg* 1941;51:662–683.
41. Morrey BF, Askew LJ, An KN, et al: Rupture of the distal tendon of the biceps brachii: A biomechanical study. *J Bone Joint Surg* 1985;67A:418–421.
42. Baker BE: Operative vs non-operative treatment of disruption of the distal tendon of biceps, letter. *Orthop Rev* 1982;11(10):71.
43. Nielsen K: Partial rupture of the distal biceps brachii tendon: A case report. *Acta Orthop Scand* 1987;58:287–288.

44. Hovelius L, Josefsson G: Rupture of the distal biceps tendon: Report of five cases. *Acta Orthop Scand* 1977;48:280–282.

45. Boyd HB, Anderson LD: A method for reinsertion of the distal biceps brachii tendon. *J Bone Joint Surg* 1961;43A:1041–1043.

46. Anderson KJ, LeCocq JF: Rupture of the triceps tendon. *J Bone Joint Surg* 1957;39A:444–446.

47. Bennett BS: Triceps tendon rupture: Case report and a method of repair. *J Bone Joint Surg* 1962;44A:741–744.

48. Farrar EL III, Lippert FG III: Avulsion of the triceps tendon. *Clin Orthop* 1981;161:242–246.

Surgical Exposure of the Elbow: A Limited Treatise on the More Valuable Exposures in Elbow Reconstruction and Trauma

Harry E. Figgie III, MD

Introduction

The elbow is a complex joint that has multiple neurovascular structures in close proximity to it. Depending on the pathologic condition and the goals of the surgical intervention, the joint or the periarticular region can be approached from anterior, posterior, medial, or lateral directions. The anteromedial approach is considered a poor surgical choice because the median nerve and the brachial artery are located in this quadrant. The most valuable approaches to the elbow joint are the three extensile approaches, and these will be described in the greatest detail. The medial extensile approach described by Bryan and Morrey[1] is one of the most widely used approaches and is excellent both for treating trauma and for reconstruction. This procedure is the best choice for exposing the medial and posterior aspects of the elbow. The extensile lateral Kocher approach is most useful for reconstruction of the lateral and anterior aspects of the joint. The extensile anterior approach of Henry is not often used, but it is a valuable procedure for release of anterolateral contractures, biceps tendon problems, and exploration of the radial nerve. Direct posterior approaches that disrupt the extensor mechanism are described. Although they can be of value, they have certain drawbacks not shared by the extensile approaches. These drawbacks will be discussed in general.

A number of limited lateral exposures have been described, but I have chosen the Kocher lateral and the Pankovich posterolateral approaches for primary discussion. I have included the limited medial approach, described by Banks in 1953, as well, although this, too, has very limited application at this time. This chapter is not meant to be an exhaustive treatise on the surgical approaches to the elbow, but rather attempts to focus on the primary extensile approaches along with useful limited exposures.

Extensile Exposures

General Principles

The basic requirements for extensile exposures to the elbow are to provide adequate visualization and to allow extension to address unforeseen circumstances safely, to preserve normal anatomy as much as possible and allow dissection along natural tissue planes, to permit satisfactory soft-tissue closure, and to allow rapid and predictable rehabilitation without disruption of the flexor or extensor mechanisms.

Extensile Approaches to the Anterior and Anterolateral Aspects of the Elbow

The anterior extensile approach, described by Henry,[2] is useful for exposure of anterior and anterolateral pathologic conditions in the elbow and periarticular regions. It is used in treating displaced fractures, biceps tendon ruptures, and radial tunnel entrapments, as well as for releasing anterior contractures (Fig. 1).

Technique The technique of the modified Henry approach begins with a skin incision that starts 5 cm proximal to the flexor crease of the elbow joint and is extended distally on the anterior margin of the brachioradialis (Fig. 1,A). The incision is carried medially across the flexor crease at a 45-degree angle and is then continued to the biceps tendon, where it is brought distally to the medial and volar aspect of the forearm, 7 cm distal to the flexion crease. The anterior exposure is between the brachioradialis laterally and the biceps and brachialis medially. This interval is identified and explored to identify the brachioradialis and the pronator teres (Fig. 1,B). The interval between the brachioradialis and pronator teres is entered after incision of its fascia, and the radial nerve is identified on the inner surface of the brachioradialis. The radial nerve at this point gives off the branch of the superficial sensory nerve. The deep motor structures of the radial nerve are retracted laterally with the brachioradialis muscle.

When the goal of the surgeon is to expose the anterior and lateral elbow joint, the brachioradialis is retracted laterally and the pronator retracted medially. The radial artery is observed at this level, and the muscular branches can be sacrificed to provide further exposure (Fig. 1,C). The mobile wad of three is retracted laterally. The brachialis muscle may be elevated and retracted medially to expose the more proximal capsule. When distal exposure is needed, the forearm is fully supinated and the insertion of the supinator muscle on the proximal radius is identified. The supinator muscle is dissected subperiosteally from the bone and is retracted laterally, protecting the posterior interosseous nerve that passes through its substance. At this point, the proximal portion of the radius is identified down to the junction of the proximal and middle thirds. Further exposure of the radius can be performed by pronating the radius at this point.

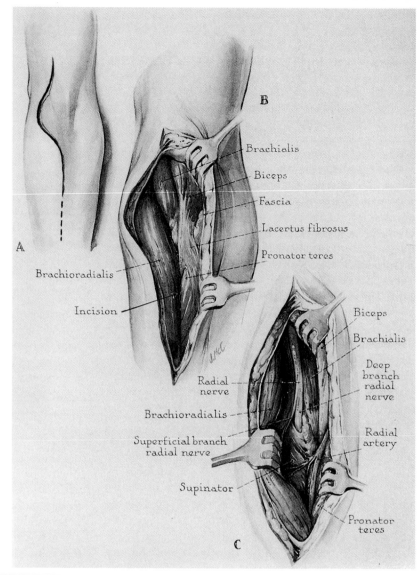

Fig. 1 The anterior Henry approach. The procedure is detailed in the text. (Reproduced with permission from Banks SW, Laufman H: *An Atlas of Surgical Exposures of the Extremities*. Philadelphia, WB Saunders, 1987, p 109.)

The Posteromedial Extensile Triceps-Sparing Exposure

Described by Bryan and Morrey[1] in 1982, this is an extremely useful approach to posterior and medial abnormalities, including damage to the ulnar collateral ligament and ulnar nerve, supracondylar fractures (including T and Y fractures), infection, and the floating elbow. It is also useful for total joint arthroplasty and can be extended to address fractures of the proximal ulna. This approach allows exposure of the medial collateral ligament and ulnar nerve, including extensive posterior and medial exposures. A more extensive anterior exposure is available by means of the extensile Kocher approach. Elbow synovectomy can be performed through this exposure, although it is more commonly done through the lateral approach (Fig. 2).

Technique The patient is placed in a supine position with a sandbag under the scapula. The procedure em-

ploys a sterile pneumatic tourniquet. The arm is brought across the chest. The elbow is approached through a posterior incision medial to the midline directly over the ulnar nerve (Fig. 2,*A*). It begins at a point 9 cm proximal and transverses to a point 8 cm distal to the tip of the olecranon. The distal limb of the exposure is brought toward the midline of the forearm. The ulnar nerve is identified proximally at the medial head of the triceps and is dissected free of the cubital tunnel (Fig. 2,*B*).

The medial triceps is elevated from the humerus along the intermuscular septum (Fig. 2,*C*). The insertion of the triceps onto the olecranon is dissected free and the superficial fascia of the forearm is incised distally to the level of the periosteum of the proximal ulna. The periosteum, fascia, and triceps insertions are all reflected laterally (Fig. 2,*D*). Care must be taken to prevent the development of discontinuity in the triceps

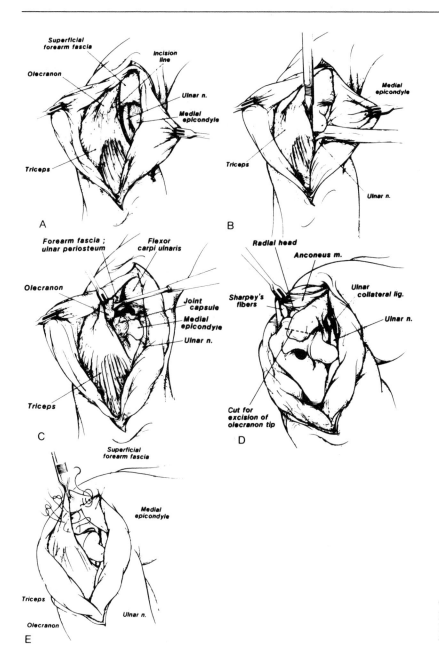

mechanism. The flap is dissected laterally and, if exposure of the radial head is desired, the anconeus is dissected subperiosteally from the proximal ulna and the flap retracted further laterally. The tip of the olecranon is removed for visualization of the trochlea. To disarticulate the olecranon from the humerus, the medial collateral ligament is released at the level of the sublimis tubercle. When closure is initiated, the extensor mechanism is returned to the anatomic position and sutured to the olecranon (Fig. 2,*E*). The periosteum and the superficial forearm fascia are repaired and, if it has been released, the medial collateral ligament is

also repaired. The tourniquet should be released before closure.

The Triceps-Sparing Approach

Described by Kocher[3] in 1911, this approach is best used for the resurfacing-style total elbow arthroplasty, surgery for ankylosis or synovectomy, and for excision of the radial head. This procedure is the extensile version of the more limited approach described below (Fig. 3).

Technique In the extensile approach, the skin incision

begins 8 cm proximal to the joint, posterior to the supracondylar ridge of the triceps (Fig. 3,A). The incision is brought distally over the anconeus and continues 6 cm distal to the tip of the olecranon. The triceps is identified and the interval between the triceps and brachioradialis and extensor carpi radialis longus at the level of the intermuscular septum is identified. The interval between the extensor carpi radialis longus and anconeus is identified proximally, and the interval between the extensor carpi ulnaris and the anconeus is identified distally (Fig. 3,B). These intervals are developed and the capsule is exposed. The anconeus is reflected subperiosteally toward the triceps, protecting its innervation (Fig. 3,C). At the insertion of the triceps tendon, the tip of the olecranon is sharply released, and the extensor mechanism composite is reflected medially. The joint can now be dislocated after subperiosteal release of the radial collateral ligament complex is performed (Fig. 3,D). The elbow is dislocated along the medial hinge of the medial epicondyle. This exposure gives excellent visualization of the elbow joint itself and provides excellent access not only to the lateral compartment, but also to the anterior portion of the elbow.

Limited Lateral Exposure

The lateral approach to the elbow joint is the one most frequently used and the one that has the largest number of variations. The approach used most often is the lateral one described by Kocher[3] in 1911, which approaches the joint between the extensor carpi ulnaris and the anconeus. It is an ideal approach for excision of the radial head or exploration of the lateral compartment of the elbow.

Advantages

This is the safest of approaches to the radial head, because it provides significant protection to the deep radial nerve as it passes close to the radius in the distal aspect of the exposure. It is preferable to the lateral approach described by Kaplan[4] in 1941 and the transepicondylar lateral approach of Campbell and associates[5] described in 1971, because it can be extended into an extensile posterolateral exposure if this becomes desirable.

Technique The skin incision is placed just proximal to the lateral epicondyle of the humerus in the avascular interval, and is extended distally and posteriorly approximately 6 cm obliquely over the fascia of the anconeus and the extensor carpi ulnaris. Dissection is carried down to the joint capsule through the interval of the anconeus and the extensor carpi ulnaris. The deep radial nerve is protected by the bulk of the extensor carpi ulnaris and the extensor digitorum communis. Adequate posterior exposure of the humerus is pro-

vided by subperiosteal dissection of the origin of the anconeus muscle. The radiocapitellar joint can be exposed at this point. If the lateral condyle is fractured, the exposure can be extended into the extensile Kocher approach described previously.

Limited Posterolateral Exposure

The Posterolateral Exposure

Described by Pankovich[6] in 1977, this approach is the most extensive posterolateral exposure available. It permits treatment of radial head or Monteggia fractures, lateral ligament reconstruction, and exposure of the lateral compartment of the elbow. With the techniques described by Boyd[7] in 1940, it can be extended to include exposure of the ulna.

Technique The patient is placed in a semilateral position with support under the scapula. The arm is brought across the chest. The incision begins 2 to 3 cm proximal to the olecranon, extends over the lateral border of the triceps tendon, and is directed 5 cm down the posterior ridge of the ulna. The extensor fascia is released from the ulna along the dorsal origin of the anconeus. The interval between the anconeus and extensor carpi ulnaris is identified, and the anconeus is reflected proximally off its ulnar insertion by subperiosteal dissection. The medial portion of the anconeus is then released as it abuts the triceps, which exposes the lateral compartment of the elbow. The anconeus muscle may be reflected in toto from distal to proximal without interruption of its innervation. At this point, the surgeon has excellent visualization of the lateral collateral ligament complex, proximal ulna, posterolateral capsule, and elbow joint compartment. Further visualization of the lateral compartment can be achieved by releasing the lateral collateral ligament complex and common extensor origin from its proximal attachment on the humerus. Dislocating the elbow joint posteriorly exposes the anterior compartment and the coronoid process. The dislocated elbow joint hinges on the intact medial collateral ligament complex. When further exposure of the ulna is required, the anconeus and extensor carpi ulnaris are stripped subperiosteally from the ulna, beginning on the lateral subcutaneous crest of the bone and reflecting the muscles in a volar direction. The supinator is released subperiosteally from its insertion on the ulna. When greater exposure of the radius is needed, the recurrent interosseous artery is divided and the muscle mass of the supinator is reflected volarward to expose the interosseous membrane.

Posterolateral Exposure of the Radial Head and Proximal Ulna

Described by Boyd[7] in 1940, this approach is perhaps more useful than the Pankovich[6] approach for the Monteggia fracture.

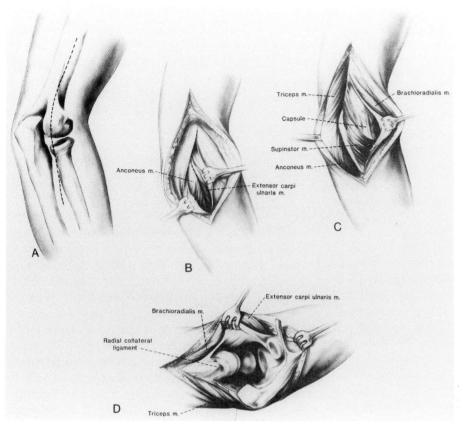

Fig. 3 The triceps-sparing approach. The procedure is detailed in the text. (Reproduced with permission from the Mayo Foundation.)

Technique The approach is begun just posterior to the lateral epicondyle and lateral to the triceps tendon and is continued along the subcutaneous border of the ulna for approximately one third of its length. The anconeus and extensor carpi ulnaris are stripped subperiosteally from the ulna, beginning on the lateral aspect of the ulna and reflecting the muscles volarly. The lateral surface of the ulna and proximal portion of the radius can be exposed adequately by this approach. When greater exposure is needed, the recurrent interosseous artery is divided and the muscle mass of this supinator, as well as the other muscle groups, is reflected further volarward.

The posterolateral approach described by Gordon[8] in 1967 attempts to combine features of both the Boyd and the Kocher approach. Although it offers theoretical benefits, I have no experience with this particular approach.

Limited Medial Approaches

Indications for a medial approach to the elbow joint are limited. The medial transepicondylar approach described independently by Molesworth[9] in 1930 and Campbell[10] in 1932 is beneficial for the treatment of

medial joint abnormalities with associated ulnar nerve symptoms. The medial approach to the proximal ulna designed by Taylor and Scham[11] in 1969 is useful for ulnar fractures. However, in most cases the extensile Mayo approach is a more useful approach for these particular problems, and the reader is encouraged to use this approach.

Banks Approach

For limited disease of the medial joint and capsule, such as the removal of loose bodies not appropriate for arthroscopic debridement, the Banks and Laufman[12] approach described in 1953 is recommended. Because this approach does not interrupt the main anterior bundle of the ulnar collateral ligament, it does not risk destabilizing the elbow.

Technique The elbow is approached through a 6-cm longitudinal incision centered over the posterior aspect of the elbow joint midway between the medial epicondyle and the olecranon process. The ulnar nerve is identified and retracted, and dissection is carried medially to the medial epicondyle. The proximal fibers of the flexor carpi ulnaris are retracted away from the ulna, and the joint capsule is exposed through the space from the flexor carpi ulnaris distally and by stripping the triceps muscle and tendon from the posterior capsule proximally. Care must be taken not to release the anterior portion of the medial collateral ligament.

Posterior Approaches That Disrupt the Extensor Mechanisms

There are a number of direct posterior approaches to the triceps. In general, I recommend the reflection of the triceps in continuity, using either of the two extensile exposures described above. When the posterior exposure of the distal humerus for intercondylar fractures is needed, the exposure described by Alonso-Llames[13] is recommended.

Triceps Splitting and Triceps Reflection

There are two primary approaches that interrupt the triceps posteriorly. The first, described by Campbell and associates[5] in 1932, is a posterior triceps-splitting incision. The second is the triceps reflection described by Campbell and associates[5] in 1932 and Van Gorder[14] in 1940. The two approaches are similar; both interrupt the triceps mechanism. The triceps reflection approach is preferable for ankylosis, in which tensioning of the triceps is beneficial. Both procedures have the complication of disrupting the continuity of the triceps. They do not allow rapid mobilization of the arm, and they limit medial and lateral exposure. Specifically, in the posterior triceps-splitting incision, care must be taken to maintain the medial portion of the triceps expansion over the forearm fascia and continuity with the flexor carpi ulnaris, which can be difficult. Failure to do this leads to triceps rupture medially. The benefit of the procedure is excellent proximal extension.

Technique For the posterior triceps-splitting approach, a skin incision is directed in the midline over the triceps 10 cm above the joint line and brought slightly medially at the tip of the olecranon and then distally over the proximal ulna for approximately 6 cm. The triceps is exposed through the proximal limb of the incision, and a midline incision is made through the triceps fascia and tendon. The triceps tendon and muscle are split longitudinally, exposing the distal humerus. The anconeus is reflected subperiosteally laterally, and the flexor carpi ulnaris is reflected medially. The insertion of the triceps is released from the olecranon, leaving the extensor mechanism in continuity with the forearm fascia and muscles medially and laterally. I recommend visualizing the ulnar nerve. The Van Gorder[14] approach is similar, except that the tendinous attachment of the triceps to the olecranon is maintained, and a V-Y turndown of the triceps performed. This approach offers the advantage of allowing subperiosteal dissection, exposing both the medial and lateral condyles. Again, the difficulty with this approach is the necessity for postoperative immobilization.

Posterior Transosseous Exposures

Several of these exposures have been described. The two most commonly used are the oblique osteotomy of the olecranon, described by Muller and associates[15] in 1970, and the transolecranon osteotomy, described by MacAusland[16] in 1915. Both are useful for the treatment of ankylosed joints and T- or Y-shaped condylar fractures. The difficulty with all of these approaches is that they necessitate healing of an additional fracture and they provide, in effect, a fracture line through the elbow joint itself. Furthermore, transolecranon osteotomies are a poor choice in rheumatoid arthritis, because the olecranon itself can be quite thin and fixation can be difficult.

Technique Both approaches recommend a posterior longitudinal approach. In the Muller approach, the incision is begun approximately 6 cm proximal and carried 8 cm distal to the tip of the olecranon. The lateral margin of the triceps is identified and reflected medially to expose the distal humerus. After the proximal ulna is drilled, an oblique extra-articular osteotomy, including the triceps attachment, is made across the proximal ulna, and the triceps attachment is reflected proximally and medially. In the MacAusland approach, both the medial and lateral margins of the triceps are identified. The ulnar nerve is protected, the ulna is osteotomized in the midportion of the sigmoid fossa, and the extensor mechanism is retracted proximally. The elbow is flexed in both procedures, and the joint is exposed. Again, the particular difficulties with these approaches include failure to achieve fixation and the need for another fracture to heal.

Summary

The focus of this chapter is the provision of some general guidelines concerning the approaches to the elbow. I recommend using extensile approaches to the elbow whenever possible. The medial extensile approach allows the surgeon to maintain the extensor mechanism in continuity and to see the distal humerus as well as the joint itself. It can be extended to address fractures of the proximal ulna. Ulnar nerve conditions may also be addressed at this time.

The extensile Kocher lateral approach, which exposes the lateral column and lateral joint complex, can be extended to deal with problems of the anterior capsule and anterior compartment of the elbow.

The anterior Henry approach has the benefit of exposing the anterolateral portions of the elbow joint. With retraction of the brachialis, it can, with some difficulty, expose a fair amount of the anterior elbow capsule. It is an excellent approach to the proximal third of the radius and to the radial nerve at its sites of entrapment. With exposure distally, pronation of the radius, and the use of subperiosteal dissection, the entire distal radius can be exposed. Approaching the anteromedial aspect of the elbow joint directly is not recommended, because of the presence of the neurovascular bundle at that point.

Posterior approaches to the elbow that interrupt the extensor mechanism have been in use for a long time. The difficulty with these approaches is that healing may be delayed and motion is frequently delayed. They also have the risk of an additional complication such as nonunion, avascular necrosis, malunion, or other intra-articular pathologic conditions. Also, the fixation devices often require later removal, necessitating a second procedure. When nonosseous procedures are performed, triceps weakness is frequently described.

The limited lateral and medial exposures described above have only isolated uses.

References

1. Bryan RS, Morrey BF: Extensive posterior exposure of the elbow: A triceps-sparing approach. *Clin Orthop* 1982;166:188–192.
2. Henry AK: *Extensile Exposure*, ed 2. Baltimore, Williams & Wilkins, 1957.
3. Kocher T: *Text-Book of Operative Surgery*, ed 3, Stiles HJ, Paul CB (trans). New York, Macmillan, 1911.
4. Kaplan EB: Surgical approach to the proximal end of the radius and its use in fractures of the head and neck of the radius. *J Bone Joint Surg* 1941;23:86–92.
5. Crehnshaw AH: Surgical approaches, in Campbell WC (ed): *Campbell's Operative Orthopedics*, ed 6. St. Louis, CV Mosby, 1971, vol 1, p 119.
6. Pankovich AM: Anconeus approach to the elbow joint and the proximal part of the radius and ulna. *J Bone Joint Surg* 1977;59A:124–126.
7. Boyd HB: Surgical approaches to the elbow joint, in Thomson JE (ed): American Academy of Orthopaedic Surgeons *Instructional Course Lectures, IV*. Ann Arbor, JW Edwards, 1948, pp 172–177.
8. Gordon ML: Monteggia fracture: A combined surgical approach employing a single lateral incision. *Clin Orthop* 1967;50:87–93.
9. Molesworth HWL: Operation for complete exposure of the elbow-joint. *Br J Surg* 1930;18:303–307.
10. Campbell WC: Incision for exposure of the elbow joint. *Am J Surg* 1932;15:65–67.
11. Taylor TK, Scham SM: A posteromedial approach to the proximal end of the ulna for the internal fixation of olecranon fractures. *J Trauma* 1969;9:594–602.
12. Banks SW, Laufman H: *An Atlas of Surgical Exposures of the Extremities*. Philadelphia, WB Saunders, 1953.
13. Alonso-Llames M: Bilaterotricipital approach to the elbow: Its application in the osteosynthesis of supracondylar fractures of the humerus in children. *Acta Orthop Scand* 1972;43:479–490.
14. Van Gorder GW: Surgical approach in supracondylar "T" fractures of the humerus requiring open reduction. *J Bone Joint Surg* 1940;22:278–292.
15. Muller ME, Allgower M, Willenegger H: *Manual of Internal Fixation: Technique Recommended by the AO Group*. Berlin, Springer-Verlag, 1970.
16. MacAusland WR: Ankylosis of the elbow with report of four cases treated by arthroplasty. *JAMA* 1915;64:312–318.

CHAPTER 6

Heterotopic Ossification About the Elbow

Jesse B. Jupiter, MD

Heterotopic ossification is a well-recognized, albeit uncommon, complication of trauma about the elbow.[1-6] The resulting loss of elbow motion can prove disabling, especially if the hand can no longer be positioned for functional tasks. Although much has been written regarding the subject of heterotopic ossification,[1,7-13] in fact, there still remains a good deal of misunderstanding and misinformation regarding its etiology, incidence, and treatment.

Definition

Part of the confusion surrounding heterotopic ossification lies in its definition. Heterotopic or ectopic bone formation reflects the sequelae of a clinical situation in which highly organized bone is formed in and about the elbow joint. This differs from myositis ossificans, in which organized bone forms within skeletal muscle, most commonly the brachialis muscle anterior to the elbow joint. The histologic appearance of heterotopic bone and myositis ossificans is similar.

Both of these entities must be contrasted to heterotopic calcification about the elbow. The radiographic appearance of the latter is an amorphous, well-circumscribed, and often globular structure without evidence of a trabecular pattern. It is commonly located in the collateral ligaments or capsule. As calcification about the elbow rarely interferes with mobility and requires no treatment, its radiographic differentiation and clinical implication are important after elbow trauma.

Confusion regarding the incidence of heterotopic ossification after elbow trauma may lie in part in its radiographic interpretation. Mikic and Vukadinovic[14] noted "periarticular ossification" in 34 of 60 patients reviewed after radial head excision, whereas Josefsson and associates[15] reported on the late sequelae of elbow dislocation, noting a 95% incidence of "periarticular calcification" in adults, while only one of their 52 patients had ectopic calcification.

Pathophysiology

Although most investigators agree that heterotopic ossification is the outcome of the differentiation of pluripotential mesenchymal cells into bone-forming cells, the initiating factors and biologic mediators remain to be defined. Craven and Urist's[9,13] earlier studies postulated a bone morphogenetic protein that would be transferred from the injured bone to surrounding soft tissues, stimulating the transformation of perivascular mesenchymal cells and osteoblasts. More recent studies have suggested that prostaglandin E_2 may be a mediator in the differentiation of the "pre-osteoblasts."[16] A centrally mediated factor has also been postulated, which would help explain the high incidence of para-articular ossification found with head or central nervous system trauma.[13]

What has been experimentally established and is of clinical relevance is the fact that the process of modulation of the pluripotential mesenchymal cells begins very soon after an injury. Tonna and Cronkite[17] observed osteoblastic differentiation from primitive stem cells as early as 16 hours after experimentally induced trauma to mice femurs. Clinically, this activity can be documented as early as two to three weeks after injury by means of a technetium Tc 99m radionuclide bone scan, and it is generally visible radiographically by the sixth week.[1,18]

Incidence

The risk of heterotopic ossification as an outcome of elbow trauma has influenced therapeutic decisions. McLaughlin,[18] for example, considered a radial head fracture associated with elbow dislocation to be a "fracture of necessity," and recommended early surgical intervention to minimize the risk of heterotopic ossification. This concept, which could well be challenged, continues to be advocated today.

How common is heterotopic ossification after elbow trauma? In order to assess its incidence accurately, one must distinguish isolated elbow trauma from that associated with central nervous system or head injury. Perhaps the most informative study of heterotopic ossification about the elbow in the absence of head trauma is that of Thompson and Garcia,[6] who reviewed 1,314 patients with elbow trauma treated at New York Orthopaedic Hospital from 1924 to 1964. Overall, they observed an incidence of 3% (41 patients) of heterotopic ossification. Among the 60 patients with isolated fracture of the radial head, two of 32 who underwent "early" surgery developed heterotopic ossification, compared with one of 28 after "late" surgery. A total of 59 patients had radial head fractures associated with elbow dislocations. Heterotopic ossification was observed in three of 14 patients treated nonsurgically, four of 32 patients with "early" surgery, and five of 13 patients treated with "late" surgery. Among the 311 patients with elbow dislocations without fracture, 11 developed heterotopic ossification. These authors concluded that heterotopic ossification after elbow trauma was more likely to be found in association with a dislocation and could be lessened by anesthesia adequate to allow an atraumatic reduction, early surgery, and the avoidance of passive manipulation to gain mobility.

The adverse effect of manipulation after elbow trauma was additionally documented in a series by Mohan,[19] who observed an unusually high incidence of heterotopic ossification in patients treated with manipulation by traditional "bone setters" of India.

An additional contemporary factor in the association of heterotopic bone with elbow trauma has been high-energy injury associated with disruption of the soft-tissue envelope. Today's trauma centers are confronted with extraordinary injuries with massive soft-tissue loss in combination with complex elbow fracture-dislocations. In this setting, heterotopic ossification is commonplace.

In the presence of head or central nervous system injury, the incidence of heterotopic ossification after elbow trauma increases dramatically. Garland and O'Hollaren,[3] in a series of 496 patients with head or central nervous system trauma, observed a 5% incidence of heterotopic ossification in the absence of elbow trauma. This incidence increased to 89% when elbow trauma was present.

These authors have advanced a radiologic grading system for heterotopic ossification, which should serve as a means of standardization of this entity. They considered the lesion to be mild when it was observed in only small amounts in the vicinity of the collateral ligaments, moderate when seen in the anterior and/or posterior tissues, and severe when present in all planes.[3]

Treatment

The approach to the problem of heterotopic ossification about the elbow can be viewed from two perspectives: prophylaxis both at the time of injury and after surgical resection and surgical excision of existing ectopic bone.

Prophylaxis

Given the fact that heterotopic ossification after elbow trauma is actually quite uncommon in the absence of central nervous system injury and passive forceful manipulation, there has been little experience with prophylactic measures administered immediately after an injury. Thus, much of the experience with prophylaxis has been generated in association with total hip ar-

throplasty or after resection of established heterotopic ossification.[7,10,12,18,20-23]

Two distinct pharmacologic measures have been applied in the prevention of heterotopic ossification. The first group is the diphosphonates (disodium etidronate and ethane hydroxydiphosphonate), which have been shown to inhibit the growth of hydroxyapatite crystals in vitro, thereby delaying the mineralization of osteoid.[7,11,24] Unfortunately, the disphosphonates have not been shown to have an effect on the formation of the osteoid matrix. Thus, calcification of the osteoid occurs once the diphosphonate therapy is discontinued.[12] If the diphosphonate is administered over a lengthy period, osteomalacia may occur, further limiting its attractiveness as a prophylactic measure.

The nonsteroidal agents, in particular ibuprofen and indomethacin, have been shown experimentally to inhibit the cyclo-oxygenase needed for the production of prostaglandin E_2.[16] The latter has been thought to be a formative agent in the inflammatory response and a

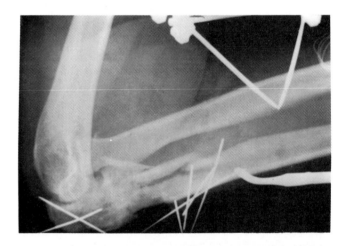

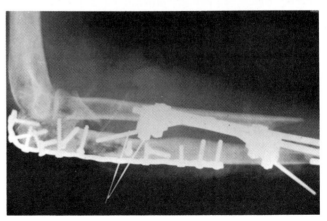

Fig. 1 A 23-year-old man was involved in a high-speed motorcycle accident associated with a complex fracture-dislocation about this elbow. Extensive soft-tissue injury was present. **Top,** An intraoperative lateral radiograph demonstrates the complex nature of the fracture. **Bottom,** The comminuted ulnar fracture was securely stabilized with external fixation applied for a more distal injury.

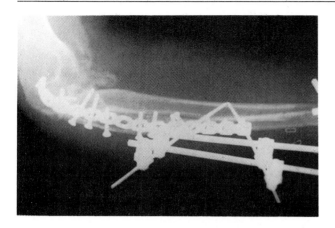
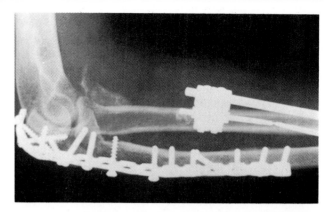
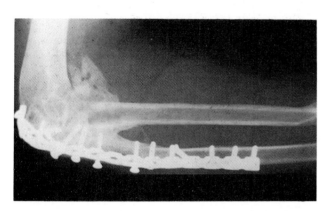
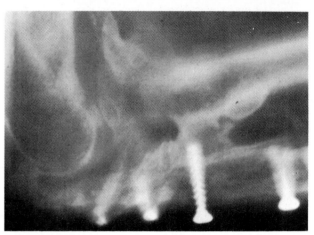

Fig. 2 The same patient shown in Figure 1. **Top left,** After three weeks, the heterotopic ossification is becoming visible. The patient was experiencing persistent pain, and his elbow remained swollen. **Top right,** At the eighth week, the heterotopic bone is becoming more mature. **Bottom left,** At four months, extensive heterotopic ossification completely blocks any mobility of the elbow. **Bottom right,** Lateral tomography clearly demonstrates extensive heterotopic ossification as well as some intrinsic damage to the articulation of the semilunar notch of the olecranon.

chemical mediator in heterotopic ossification.[25] These agents may also inhibit the differentiation of pluripotential cells into osteoblasts.[26] Their clinical efficacy has been documented in several studies associated with total hip arthroplasty.[21,22]

A third modality that offers promise as a prophylactic measure is low-dosage radiation therapy. Ionizing radiation has been shown to be effective in preventing bone formation in the rat.[17] Clinical trials in high-risk patients undergoing total hip replacement or acetabular surgery have offered encouraging results even with dosages as low as 10 Gy in five fractions, provided it is initiated as early as possible (before postoperative day 4).[7,8,20,23] Although radiation has been associated with the development of sarcomatous changes, several studies have found no radiation-induced sarcomas at doses below 30 Gy over a three-week period.[27,28] By the same token, given the fact that elbow trauma is more common in young adults, the long-term consequences of any radiation must be contemplated as well as immediate risk to wound healing about the elbow.

Treatment for heterotopic ossification need not be considered unless function is significantly impaired. If surgical excision is thought to be warranted, the timing becomes crucial. It has long been taught that excision should not be considered until the heterotopic bone has "matured." Several difficulties exist in adhering to this guideline. In the first place, radiographs, serum alkaline phosphatase levels, and even technetium Tc 99m bone scans have proven unreliable in quantifying the maturity of the process.[1] Secondly, extensive delay in the restoration of some elbow mobility can well lead to the development of intrinsic problems, such as capsular or ligamentous contracture or even articular cartilage degeneration (Figs. 1 and 2).[4]

In the absence of head or central nervous system injury, surgical excision of heterotopic bone about the elbow can be considered as early as six to nine months after injury. Although capsular or ligamentous release may be necessary, I strongly recommend against additional procedures such as osteotomies or even implant removal that would leave raw bony surfaces and a greater likelihood of reformation of ectopic bone. Hemostasis, suction drainage, and continuous passive motion are also important.

The surgical approach to heterotopic ossification in patients with associated head or central nervous system trauma is considerably different. Patient selection is critical. Garland and associates,[2] in a series of 23 elbow resections performed in patients with head trauma, noted that most patients with minimum cognitive disability, a normal level of alkaline phosphatase, and lesions that were "mature" approximately 18 months after injury, had improved motion and limb function with fewer complications and less recurrence of heterotopic ossification.

The four complications noted in their series of 23 elbows included three postoperative infections and one ulnar nerve laceration. They also noted recurrence of the lesion in all five elbows in patients with severe cognitive and physical defects, suggesting that the heterotopic ossification, despite a "mature" appearance radiographically, is not always self-limited in patients with severe neural deficits.

Summary

Heterotopic ossification, a dreaded complication of trauma about the elbow, is, in fact, uncommon in the absence of head trauma, severe soft-tissue injury, and postoperative passive manipulation. If it does occur and proves to be functionally disabling, consideration can be given to surgical resection, which should be as atraumatic as possible and not associated with other skeletal procedures such as osteotomy or implant removal. Prophylaxis against recurrence remains unpredictable, but, at present, indomethacin and low-dose radiation therapy, both instituted immediately after injury or surgery, appear to offer some help.

Heterotopic ossification about the elbow in the presence of brain or central nervous system injury is extremely common. In this setting, if resection is considered, patients with minimal cognitive disability, a normal alkaline phosphatase level, and a longer interval from injury to surgery are the ones most likely to have a favorable outcome.

References

1. Coventry MB: Ectopic ossification about the elbow, in Morrey BF (ed): *The Elbow and Its Disorders.* Philadelphia, WB Saunders, 1985, pp 464–471.
2. Garland DE, Hanscom DA, Keenan MA, et al: Resection of heterotopic ossification in the adult with head trauma. *J Bone Joint Surg* 1985;67A:1261–1269.
3. Garland DE, O'Hollaren RM: Fractures and dislocations about the elbow in the head-injured adult. *Clin Orthop* 1982;168:38–41.
4. Plasmans CM, Kuypers W, Slooff TJ: The effect of ethane-1-hydroxy-1, 1-diphosphonic acid (EHDP) on matrix-induced ectopic bone formation. *Clin Orthop* 1978;132:233–243.
5. Roberts PH: Dislocation of the elbow. *Br J Surg* 1969;56:806–815.
6. Thompson HC III, Garcia A: Myositis ossificans: Aftermath of elbow injuries. *Clin Orthop* 1967;50:129–134.
7. Ayers DC, Evarts CM, Parkinson JR: The prevention of heterotopic ossification in high-risk patients by low-dose radiation therapy after total hip arthroplasty. *J Bone Joint Surg* 1986;68A:1423–1430.
8. Bosse MJ, Poka A, Reinert CM, et al: Heterotopic ossification as a complication of acetabular fracture: Prophylaxis with low-dose irradiation. *J Bone Joint Surg* 1988;70A:1231–1237.
9. Craven PL, Urist MR: Osteogenesis by radioisotope labelled cell populations in implants of bone matrix under the influence of ionizing radiation. *Clin Orthop* 1971;76:231–233.
10. Jowsey J, Coventry MB: Heterotopic ossification: Theoretical considerations, possible etiologic factors, and a clinical review of total hip arthroplasty patients exhibiting this phenomenon. *Orthop Times* 1977;1:69.
11. McLaren AC: Prophylaxis with indomethacin for heterotopic bone: After open reduction of fractures of the acetabulum. *J Bone Joint Surg* 1990;72A:245–247.
12. Thomas BJ, Amstutz HC: Results of the administration of diphosphonate for the prevention of heterotopic ossification after total hip arthroplasty. *J Bone Joint Surg* 1985;67A:400–403.
13. Urist MR: New bone formation induced in postfetal life by bone morphogenic protein, in Becker RO (ed): *Mechanisms of Growth Control.* Springfield, Charles C Thomas, 1981, pp 406–434.
14. Mikic ZD, Vukadinovic SM: Late results in fractures of the radial head treated by excision. *Clin Orthop* 1983;181:220–228.
15. Josefsson PO, Johnell O, Gentz CF: Long-term sequelae of simple dislocation of the elbow. *J Bone Joint Surg* 1984;66A:927–930.
16. Ho SSW, Stern PJ, Bruno LP, et al: Pharmacological inhibition of prostaglandin E_2 in bone and its effect on pathological new bone formation in a rat burn model. *Trans Orthop Res Soc* 1988;13:536.
17. Tonna EA, Cronkite EP: Autoradiographic studies of cell proliferation in the periosteum of intact and fractured femora of mice utilizing DNA labeling with H_3 thymidine. *Proc Soc Exp Biol Med* 1961;107:719–721.
18. McLaughlin HL: Symposium on critical emergencies: Some fractures with a time limit. *Surg Clin North Am* 1955;35:553–561.
19. Mohan K: Myositis ossificans traumatica of the elbow. *Int Surg* 1972;57:475–478.
20. Coventry MB, Scanlon PW: The use of radiation to discourage ectopic bone: A nine-year study in surgery about the hip. *J Bone Joint Surg* 1981;63A:201–208.
21. Ritter MA, Sieber JM: Prophylactic indomethacin for the prevention of heterotopic bone formation following total hip arthroplasty. *Clin Orthop* 1985;196:217–225.
22. Schmidt SA, Kjaersgaard-Andersen P, Pedersen NW, et al: The use of indomethacin to prevent the formation of heterotopic bone after total hip replacement: A randomized, double-blind clinical trial. *J Bone Joint Surg* 1988;70A:834–838.
23. Sylvester JE, Greenberg P, Selch MT, et al: The use of postoperative irradiation for the prevention of heterotopic bone formation after total hip replacement. *Int J Radiat Oncol Biol Phys* 1988;14:471–476.
24. Fleisch HA, Russell RG, Bisaz S, et al: The inhibitory effect of phosphonates on the formation of calcium phosphate crystals in vitro and on aortic and kidney calcification in vivo. *Eur J Clin Invest* 1970;1:12–18.
25. Stern PJ, Bruno LP, Hopson CN: Skeletal deformities after burn injuries: An animal model. *Trans Orthop Res Soc* 1985;10:175.
26. Rosenoer LML, Gonsalves MR, Roberts WE: Indomethacin inhibition of preosteoblast differentiation associated with mechanically induced osteogenesis. *Trans Orthop Res Soc* 1989;14:64.
27. Brady LW: Radiation-induced sarcomas of bone. *Skeletal Radiol* 1979;4:72–78.
28. Kim JH, Chu FC, Woodard HQ, et al: Radiation-induced soft-tissue and bone sarcoma. *Radiology* 1978;129:501–508.

The Rehabilitation of the Elbow After Injury

Allan E. Inglis, MD

Few therapeutic modalities challenge the orthopaedic surgeon, the therapist, and the patient more seriously than elbow stiffening after an injury. The patient, finding that the elbow does not bend to raise the hand to the face or lower it to the feet, becomes frustrated and, in many cases, angry. The painless flexibility of the normal elbow is such an unconscious function that the patient is rarely aware of the fact that it is this flexibility that makes it possible to posture the hand in space. The great value of this function is often fully appreciated only after it is lost.

Caring for patients whose initial treatment was performed elsewhere can put the orthopaedic surgeon or the treating physician at a disadvantage. In such a case, the patient must make the adjustment to a new physician and a new treatment location. Treatment must start over again, with new concerns regarding prognosis, likelihood of success, and, on the physician's part, compliance levels.

Therapeutic Problems

Successful elbow function occurs through multiple articulations. The ulnohumeral joint must remain stable. This is accomplished both through its grooved surface contacts and through the anterior medial ligament. The tip of the olecranon process and also the coronoid process must have sufficient space in the coronoid and the olecranon fossae of the humerus to allow full flexion and full extension. The radiocapitellar joint, although normally lightly loaded (no more than 50% except pathologically), must be congruous to prevent impingement. A fracture of the radial head or of the capitellum that leaves an elevated or prominent surface can lead to impingement and reduced function (Fig. 1). The radioulnar articulation must be perfectly congruous. The annular ligament stabilizes and holds the radial head tightly against the ulna, so that any irregularity in the radial head immediately restricts rotation of the forearm. Damage to any of its articulations restricts the function of the elbow (Fig. 2).

Counterproductive stretch reflexes in the triceps and the elbow flexor muscles can be difficult to manage. When the elbow is painful, these stretch reflexes become hyperreactive. If the therapist is gently using an assisted exercise program for a painful elbow, the antagonist muscle invariably begins to resist with great force. Even such activities as carrying a heavy weight

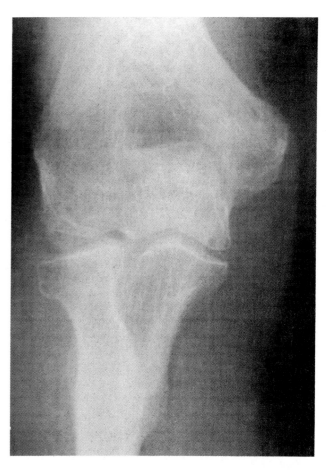

Fig. 1 This patient, who had fractured the radial head a year earlier, complained of poor pronation and restricted flexion. Removal of the radial head allowed greater flexion and 45 degrees of pronation.

to stretch the elbow out can increase the flexion contracture caused by these counterproductive stretch reflexes.

Defining precisely the functional needs of the patient can help in setting realistic goals. The patient's needs may be very different from the goals sought by the physician and the therapist. Conversely, the goals the patient desires may be unrealistic in view of the condition of the injured joint. There is frequently a very aggressive repair phenomenon in the capsular structures about the elbow joint. The normally thin anterior capsule of the elbow becomes dense and thickened and appears to grow worse with each therapy session. Ex-

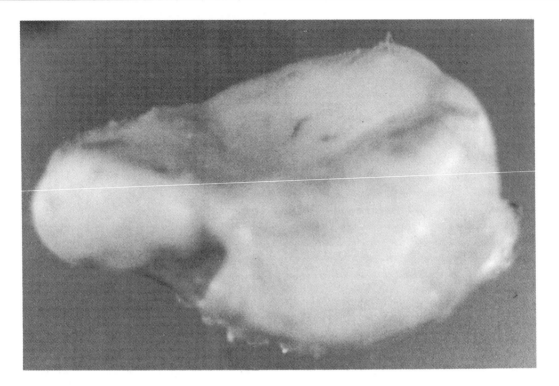

Fig. 2   The excised radial head of the patient in Figure 1. The large extruded fracture fragment that impinged on the anterior border of the capitellum, preventing flexion, also impinged against the ulna, restricting pronation.

cessive fibroplasia and contracture are difficult problems.

With any injury to the elbow joint, energy released in the joint is transmitted to the surrounding tissues. This energy causes gross disruption of the tissues, and is also dissipated into the tissues at a cellular level. These forces can initiate such cellular reactions as edema (Fig. 3), inflammation, and fibroplasia. The extremes of these reactions may be seen in myositis ossificans and the faint calcifications and ossifications within the capsule and ligaments. A rehabilitation program must consider these risks and moderate the therapy to keep from initiating additional tissue reactions.

Assessment of Injury

Even for a patient transferred to the physician's care for follow-up treatment and rehabilitation, a detailed history and physical examination must be performed, including precise information about the cause of the injury. A careful examination of the contralateral upper extremity for comparison and a detailed examination of the shoulder, elbow, wrist, and hand on the injured side are required. All elements of the injury, including signs and symptoms of reflex sympathetic dystrophy, reduced neurofunction, joint effusions, and soft-tissue edema, must be assessed carefully. It is also essential to obtain new radiographs. If there is any difficulty assessing normal radiographs, computed axial tomography can be very helpful. Other laboratory data, including erythrocyte sedimentation rate, uric acid level, and, at times, an evaluation for Lyme disease or inflammatory arthritis, can also be of use. During this time, the physician can also assess the patient's personality and determine the patient's pain threshold, compliance commitments, and employment demands. With this information a rehabilitation program can be designed with the help of a therapist, who should conduct a separate profile and therapeutic assessment.

Therapeutic Goals

After the initial evaluation, the physician should meet with the patient to redefine the patient's vocational and avocational needs. The physician should be conservative in predicting the final therapeutic result. In some cases, the avocational needs of the patient may take precedence over the vocational requirements. For example, the avid golfer must have a flexible right elbow, while the left elbow can be fairly stiff in extension. In addition to determining needs, a conservative time frame for achieving these goals should be established.

Problem Injuries

Rehabilitation must consider soft tissue, bone, and combinations of the two. Some injuries, for example, tennis elbows and overuse syndromes involving the medial side of the elbow such as the pronator teres, may involve only muscle and tendon. Others may involve the capsule and the ligamentous support. Many injuries respond to rest followed by a stretching and strengthening program. If soft-tissue injuries require surgery, there will be an inflammatory response as the wounds heal. It is, therefore, necessary to consider both the surgery and the primary injury in designing a rehabilitation program. Fractures and dislocations with attendant fragmentation and instability also require study and planning. Again, surgery to correct fractures and dislocations adds another dimension to the healing and rehabilitation process.

Subjects

Rehabilitation of injuries in children may be helped by the greater flexibility of their young tissues. Additionally, growth potential may gradually improve a flexion or extension contracture. In general, children have a relatively high threshold for pain. On the other hand, although their tissues are less flexible, adults are often more cooperative and, if motivated, remain more compliant during a long and tedious rehabilitation program.

Problem Avoidance

Elbow swelling must be controlled. Any edema in the soft tissues about the elbow results in a concomitant joint effusion, which will distend the capsule and restrict motion (Fig. 3). Elastic bandages, compression dressings, or elastic elbow stockings are very helpful. A warm whirlpool, although it may feel good, generally only aggravates the swelling of the entire extremity. During therapy, analgesics should be administered generously. These can be nonsteroidal anti-inflammatory drugs, salicylates, or even low-dose narcotics. It is extraordinarily difficult, if not impossible, to rehabilitate the traumatic elbow if the patient is in pain throughout the rehabilitation session. The entire elbow should be immersed in an ice bath after the therapy session to reduce swelling and inflammation. A small ice bag placed on one side of the elbow is insufficient. Resting splints are nearly always mandatory. When the elbow is not being exercised it should be rested. Dynamic splints are not useful because their continuous flexion or extension of the elbow causes inflammation, and the elbow muscles, which need rest, constantly fight these splints. It is also essential that night splints, usually in

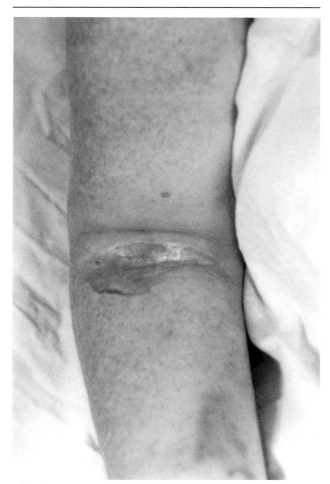

Fig. 3 This patient had a simple epicondylar fracture. A tight elbow cylinder cast caused an antecubital skin slough and moderately severe elbow and forearm swelling. Although the fracture healed, rehabilitation was slow and in the end achieved only 45 degrees of extension while obtaining full flexion and rotation.

extension, be employed (Fig. 4). All elbows, whether injured or normal, tend to assume a flexed posture at night, in effect giving the fibroblast a six- to eight-hour head start each night. In my experience, extension splints may be needed for many months after an elbow injury. Ground gained during rehabilitation may very well be lost each night if the elbow is allowed to relax into a flexed posture.

During elbow rehabilitation, other serious problems can appear. If the elbow is kept in a sling or if an exercise program is not prescribed and developed for the shoulder as well as the elbow, adhesive capsulitis of the shoulder can result. This problem can be avoided by putting the shoulder through a complete range of motion twice a day. During elbow rehabilitation, there can also be loss of wrist and digital flexion and extension and loss of grasp. Patients should be encouraged to exercise the wrist and to exercise the hand with a grasp-and-release program. Subliminal compartment syndromes may be present, especially in children. These

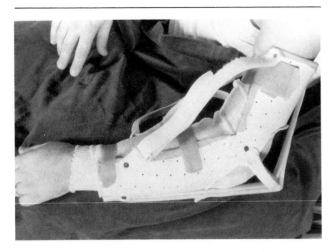

Fig. 4 An adjustable splint fabricated to fit the individual patient. The adjustable posterior strap, which holds the splint in extension, can be released to allow active flexion and extension. Anterior straps are used to hold the elbow in flexion.

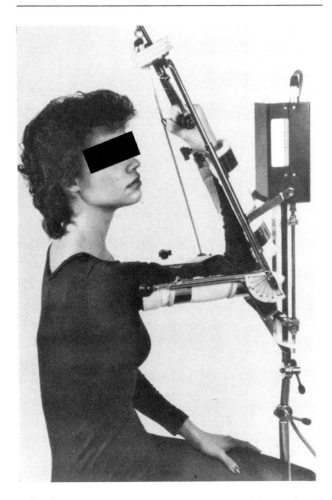

Fig. 5 This elbow constant passive motion machine can be adjusted for any size arm. The speed is variable and the angles of flexion and extension can be adjusted to tolerance and comfort. It also can be used at the bedside at night.

can be identified very simply by asking the child to open and close the hand and to extend the fingers fully in a passive fashion. Reflex sympathetic dystrophy is rare, but it is a devastating problem when it occurs. This should be treated almost as an emergency. Stellate blocks, medications, and therapy are used to control this serious problem.

Personnel

Both occupational and physical therapists are trained to treat patients with elbow injuries. Occupational therapists have a special interest in upper-extremity rehabilitation problems because they recognize the need for coordinating the function of the shoulder, elbow, and hand. Therapists who have treated a number of patients with elbow problems are of particular value when assisted exercises are needed, because they have the experience and patience to know how much gentle stretching and resistance are required. Occupational therapists use a wide range of equipment, including rolling pins, wheels and axles, and continuous passive motion devices, designed for treating adjacent elbow and shoulder problems (Figs. 5 and 6). My experience with physical therapists has also been excellent and, in many cases, patients find it easier and more convenient to schedule time with them than with their physician. Detailed instruction and follow-up by the physician helps both patient and therapist. This team approach promotes successful upper-extremity and elbow reha-

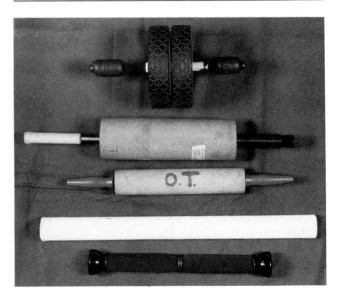

Fig. 6 Essential occupational therapy tools. The upper three devices allow active elbow flexion with varying degrees of resistance. The lower two use the opposite extremity to assist flexion and extension, and, when used in one hand, function to improve pronation and supination. The patient can start by using these during supervised therapy and then improvise for home use.

bilitation and avoids territorial problems among those providing care.

Critical Time Frame

Whenever possible, the rehabilitation program should be initiated within the first three weeks after an injury. Earlier is better. At times, however, the soft tissues need time to rest and recover from the initial shock of the injury before therapy is started. Rigid flexion and extension contractures develop rapidly after the three-week window. Surgical therapy should always be designed so that the rehabilitation process can be initiated within this three-week time period.

Complications

Complications can arise both as a result of the injury and as the result of the treatment program. Little can be done for myositis ossificans or pericapsular calcifications resulting from the injury. Rest and control of swelling are of some benefit. Overzealous therapy can increase the inflammatory reaction, causing pain, swelling, local heat, and reduced motion. In this situation the elbow should be rested and cooled with ice.

Adjunct Measures

Diathermy and ultrasound have been recommended by physiatrists and physical therapists. These can be safely administered in low doses and for short periods, but, because of the risk of increased inflammation, these modalities should be used with caution. Transcutaneous electrical stimulation can be helpful after therapy, but, in my experience, splints and ice, along with modest analgesics, are simpler to use and equally effective. Manipulation under anesthesia may also be considered in certain recalcitrant cases. I have been rather disappointed with this treatment, as the elbow appears to return rapidly to its premanipulation state. Turnbuckle splints or splints adjusted with Velcro (Fig. 4) are gentler and are effective.

I find continuous passive motion machines to be very useful. Hospital units are effective and can be used both in the therapy departments and at the bedside (Fig. 5). These units can be adjusted to provide gradual elbow flexion and extension, as well as pronation and supi-

nation, and can be rented for outpatient use. The units are usually delivered to the home, where they are set up and monitored by the therapists. The therapists either instruct the patient in their use or come by and adjust the units themselves.

Splints

There are two basic types of elbow splints. The dynamic elbow splint is expensive and I have not found it to be very effective. Its use can overstress a recovering elbow that actually needs rest, in which case its spring-loaded system produces pain and inflammation. I prefer using static splints. The fixed, right-angle splint can be individually fabricated and adjusted for comfort by the occupational therapist. Splints are particularly useful immediately after an injury. As therapy progresses, the movable static splint can be refabricated and modified by the occupational therapist. This splint has Velcro straps for adjusting extension and flexion. If more flexion is required, the splint is gently flexed and secured with the Velcro strap. If more extension is required, the extension strap is tightened. Flexion and extension straps can be used on alternating nights as a night splint. This splint has a high compliance rate with patients because it is easily adjusted, is not painful, and allows active flexion and extension. It can easily be removed for pronation and supination exercises. The splint also protects the elbow from being bumped against doors, furniture, or other objects, which, by causing pain, can interfere with the rehabilitation program.

Conclusion

Success can be achieved if the four following principles are adhered to: (1) The surgeon must accurately assess the physiologic and anatomic problems to know the precise nature of the injury and the problem. (2) The surgeon must correctly assess the patient's vocational and avocational needs and motivation for success. (3) There must be clearly defined goals that are both realistic and conservative. Any gain in excess of these goals should be viewed as a dividend. (4) The therapeutic effort requires communication and cooperation among the orthopaedic surgeon, the patient, and the therapist, because successful rehabilitation of elbow injuries requires great determination and patience on the part of the entire team.

Comments on the Historical Milestones in the Development of Elbow Arthroplasty: Indications and Complications

Ralph W. Coonrad, MD

The significant loss of function in an upper extremity resulting from ankylosis, loss of stability, or painful motion at the elbow has produced a variety of arthroplastic approaches that attempt to solve all three problems. Swanson[1] suggested that any ideal prosthetic replacement must have six basic features: It should be (1) pain-free, (2) stable, (3) durable, (4) mobile, (5) retrievable, and (6) reproducible. Additionally, arthroplasty should be considered only after conservative measures have failed.

The primary indications for elbow arthroplasty are pain, instability, and bilateral ankylosis. If these are extrapolated into pathologic entities, most arthroplasties performed in the United States at present are for elbows with articular destruction from rheumatoid arthritis; approximately one-third that number are performed for traumatic arthrosis, a few for degenerative arthrosis, and a very few when en bloc excision has been done for bone tumor.

Examples of the types of joint destruction for which arthroplasty may be considered include (1) advanced stage III or IV rheumatoid arthrosis, unresponsive to good medical management; (2) rheumatoid arthrosis in which synovectomy and radial head excision have failed; (3) degenerative arthrosis after failed debridement and loose body excision; (4) traumatic arthrosis resulting from bone stock loss or articular destruction; (5) failed interpositional or anatomic arthroplasty; (6) failed prosthetic arthroplasty; (7) arthrodesis in poor functional position, or with ankylosis of the opposite elbow; and (8) after en bloc resection for tumor.

Strict contraindications for elbow arthroplasty are (1) active infection; (2) absent flexors, or a flail elbow from motor paralysis; (3) a noncompliant patient with respect to activity limitations; (4) inadequate posterior skin quality resulting from previous surgery, burn, or other trauma; (5) inadequate bone stock or ligamentous instability with resurfacing implants; and (6) a neurotrophic joint. The functional range of motion required for the majority of activities of daily living has been reported by Morrey and associates[2] as 30 to 130 degrees of flexion. However, a lesser range of motion in the absence of pain or instability may well be satisfactory, particularly when the opposite upper extremity is normal.

Developmental milestones in the history of elbow arthroplasty can be divided into five eras or periods. They are summarized only briefly here because they have been well described elsewhere.[3-5]

The first period, from 1885 to 1947, included the development of resection, interposition, and anatomic arthroplasty. Resection arthroplasty[6] was never functionally acceptable because of the profound instability it created. On the other hand, interposition[7] and anatomic arthroplasty remain a current salvage option after prosthetic failure or infection, in preference to the handicapping restriction imposed by arthrodesis. As a primary procedure for pain relief in the stable elbow, interposition arthroplasty has produced 70% satisfactory results in some reports.[5,8-10]

The second period, from 1947 to 1970, was one primarily of custom-designed prostheses with an occasional constrained metal-to-metal hinge being reported.[11-23] Twenty-one custom implants, including those of Barr and Eaton,[24] Mellen and Phalen,[25] Robineau,[26] and Venable,[27] had been reported by 1967. Follow-up examinations after eight months to 23 years noted satisfactory early pain relief and a functional range of motion, but high rates of complication, progressive loosening, and instability.

The third period, from 1970 to 1975, called the modern era by Bryan and associates,[28,29] was one of constrained, metal-to-metal hinges held in place by polymethylmethacrylate cement,[3,30-33] a contribution from hip replacement experience by Sir John Charnley.[34] The universal failure rate in this period, caused by interface loosening resulting from hinge constraint, was inevitable because unrecognized forces of as much as three times body weight develop across the elbow joint.

The fourth period, from 1975 to 1980, saw changes in prosthetic design toward normal joint laxity, which alone nearly eliminated the problem of interface loosening. The second major contribution of Sir John Charnley in this period, that of a low-friction, metal-on-polyethylene bearing,[35] plus the major biomechanical and kinematic contributions of Morrey and associates,[36,37] Volz,[38] Inglis,[39] and others,[40-45] served to improve the longer-term results of elbow replacements significantly. The stability of implants was further increased in this period by improvement in cement technique, salvaging as much condylar bone stock as possible, and protecting the integrity of the collateral ligaments, particularly the medial. In addition, the triceps-sparing surgical approach, developed by Bryan and Morrey[46] in 1978, permitted earlier mobilization of the elbow and reduced the complications of wound healing, triceps insufficiency, and ulnar nerve prob-

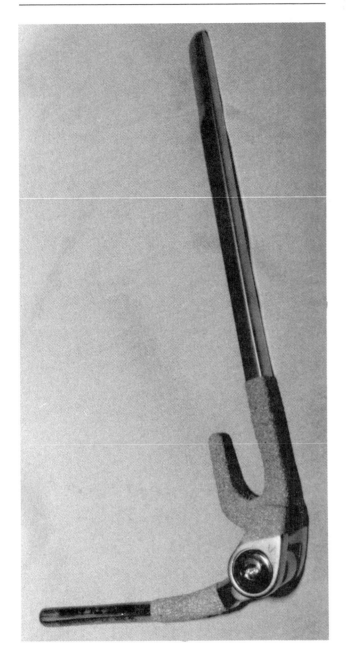

Fig. 1 Coonrad-Morrey total elbow prosthesis with band of porous beading for bio-ingrowth and anterior stabilizing flange.

lems. This approach has almost become the standard utility exposure for extensive elbow procedures.

During this period, unconstrained resurfacing prostheses used in the United States included those described by Ewald and associates,[47,48] London,[49] Wadsworth,[50,51] Street and Stevens,[52] Kudo and associates,[53] Tuke,[54] and others. Semiconstrained "snap-fit" prostheses included the Volz,[3,38,47,55] Mayo,[44,47,56–58] Pritchard-Walker,[59–61] and Tri-Axial types.[39,62,63] The semiconstrained hinge-type, the Coonrad,[58,64–69] underwent revision to a less constrained hinge and alternative longer stems. Also, during this period, the silicone implants of Niebauer and Swanson were discontinued because of a high breakage rate.

The fifth period, beginning about 1980, has seen further design changes that have improved the stability of the available prosthetic implants. Modifications of both stem length and articulating surfaces of some of the unconstrained implants, such as those of Ewald and associates and London, and the addition to the Coonrad prosthesis by Morrey of an anterior stabilizing flange and band of porous beading for bio-ingrowth (Fig. 1) appear to have further decreased the incidence of loosening with these implants. Design modifications of the Tri-Axial and Pritchard-Walker prostheses have almost eliminated the complication of dislocation with these snap-fit devices. Attempts to compensate for the normal radial-ulnar load-bearing forces across the elbow (50% to 52%) in the design of the three-part Volz,[3,39,47,55] Mayo,[3,55] and capitellocondylar (Ewald) implants were abandoned during this period because of the technical difficulty of equalizing forces on both the medial and lateral sides of the joint, even though the theoretical basis for this trend in design appeared to be, and may still be, important.

In this latest and continuing period, cadaver allograft replacement has been carried out in a small prospective study at several centers in the United States, with follow-up periods that have now reached 13 to 15 years. All the implants show progressive articular destruction, which has been compared to neurotrophic or "Charcot" joints, but the success rate is reasonable in younger individuals in whom the goal is to restore bone stock for possible implant arthroplasty at a later time. The complication rate, however, has been high, primarily from infection. In one study of 13 patients followed up for 13 years, the rate was 23% (J.R. Urbaniak, personal communication, 1990). Other complications, in addition to the joint destruction in Urbaniak's series, include nonunion, instability, and fracture; however, ten implants remain in place.

Although both resurfacing and semiconstrained hinge-type prostheses have reached a stage of development that can be considered 90% successful in the presence of good bone stock, neither type accepts the sustained force loads demanded of the normal elbow. Both types, however, allow most of the important activities of daily living, excluding sports.

Complications

The major complications after total elbow arthroplasty have included loosening of constrained prostheses, dislocation of the nonconstrained or resurfacing designs, infection, triceps insufficiency, neuropraxia, ankylosis, delay in wound healing, and intraoperative fractures.[44,55,65,68,70] Historically, complication rates from elbow arthroplasty have been higher than for the hip and knee, and during the early years[29] were reported to be 23% to 59%. The early problem of loosening is now rare in both semiconstrained and unconstrained prostheses, primarily because of added laxity in the design of the former and somewhat longer stems in the latter. Dislocation of the snap-fit, semiconstrained implants has been almost eliminated by modifications in design constraint (M.P. Figgie, personal communication) and in the resurfacing devices by a lateral triceps-sparing exposure, by a longer period of immobilization after surgery, and by design changes in articular congruency.

The catastrophic complication of deep infection has become the problem of most concern with elbow arthroplasty. When implant and total cement removal are necessary to control infection, the resultant loss of stability, extremity function, and associated vocational interruption or change can be disastrously disruptive. Financial costs for a single infection have exceeded $100,000 to $400,000 in medical expenses alone. Our increasing knowledge of antibiotic characteristics[71,72] and improvements in surgical precautions[73] and technique[74] have reduced the incidence of infection at the elbow from between 3% to 11% in 1966 to between 1% and 3% in 1990. Recent figures reported are summarized in Table 1.[75-80]

In considering total elbow arthroplasty, the criteria for patient selection, beyond the functional and pathologic status alone, are of great importance. Predisposing conditions[81] associated with elbow replacement include previous infection about the elbow; a history of musculoskeletal sepsis elsewhere in the body; nutritional depletion; severe immunosuppression; a concomitant urinary, pulmonary, dental-oral, or systemic infection; previous or anticipated surgery; advanced rheumatoid grade IV disease; and steroid administration. Patients who have ipsilateral shoulder ankylosis and are unable to maintain extremity elevation after surgery have been shown to be at higher risk. Age, sex,

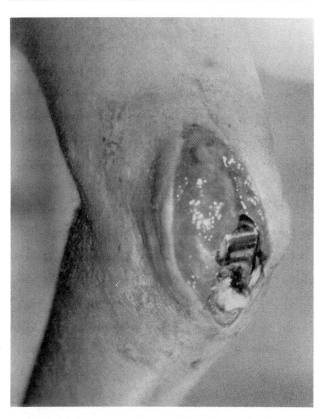

Fig. 2 Open elbow wound two weeks after first debridement and just before abdominal flap closure in a 38-year-old woman with a hematogenous inoculation infection. She had undergone surgery three months after elbow replacement. Nine years later, the patient has a functional range of motion and is pain-free.

and duration of arthroplastic surgery have not been shown to be predisposing factors. Drainage after surgery carries an increased risk, as does poor-quality or scarred skin in the area of elbow exposure.

A discussion of the pathogenesis and treatment of infection involving total joint replacement is beyond the scope of this chapter, but it is important to point out that the earlier a definite diagnosis of infection can be made, the greater the likelihood that the implant can be salvaged. Infection within 12 weeks of surgery, during the acute or "arthritic" stage and before the cement interface becomes involved, often responds to prompt debridements with the wound left open or with the wound closed under suction drainage (Fig. 2). If the wound is treated in an open fashion until cultures are negative and the active, acute phase has subsided, which I prefer, a local or pedicle flap is usually necessary to achieve a tension-free closure.

Subacute infections occurring within a year or late infections occurring after a year have a high association with bacteremia and embolic spread and a greater likelihood of cement interface involvement warranting complete removal of cement and the implant. The most common organisms implicated in implant replacements

Table 1
Comparison of infection rates reported in total elbow arthroplasty

Authors	Year	Rate
Morrey[69]	1985	9%
	1990*	1% to 2%
Ewald et al[47,77]	1980	4.3%
	1990	1.5%
Inglis[39]	1982	4.5%
Wolfe et al[78]	1990	4.7%
Trancik et al[79]	1987	8.5%
Coonrad[64]	1982	3%
	1990†	2%
R. W. Pritchard*		
Semiconstrained	1990	10%
Resurfacing	1990	0%

*Personal communication, 1990.
†Current incidence.

at the elbow are *Staphylococcus aureus* and coagulase-negative staphylococci.[82] Other organisms are sometimes involved. With coagulase-negative staphylococci, a limited period of appropriate antibiotic therapy, usually six weeks, may be appropriate. *S aureus* infections can require suppressive therapy for life.

References

1. Swanson AB: *Flexible Implant Resection Arthroplasty in the Hand and Extremities.* St. Louis, CV Mosby, 1973.

2. Morrey BF, Askew LJ, Chao EY: A biomechanical study of normal functional elbow motion. *J Bone Joint Surg* 1981;63A:872–877.

3. Dee R: Total replacement arthroplasty of the elbow for rheumatoid arthritis. *J Bone Joint Surg* 1972;54B:88–95.

4. Morrey BF, Bryan RS: Total joint replacement, in Morrey BF (ed): *The Elbow and Its Disorders.* Philadelphia, WB Saunders, 1985, pp 546–569.

5. Knight RA, Van Zandt IL: Arthroplasty of the elbow: An end-result study. *J Bone Joint Surg* 1952;34A:610–618.

6. Ollier L: *Traite des resections et des operations conservatrices qu'on peut pratiquer sur le systeme osseux.* Paris, G Masson, 1885–1889.

7. Baer WS, cited in McGehee FO: *Elbow Arthroplasty*, thesis. American Orthopaedic Association, 1959.

8. Wright PE II, Steward MJ: Fascial arthroplasty of the elbow, in Morrey BF (ed): *The Elbow and Its Disorders.* Philadelphia, WB Saunders, 1985, pp 530–539.

9. Wright PE II: The elbow IV: Adult; elbow arthroplasty. Presented at the 57th Annual Meeting of the American Academy of Orthopaedic Surgeons, New Orleans, Feb 8–13, 1990.

10. Campbell WC: Arthroplasty of the knee: Report of cases. *J Orthop Surg* 1921;3:430–434.

11. Boerema I, de Waard DJ: Osteoplastische verankerung von metall prothesen bei pseudarthrose und bei arthroplastik. *Acta Chir Scand* 1942;86:511–524.

12. Carr CR, Howard JW: Metallic cap replacement of the radial head following fracture. *West J Surg* 1951;59:539–546.

13. Cavendish ME, Elloy MA: A simple method of total elbow replacement, in *Joint Replacement in the Upper Limb.* London, Mechanical Engineering Publications, 1977, pp 93–98.

14. Chatzidakis C: Arthroplasty of the elbow joint using a vitallium prosthesis. *Int Surg* 1970;53:119–122.

15. Cherry JC: Use of acrylic prosthesis in the treatment of fracture of the head of the radius. *J Bone Joint Surg* 1953;35B:70–71.

16. Driessen APPM: Thirty years with a complete elbow prosthesis. *Arch Chir Neer* 1972;24–11:87–92.

17. Johnson EW Jr, Schlein AP: Vitallium prosthesis for the olecranon and proximal part of the ulna: Case report with 13-year follow-up. *J Bone Joint Surg* 1970;52B:721–724.

18. MacAusland WR: Replacement of the lower end of the humerus with a prosthesis: A report of four cases. *West J Surg* 1954;62:557–566.

19. Morrey BF, Askew L, Chao EY: Silastic prosthetic replacement for the radial head. *J Bone Joint Surg* 1981;63A:454–458.

20. Schlein AP: Semiconstrained total elbow arthroplasty. *Clin Orthop* 1976;121:222–229.

21. Souter WA: Arthroplasty of the elbow: With particular reference to metallic hinge arthroplasty in rheumatoid patients. *Orthop Clin North Am* 1973;4:395–413.

22. Souter WA: Total replacement of the elbow joint, abstract. *J Bone Joint Surg* 1977;59B:99–100.

23. Souter WA: Total replacement arthroplasty of the elbow, in *Joint Replacement in the Upper Limb.* London, Mechanical Engineering Publications, 1977, pp 99–106.

24. Barr JS, Eaton RG: Elbow reconstruction with a new prosthesis to replace the distal end of the humerus: A case report. *J Bone Joint Surg* 1965;47A:1408–1413.

25. Mellen RH, Phalen GS: Arthroplasty of the elbow by replacement of the distal portion of the humerus with an acrylic prosthesis. *J Bone Joint Surg* 1947;29:348–353.

26. Robineau: Contribution à l'étude des prosthèsis osseuses. *Bull Mem Soc Nat Chir* 1927;53:886–896.

27. Venable CS: An elbow and an elbow prosthesis: Case of complete loss of the lower third of the humerus. *Am J Surg* 1952;83:271–275.

28. Bryan RS, Dobyns JH, Linsheid RL, et al: Preliminary experiences with total elbow arthroplasty, in American Academy of Orthopaedic Surgeons *Symposium on Osteoarthritis.* St. Louis, CV Mosby, 1976, pp 246–257.

29. Bryan RS: Total replacement of the elbow joint. *Arch Surg* 1977;112:1092–1093.

30. Dee R: Total replacement of the elbow joint. *Orthop Clin North Am* 1973;4:415–433.

31. Dee R: Revision surgery after failed elbow endoprosthesis, in Inglis AE (ed): American Academy of Orthopaedic Surgeons *Symposium on Total Joint Replacement of the Upper Extremity.* St. Louis, CV Mosby, 1982, pp 126–140.

32. Garrett JC, Ewald FC, Thomas WH, et al: Loosening associated with G.S.B. hinge total elbow replacement in patients with rheumatoid arthritis. *Clin Orthop* 1977;127:170–174.

33. Gschwend N, Scheier H, Bähler A: GSB elbow-, wrist-, and PIP-joints, in *Joint Replacement in the Upper Limb.* London, Mechanical Engineering Publications, 1977, p 107–116.

34. Charnley J: *Acrylic Cement in Orthopaedic Surgery.* Baltimore, Williams & Wilkins, 1970.

35. Charnley J: Total hip replacement by low-friction arthroplasty. *Clin Orthop* 1970;72:7–21.

36. Morrey BF, Chao EY, Hui FC: Biomechanical study of the elbow following excision of the radial head. *J Bone Joint Surg* 1979;61A:63–68.

37. Morrey BF, Chao EYS: Passive motion of the elbow joint. *J Bone Joint Surg* 1976;58A:501–508.

38. Volz RG: Development and clinical analysis of a new semicon-strained total elbow prosthesis, in Inglis AE (ed): American Academy of Orthopaedic Surgeons *Symposium on Total Joint Replacement of the Upper Extremity.* St. Louis, CV Mosby, 1982, pp 111–125.

39. Inglis AE (ed): American Academy of Orthopaedic Surgeons *Symposium on Total Joint Replacement of the Upper Extremity.* St. Louis, CV Mosby, 1982.

40. Torzilli PA: Biomechanics of the elbow, in Inglis AE (ed): American Academy of Orthopaedic Surgeons *Symposium on Total Joint Replacement of the Upper Extremity.* St. Louis, CV Mosby, 1982, pp 150–168.

41. Amis AA, Dowson D, Wright V: Muscle strengths and musculoskeletal geometry of the upper limb. *Eng Med* 1979;8:41.

42. Amis AA, Dowson D, Wright V: Elbow joint force predictions for some strenuous isometric actions. *J Biomech* 1980;13:765–775.

43. Amis A, Miller JH, Dowson D, et al: Biomechanical aspects of the elbow. Joint forces related to prosthesis design. *Eng Med* 1981;10:65.

44. Davis PR: Some significant aspects of normal upper limb functions. Presented at the Conference on Joint Replacement of the Upper Extremity, London, 1977.

45. Youm Y, Dryer RF, Thambyrajah K, et al: Biomechanical analyses of forearm pronation-supination and elbow flexion-extension. *J Biomech* 1979;12:245–255.

46. Bryan RS, Morrey BF: Extensive posterior exposure of the elbow: A triceps-sparing approach. *Clin Orthop* 1982;166:188–192.

47. Ewald FC, Scheinberg RD, Poss R, et al: Capitellocondylar total elbow arthroplasty: Two to five-year follow-up in rheumatoid arthritis. *J Bone Joint Surg* 1980;62A:1259–1263.

48. Ewald FC, Jacobs MA: Total elbow arthroplasty. *Clin Orthop* 1984;182:137–142.

49. London JT: Resurfacing total elbow arthroplasty. Presented at the 45th Annual Meeting of the American Academy of Orthopaedic Surgeons, Dallas, Feb 23–28, 1978.

50. Wadsworth TG (ed): *The Elbow.* Edinburgh, Churchill Livingstone, 1982.

51. Wadsworth TG: A new technique of total elbow replacement. *Eng Med* 1980;10:69.

52. Street DM, Stevens PS: A humeral resurfacing prosthesis for the elbow. Presented at the 55th Annual Meeting of the American Academy of Orthopaedic Surgeons, Atlanta, 1988.

53. Kudo H, Iwano K, Watanabe S: Total replacement of the rheumatoid elbow with a hingeless prosthesis. *J Bone Joint Surg* 1980; 62A:277–285.

54. Tuke MA: The ICLH Elbow. *Eng Med* 1981;10:75.

55. Brumfield RH Jr, Volz RG, Green JF: Total elbow arthroplasty: A clinical review of 30 cases employing the Mayo and AHSC prostheses. *Clin Orthop* 1981;158:137–141.

56. Morrey BF, Bryan RS: Complications of total elbow arthroplasty. *Clin Orthop* 1982;170:204–212.

57. Morrey BF, Bryan RS: Prosthetic arthroplasty of the elbow, in Evarts CM (ed): *Surgery of the Musculoskeletal System.* New York, Churchill Livingstone, 1983, vol 2, pp 3:273–3:301.

58. Morrey BF, Bryan RS, Dobyns JH, et al: Total elbow arthroplasty: A five-year experience at the Mayo Clinic. *J Bone Joint Surg* 1981; 63A:1050–1063.

59. Rosenfeld SR, Anzel SH: Evaluation of the Pritchard total elbow arthroplasty. *Orthopedics* 1982;5:713.

60. Pritchard RW: Semiconstrained elbow prosthesis: A clinical review of five years of experience. *Orthop Rev* 1979;8:33–43.

61. Pritchard RW: Long-term follow-up study: Semiconstrained elbow prosthesis. *Orthopedics* 1981;4:151.

62. Inglis AE: Tri-Axial total elbow replacement: Indications, surgical technique, and results, in Inglis AE (ed): American Academy of Orthopaedic Surgeons *Symposium on Total Joint Replacement of the Upper Extremity.* St. Louis, CV Mosby, 1982, pp 100–110.

63. Inglis AE, Pellicci PM: Total elbow replacement. *J Bone Joint Surg* 1980;62A:1252–1258.

64. Coonrad RW: Seven-year follow-up of Coonrad total elbow replacement, in Inglis AE (ed): American Academy of Orthopaedic Surgeons *Symposium on Total Joint Replacement of the Upper Extremity.* St. Louis, CV Mosby, 1982, pp 91–99.

65. Coonrad RW, Bryan RS: Technique of Coonrad elbow arthroplasty. Warsaw, IN, Zimmer, 1974.

66. Cofield RH, Morrey BF, Bryan RS: Total shoulder and total elbow arthroplasties: The current state of development. *J Contin Educ Orthop* 1979;11:17–25.

67. Cooney WP III: Total joint arthroplasty: Introduction to the upper extremity. *Mayo Clin Proc* 1979;54:495–499.

68. Cooney WP III, Bryan RS: Rheumatoid arthritis: Part I. Rheumatoid arthritis in the upper extremity. Treatment of the elbow and shoulder joints, in American Academy of Orthopaedic Surgeons *Instructional Course Lectures, XXVIII.* St. Louis, CV Mosby, 1979, pp 247–262.

69. Morrey BF (ed): *The Elbow and Its Disorders.* Philadelphia, WB Saunders, 1985.

70. Coonrad RW: History of total elbow arthroplasty, in Inglis AE (ed): American Academy of Orthopaedic Surgeons *Symposium on Total Joint Replacement of the Upper Extremity.* St. Louis, CV Mosby, 1982.

71. Hughes SPF: The use of antibiotics in orthopaedic surgery: Total joint, single- v multiple-dose prophylaxis. *Orthop Rev* 1987;16(4): 209–214.

72. Hughes SPF: Treatment of infected implants, antibiotic acrylic composites. *Orthop Rev* 1987;16(4):233–235.

73. Moggio M, Goldner JL, McCollum DE, et al: Wound infections in patients undergoing total hip arthroplasty: Ultraviolet light for the control of airborne bacteria. *Arch Surg* 1979;114:815–823.

74. Ritter MA, Marmion P: Exogenous sources and controls of microorganisms in operating room. *Orthop Rev* 1987;16(4):224–232.

75. Morrey BF, Bryan RS: Infection after total elbow arthroplasty. *J Bone Joint Surg* 1983;65A:330–338.

76. Morrey BF, Bryan RS: Total joint arthroplasty: The elbow. *Mayo Clin Proc* 1979;54:507–512.

77. Ewald FC, Simmons ED, Sullivan JA: Long term review of the capitellocondylar total elbow replacement. Presented at the 57th Annual Meeting of the American Academy of Orthopaedic Surgeons, New Orleans, Feb 8–13, 1990.

78. Wolfe SW, Figgie MP, Inglis AE, et al: Management of the septic total elbow replacement. Presented at the 57th Annual Meeting of the American Academy of Orthopaedic Surgeons, New Orleans, Feb 8–13, 1990.

79. Trancik T, Wilde AH, Borden LS, et al: Capitellocondylar total elbow arthroplasty: Two- to eight-year experience. *Clin Orthop* 1987;223:175–180.

80. Pritchard RW: Anatomic surface elbow arthroplasty: A preliminary report. *Clin Orthop* 1983;179:223–230.

81. Bohn WW, Wolfe SW, Figgie MP, et al: Infection in total elbow arthroplasty: An analysis of risk factors. Presented at the 57th Annual Meeting of the American Academy of Orthopaedic Surgeons, New Orleans, Feb 8–13, 1990.

82. Sugarman B, Young EJ (eds): *Infections Associated With Prosthetic Devices.* Boca Raton, CRC Press, 1984.

Resection and Anatomic Elbow Arthroplasty With and Without Interposition: Indications and Results

Phillip E. Wright II, MD

E. Brantley Burns, MD

Introduction

An understanding of resection and anatomic arthroplasty of the elbow requires a brief look at history, because many aspects of these procedures are primarily of historical interest. Anatomic interpositional arthroplasty, however, is still a preferred procedure in certain situations.

Resection Arthroplasty

Historical Review and Indications

According to Dee,[1] Ollier credits Park of Liverpool and Moreau of France with the first use, in 1780, of elbow resection arthroplasty. They reportedly performed an extraperiosteal excision of the elbow joint, leaving none of the anatomic architecture of the elbow intact (Fig. 1). Ollier[2] noted unsatisfactory instability after this procedure and advocated subcapsular excision of the elbow, leaving more of the distal humerus and olecranon. He reported satisfactory results in more than 100 patients, most with tuberculous arthritis, using this modification. Since this early report, other authors, including Buzby,[3] Kirkaldy-Willis,[4] and Hurri and associates,[5] have indicated that resection arthroplasty is most suitable for ankylosis of the elbow after trauma, pyogenic infection, or tuberculosis. More recently, Vainio,[6] among others, found resection arthroplasty of the elbow useful for patients with rheumatoid arthritis.

Results

Although Ollier[2] believed gross instability to be inevitable after resection arthroplasty of the elbow, Buzby[3] reported "quite satisfactory" results in 13 of his 15 patients. His technique involved extensive resection of the elbow, leaving few stabilizing structures. Hass[7] reported excellent or good results in 11 of 14 patients; the best results were in patients with posttraumatic ankylosis. Hass modified the technique by forming the distal end of the humerus into a pointed, triangular shape to create a fulcrum for the olecranon to improve flexion and extension. This minimized bone contact, preventing re-ankylosis. Despite the considerable resection required by this technique, bone remodeling occurred over the years and some of these resection arthroplasties eventually resembled anatomic arthroplasties. Kirkaldy-Willis[4] reported that resection arthroplasty achieved excellent or good results in five of eight patients with posttraumatic ankylosis and in

four of six patients with tuberculous ankylosis. Hurri and associates[5] used resectional arthroplasty, with and without skin interposition, in the treatment of 73 patients with rheumatoid arthritis and reported that 64% of the 51 with resection arthroplasties and 40% of the 22 with skin interposition were pain-free. The patients could perform activities of daily living and relatively strenuous labor. Unander-Scharin and Karlholm[8] reported good results in 15 of 19 patients after resectional arthroplasty with fat interposition. Dee[1] evaluated 18 patients who had undergone resection or anatomic arthroplasties and found that nine patients with excisional arthroplasties had "generally unsatisfactory" results.

All reports indicate instability after resection arthroplasty and it may, at best, be considered a salvage procedure, especially after infection or to preserve elbow function after failed implant arthroplasty. With a vigorous exercise program, many patients with resectional arthroplasties achieve satisfactory function, although

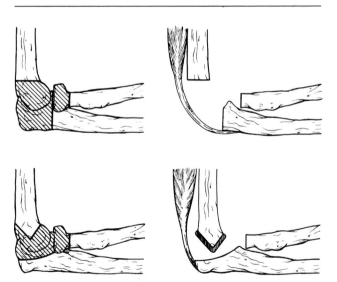

Fig. 1 Two types of excision arthroplasty of the elbow. **Top right** and **top left**, Extraperiosteal excisional arthroplasty of the elbow. (Reproduced with permission from Wadsworth TG (ed): *The Elbow*. Edinburgh, Churchill Livingstone, 1982.) **Bottom,** Subcapsular excisional arthroplasty of the elbow with triangularly shaped distal humerus advocated by Hass (**left**) and with interposition of material (skin, fascia) (**right**). (Reproduced with permission from Wadsworth TG (ed): *The Elbow*. Edinburgh, Churchill Livingstone, 1982.)

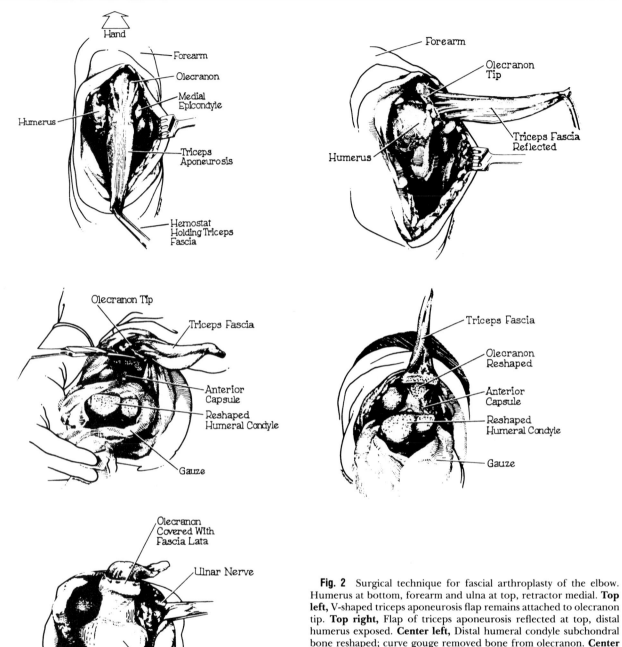

Fig. 2 Surgical technique for fascial arthroplasty of the elbow. Humerus at bottom, forearm and ulna at top, retractor medial. **Top left,** V-shaped triceps aponeurosis flap remains attached to olecranon tip. **Top right,** Flap of triceps aponeurosis reflected at top, distal humerus exposed. **Center left,** Distal humeral condyle subchondral bone reshaped; curve gouge removed bone from olecranon. **Center right,** Bony surfaces of distal humerus and olecranon prepared for application of fascia lata. **Bottom,** Fascia lata covers articular surfaces of distal humerus and olecranon. (Reproduced with permission from Wright PE II, Steward MJ: Fascial arthroplasty of the elbow, in Morrey BF (ed): *The Elbow and Its Disorders.* Philadelphia, WB Saunders, 1985, pp 530–539.)

most will have some instability with passive stressing, often necessitating bracing.

Anatomic and Interpositional Arthroplasty

Historical Review and Indications

Anatomic arthroplasty attempts to preserve most of the anatomic structures about the elbow and to main-

tain the relationship of the distal humerus with the olecranon. Defontaine[9] reportedly introduced this technique in 1887, and in the United States Murphy[10] popularized anatomic arthroplasty with interposition of fat and fascia. MacAusland,[11] Henderson,[12,13] and Campbell[14] were early advocates of fascial arthroplasty. Their indications for anatomic arthroplasty included bony ankylosis and painful fibrous ankylosis resulting from trauma, pyogenic infection, congenital deformity, or rheumatoid arthritis.

The use of this procedure in the presence of active tuberculosis in the elbow joint has been controversial. Most authors consider active tuberculosis a contraindication. However, anatomic arthroplasty with interposition of biologic material has been used successfully for ankylosis in malposition after tuberculous infection. The presence of active pyogenic infection or chronic osteomyelitis is generally agreed to be a contraindication to anatomic interposition arthroplasty.

Patients with atrophic bone (osteopenia) or severe distortion of the bony architecture, particularly after trauma, are not good candidates for anatomic arthroplasty because the unsatisfactory bone structure limits shaping of the bony surfaces. Marked muscle weakness or paralysis interferes with postoperative rehabilitation, and crutch ambulation may be difficult after elbow arthroplasty. However, crutch or walker modifications allow most patients to use these ambulatory aids if necessary. Most authors agree that anatomic or interposition arthroplasty is contraindicated in skeletally immature patients.

The best results seem to be achieved in highly motivated patients between 20 and 50 years of age who will cooperate in an intensive postoperative rehabilitation program. Even those with good results, however, cannot expect to return to heavy labor.

Interposition Materials and Technique

A wide variety of materials has been used for interposition in anatomic elbow arthroplasty, including fat and fascia,[10] pig bladder, tin, zinc, silicone, celluloid, rubber,[15] fascia alone,[11,14] absorbable gelatin sponge,[16] deep dermis of the skin,[5,17,18] and chromicized autogenous fascia.[19] Fascia lata has been the most popular interposition material.

In the technique described by Campbell,[20] a straight posterior skin incision is used and the elbow joint is approached by one of two methods: splitting of the triceps or elevating a tongue of the triceps aponeurosis from the distal olecranon (Fig. 2, *top left*). The triceps aponeurosis tongue can be used as part of the interposition material or left to aid elbow flexion in patients with severe extension ankylosis (Fig. 2, *top right*). The articular surfaces of the humerus and olecranon are then removed (Fig. 2, *center left*). Although Campbell advocated fashioning the distal end of the humerus into a single condyle (Fig. 2, *center right*), this may increase instability. The usual method is to form an olecranon concavity that matches the convex humeral condyle before covering the bone with fascia lata. Sufficient fascia lata is harvested from the thigh to cover the distal humerus, anterior capsule, and olecranon and is secured with absorbable sutures in the anterior capsule and soft tissues of the joint margins. The apposing surfaces of the arthroplasty are the deep surfaces of the fascia lata,

which create a smooth surface for the underlying vastus lateralis in its normal anatomic position (Fig. 2, *bottom*). Additional stability can be obtained by making an inverted V in the distal humerus and maintaining a matching recess in the articular surface of the olecranon (Fig. 3).[21] After the bony surfaces are covered with fascia lata, the joint is closed, taking care to protect the ulnar nerve. This technique restores motion in elbows ankylosed in a nonfunctional position, especially those with painful partial ankylosis.

Results

Henderson[12] reported 68% good or fair results after fascial arthroplasty in 21 of his patients and 94% good or fair results in 126 patients reported to him in a mail survey of 54 other surgeons. Putti[22] reported satisfactory results in 38 elbows after fascial arthroplasty. MacAusland[11] reported that four of 31 patients with fascial arthroplasty had recurrence of the ankylosis and two had persistent infection with drainage; the other 25 patients however, had "perfect" results. Campbell's[14] excellent or good results in six of 14 patients encouraged him to continue to use fascial arthroplasty. Of the 45 patients evaluated by Knight and Van Zandt[23] in 1952, 80% had good or fair results after an average follow-up of 14 years. Poor results were caused by sepsis, instability, or re-ankylosis. Richard[24] and Oyemade[25] reported good results in 78% and 76%, respectively, of patients in Nigeria and suggested that

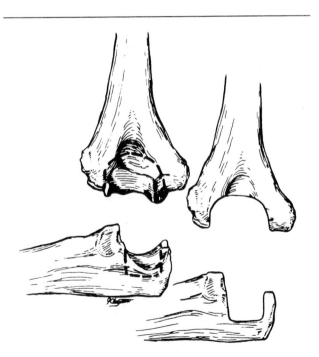

Fig. 3 Optional method of preparing distal humerus and olecranon to provide a more stable joint. (Reproduced with permission from Ferlic DC: Rheumatoid arthritis in the elbow, in Green DP (ed): *Operative Hand Surgery*, ed 2. New York, Churchill Livingstone, 1988, p 1775.)

fascial arthroplasty was appropriate treatment of elbow ankylosis in developing countries. Wright and Stewart[26] found satisfactory results in 26 of 37 patients reviewed in 1985. Dee[1] reported good results in only three of eight patients with anatomic arthroplasties without interposition. Eight of ten patients had satisfactory results after Rockwell's[16] absorbable gelatin sponge interposition arthroplasties, as did four of five patients treated with skin interposition arthroplasty reported by Froimson and associates.[18] Uuspää[27] performed 51 skin interposition arthroplasties in 48 patients with rheumatoid arthritis and reported that the procedure relieved flexion contractures and improved motion in all.

Because of the variety of grading systems used, it is difficult to compare results of different authors, but the overall average of satisfactory results from these series is approximately 65%. The best candidates for anatomic and fascial interposition arthroplasty are young, cooperative, highly motivated patients with posttraumatic bony or fibrous ankylosis causing pain or limitation of motion. Satisfactory results also may be obtained in carefully selected patients with rheumatoid arthritis.

Summary

Although resection arthroplasty is primarily of historical interest and is considered a salvage procedure for severely damaged or ankylosed, painful elbows, anatomic interpositional arthroplasty may be indicated for selected patients with posttraumatic elbow deformity or rheumatoid arthritis. Anatomic elbow arthroplasty using fascia lata as the interpositional material can alleviate pain and improve function in a significant number of patients and is often preferable to implant arthroplasty or arthrodesis, particularly in cooperative, motivated, young patients (aged 20 to 50 years) who do not require the degree of stability needed for heavy labor.

References

1. Dee R: Elbow arthroplasty. *Proc R Soc Med* 1969;62:27–31.
2. Ollier L: *Traite des resections et des operations conservatrices qu'on peut practiquer sur le systeme osseaus.* Paris, Masson, 1885.
3. Buzby BF: End-results of excision of the elbow. *Ann Surg* 1936;103:625–634.
4. Kirkaldy-Willis WH: Excision of the elbow-joint. *Lancet* 1948;1:53–57.
5. Hurri L, Pulkki T, Vainio K: Arthroplasty of the elbow in rheumatoid arthritis. *Acta Chir Scand* 1964;127:459–465.
6. Vainio K: Arthroplasty of the elbow and hand in rheumatoid arthritis: A study of 131 operations, in Chapchal G (ed): *Synovectomy and Arthroplasty in Rheumatoid Arthritis.* Stuttgart, Thieme-Verlag, 1967, pp 66–70.
7. Hass J: Functional arthroplasty. *J Bone Joint Surg* 1944;26:297–306.
8. Unander-Scharin L, Karlholm S: Experience of arthroplasty of the elbow. *Acta Orthop Scand* 1965;36:54–61.
9. Defontaine L: Ostéotomie trochléiforme: Nouvelle méthode pour la cure des ankyloses osseuses du coude. *Rev Chir* 1887;7:716–726.
10. Murphy JB: Arthroplasty. *Ann Surg* 1913;57:593–647.
11. MacAusland WR: Mobilization of the elbow by free fascia transplantation with report of thirty-one cases. *Surg Gynecol Obstet* 1921;33:223–245.
12. Henderson MS: What are the real results of arthroplasty? *Am J Orthop Surg* 1918;16:30–33.
13. Henderson MS: Arthroplasty. *Minn Med* 1925;8:97–103.
14. Campbell WC: Mobilization of joints with bony ankylosis: An analysis of one hundred and ten cases. *JAMA* 1924;83:976–981.
15. Baer WS: Arthroplasty with the aid of animal membrane. *Am J Orthop Surg* 1918;16:1–29, 94–115, 171–199.
16. Rockwell M: Arthroplasty of the elbow, abstract. *J Bone Joint Surg* 1963;45A:664.
17. Mills K, Rush J: Skin arthroplasty of the elbow. *Aust N Z J Surg* 1971;41;179–181.
18. Froimson AI, Silva JE, Richey D: Cutis arthroplasty of the elbow joint. *J Bone Joint Surg* 1976;58A:863–865.
19. Kita M: Arthroplasty of the elbow usking J-K membrane: An analysis of 31 cases. *Acta Orthop Scand* 1977;48:450–455.
20. Campbell WC: *Operative Orthopedics.* St. Louis, CV Mosby, 1939, pp 390–393.
21. Ferlic DC, Clayton ML, Parr PL: Synovectomy and arthroplasty of the elbow in rheumatoid arthritis. *Orthop Dig* 1977;5:1–14.
22. Putti V: Arthroplasty. *J Orthop Surg* 1921;3:421–430.
23. Knight RA, Van Zandt IL: Arthroplasty of the elbow: An end-result study. *J Bone Joint Surg* 1952;34A:610–618.
24. Richard D: Arthroplasty of the elbow, abstract. *J Bone Joint Surg* 1967;49B:594.
25. Oyemade GAA: Fascial arthroplasty for elbow ankylosis. *Int Surg* 1983;68:81–84.
26. Wright PE, Stewart MJ: Fascial arthroplasty of the elbow, in Morrey BF (ed): *The Elbow and Its Disorders.* Philadelphia, WB Saunders, 1985, pp 530–539.
27. Uuspää V: Anatomical interposition arthroplasty with dermal graft: A study of 51 elbow arthroplasties on 48 rheumatoid patients. *J Rheumatol* 1987;46:132–135.

Current Concepts in Snap-Fit, Sloppy-Hinge Total Elbow Arthroplasty

Harry E. Figgie III, MD

Allan E. Inglis, MD

Mark P. Figgie, MD

Victor M. Goldberg, MD

Matthew J. Kraay, MD

Introduction

Elbow arthroplasty has evolved from the use of a simple single-axis hinge joint to a complex unconstrained anatomic resurfacing arthroplasty. These changes have been made possible by a better understanding of anatomic and biomechanical concepts of the elbow joint.

Key Anatomic and Biomechanical Considerations

The elbow joint consists of three articulations: the trochleoulnar, the radiocapitellar, and the radioulnar joints. Load transmission from the hand to the shoulder occurs primarily at the trochleoulnar joint. The radioulnar joint functions primarily for forearm rotation, but also transmits compressive loads from the hand to the arm when the elbow is flexed.[1-5]

The normal elbow has an arc of 160 degrees of flexion from full extension, 80 degrees of pronation, and 85 degrees of supination.[1,6] However, the majority of activities of daily living[7] can be performed within a flexion arc of 40 to 130 degrees, and a 105-degree arc of rotation—55 degrees of pronation and 50 degrees of supination. The primary functions of the elbow include positioning of the hand in space, providing an axis for the forearm lever, and functioning as a weightbearing joint for patients who use assistive devices for walking.[8]

The distal humerus is a bicondylar articular surface consisting of the trochlea and the capitellum.[9,10] The trochlea has a 6-degree valgus inclination[7,11-13] with respect to the long axis of the humerus and a 5- to 7-degree internal rotation attitude with respect to the epicondylar axis.[7,11,13-15] The center of rotation of the trochlea is inclined anteriorly at 40 degrees[9,11,13,16] and remains essentially unchanged with flexion and extension of the elbow, although some mild variations occur at the extremes of motion.[1,7,13,17,18] In the anatomic position of full extension, the forearm is in 8 to 11 degrees of valgus in relation to the upper arm and in 6 degrees of varus when the elbow is fully flexed.[2,7,13,19]

The central depression in the head of the radius allows precise articulation with the capitellum and rotation of the forearm. The surface of the proximal ulna conforms closely to the distal humerus and resists varus, valgus, and torsional loads.[1,5] The coronoid and olecranon processes serve to resist dislocation throughout the arc of flexion. The medial collateral ligament consists of three parts, designated the anterior, posterior, and transverse bundles. The anterior bundle, the largest and clinically most important, inserts into the coronoid process along the sublimis tubercle.[9,10,13,20] The anterior bundle is taut in both flexion and extension and serves as the primary static restraint to valgus loads. Dynamic restraints to valgus dislocation forces are provided by the flexor-pronator group of muscles, but are relatively unimportant compared to the static ligamentous restraints.[1,8,11]

Forces About the Elbow Joint

In general, the muscle force and the magnitude and direction of the joint reaction force depend on the size, moment arm, and line of action of the muscles used in the activity; the position of the forearm; and the magnitude, direction, and point of application of the external load.[2,4,7,18,21-25]

Most electromyographic studies indicate that the brachialis is the primary elbow flexor, with the biceps functioning in flexion and forearm supination primarily as a deaccelerator of forearm extension. The primary elbow extensors are the anconeus and the medial head of the triceps. The lateral and long heads of the triceps are secondary elbow extensors. The maximum strength on flexion of the elbow occurs at 90 degrees and the maximum joint reaction force occurs at 30 to 60 degrees of flexion.

Varus, valgus, and rotational loads are generated under dynamic conditions such as carrying objects, rising from a sitting position with the aid of the arms, or when using devices to assist in walking. Loads caused by such activities transmit torque and shear forces to an implant-bearing mechanism and implant-bone composites.[23] Under static loading conditions, the forces produced by these activities can reach three times body weight. Dynamic loading, such as occurs in throwing and pounding, can generate peak loads in excess of six times body weight. The elbow therefore must be considered a weightbearing joint for the purpose of implant design.

Indications for Elbow Arthroplasty

The relief of pain is the primary indication for elective arthroplasty of the elbow, and restoration of stability of the elbow is the secondary indication. The restoration of motion is rarely the indication for arthroplasty.[26]

The timing of total elbow arthroplasty must take into account not only the status of the elbow but also the status of all upper- and lower-extremity joints.[11,26] When only the upper extremity requires surgery, several guidelines should be followed. The primary goal for a functional upper extremity is to restore hand function. To achieve this goal a patient must have a pain-free stable wrist and pain-free and stable metacarpophalangeal and proximal interphalangeal joints. If the hand and wrist have satisfactory function, attention may then be directed to the elbow and then the shoulder. When the elbow and shoulder are both involved with disease, the elbow should be operated on first.[27] If the shoulder has little or no rotation, however, the shoulder should be operated on before the elbow, because the substantial varus, valgus, or rotary loads that an immobile shoulder places on the elbow can lead to early failure.

When both the upper and lower extremities are involved, surgery in the lower extremity generally has priority. However, if the status of the elbows precludes the use of walking aids, elbow arthroplasty with an inherently stable prosthesis may be indicated, either before the lower-extremity surgery or at the same time.[11]

Contraindications to Total Elbow Arthroplasty

The presence of active sepsis is an absolute contraindication to an initial total elbow arthroplasty. Revision surgery for sepsis involving previous implants, however, may be necessary.

Neuropathic joints caused by diabetes, syringomyelia, or other peripheral neuropathies are relative contraindications to total elbow arthroplasty, although parkinsonism is not. Nutritional deficiencies that delay prompt healing of the surgical wound are relative contraindications to implant arthroplasty. Minor skin losses or delayed wound healing can lead to potentially disastrous deep infections or can require prolonged immobilization of the elbow with the resulting risk of stiffness. Total elbow arthroplasty in the presence of existing heterotopic ossification may stimulate still more ossification, leading to a diminished range of motion and a decreased functional score.[15,28]

Historical Perspective

The current status of total elbow arthroplasty can be traced to the introduction between 1972 and 1974 of minimally constrained cemented implants using metal and polyethylene bearing surfaces.[29–39] Semiconstrained implants developed at that time included the Schlein,[40] Pritchard-Walker (R.W. Pritchard, unpublished data), Coonrad,[31,32] AMC (R.G. Volz, unpublished data), GSB[41] and the Tri-Axial prosthesis.[8,42,43] In general, the implants that had the fewest constraints and had kinematics that most nearly approached those of the anatomic elbow had the highest degree of success.[44] In the attempt to further minimize restraint, resurfacing metal-on-plastic implants such as the Kudo,[17] London,[14] Souter, and Capitello-Condylar prostheses were developed.[45]

Description of Currently Available Snap-Fit, Sloppy-Hinge Elbow Implants

Semiconstrained Implants

These implants, consisting of stemmed humeral and ulnar components with polyethylene at the articulating surface, include the Osteonics Trispherical and the Tri-Axial.[8,42,43,46] Custom components[46] are designed to provide optimal load transfer to metaphyseal bone and positioning of the implant center of rotation. The articulating surface must be designed to resist varus, valgus, or rotational loads. These semiconstrained prostheses can tolerate soft-tissue insufficiency and metaphyseal bone stock loss better than the resurfacing implants can.

Implants That Resurface the Radial Head

Prostheses that resurface the radial head attempt to gain the benefits of load transmission stability afforded by the radiocapitellar articulation. Such designs include the ERS.[47] These prostheses have had varying results because of difficulties in balancing the radiocapitellar, radioulnar, and the trochleoulnar joints at the time of surgery.

Surgical Technique

The authors' preferred technique is the modified Bryan approach.[43,48] This is a medial approach that lifts the extensor mechanism and flexor-pronator fascia off as a single flap, exposing the distal humerus, proximal ulna, and ulnar nerve. The medial collateral ligament is released from its origin on the humerus as a part of the procedure. This approach, which is analogous to the anterior approach to the knee for total knee arthroplasty, allows for early mobilization.

Technical Considerations in Total Elbow Arthroplasty

The position of the components, as in any total joint replacement, is critical to the function and durability of the prosthesis.[16,45,49] The center of rotation of the prosthesis must be approximately equal to the normal center of rotation of the natural elbow. The neutral range of positioning of a "sloppy-hinge" style prosthesis such as the Tri-Axial or Osteonics prostheses is narrow and allows for placement variation of no more than 4 degrees anteriorly and 8 degrees posteriorly and no increase in the distal offset of the humerus relative to the anatomic center of rotation (Fig. 1). Proximal placement of the center of rotation of the humerus with this type of prosthesis is not associated with functional loss or complications if the anteroposterior placement variations are maintained. The ulnar component should be placed as far posteriorly and distally as practical. Excessive anterior and proximal positioning of the implant functionally lengthens the arm and puts excessive tension on the triceps, the posterior skin, and the ulnar nerve. In one study,[49] after an average follow-up of eight years, none of the implants aligned within the neutral alignment ranges had failed.

Improvement in strength can also be predicted if the center of rotation is in the optimal location. In a recent study,[16] there was an average 75% improvement in strength in the elbows of patients with rheumatoid arthritis when the center of rotation was properly located.[16]

Metaphyseal bone atrophy, seen in stemmed implants, is related to surgical considerations imposed by the design of the implant. If the implant stem is not parallel to the cortices of the medullary canal, me-

taphyseal atrophy and hypertrophy of the cortical bone about the stem tip are more likely (Fig. 2). Also, if the implant stem is so stiff that it fails to load the metaphyseal bone, this also can lead to load bypass and stress shielding.[50] However, the complications of this stress shielding have to date been limited to fractures through atrophic metaphyseal pillars and have not affected implant durability.

Outcome of Snap-Fit, Sloppy-Hinge Devices That Do Not Resurface the Radial Head

Sloppy-hinge-type prostheses such as the Tri-Axial[8,26,42,43,49] and the Osteonics[46,51] prostheses are indicated for all patients who meet the criteria for total

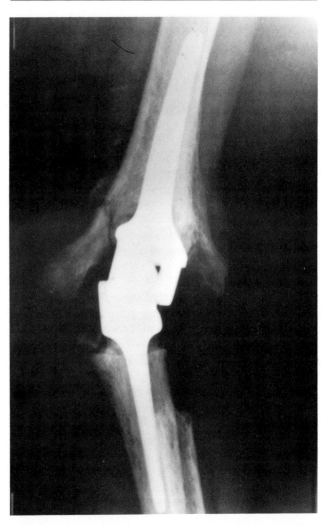

Fig. 2 Metaphyseal bony atrophy seen after cemented total elbow arthroplasty. At two years after surgery the patient had an excellent score. (Note the off-center positioning of the humeral stem.) A minimally displaced crack through an atrophic medial condyle is seen at two years after surgery after the patient lifted a frying pan. Symptomatic management only was required to restore the prefracture outcome.

5 mm

4° anterior   8° posterior

Natural Center of Rotation

Fig. 1 Range of proper positioning of the humeral center of rotation.

elbow replacement. Such implants have been used successfully in patients without ligamentous or soft-tissue competence and in revision arthroplasty.

Surgery for Rheumatoid Arthritis

When patient selection and surgical techniques are satisfactory, more than 90% of patients with rheumatoid arthritis have been described as achieving good or excellent results.[8,31,42,43,46,49,51,52] Pain relief is predictably satisfactory. Motion is more predictably achieved than with the resurfacing prostheses, in part perhaps because the soft-tissue releases can be more complete. Most implants develop a useful arc of flexion of 90 to 100 degrees and a rotation arc of 100 to 120 degrees. A flexion arc of 80 degrees and a rotational arc of 100 degrees can be restored in most elbows with complete ankylosis using such prostheses.[43]

The dislocation rate for the Tri-Axial device is 4% to 6%. One percent of the dislocations occur within the first six months and are related to component malposition and/or shoulder stiffness. Late dislocation appears to develop at the rate of approximately 0.3% to 0.5% per year of implantation. To date, dislocation has occurred only in devices aligned outside of the neutral range and is thought to be related to altered kinematics caused by component malposition and accelerated creep at the polyethylene interface (Fig. 3). No component aligned within the neutral range has become dislocated.

During intermediate to long-term follow-up, there have been no dislocations in the Trispherical or the custom devices. This improvement is thought to result in part from improved precision in implantation, metal backing of the polyethylene to resist creep, diminished constraint relative to the Tri-Axial device, and a non-loadbearing block to catastrophic disarticulation. The incidence of aseptic loosening is generally higher in snap-fit devices than with the resurfacing type of prostheses. Although the earlier hinged prostheses had aseptic loosening rates of as much as 8%, more recent series have shown an average rate of aseptic loosening of 1% to 2% in patients with rheumatoid arthritis after long-term follow-up.[49,53] Therefore, in patients with rheumatoid arthritis, the recent reported results with the sloppy-hinge and the resurfacing prostheses are similar. Most of the centers using these implants and who employ the Kocher or modified Bryan surgical approach report an infection rate of 1% to 3%.[54] Persistent peripheral neuropathy averages less than 2% for all types of implants.

Surgery for Posttraumatic Arthritis

The results of surgery for posttraumatic arthritis are less predictable than for rheumatoid arthri-

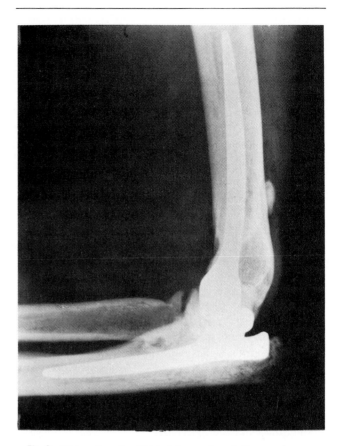

Fig. 3   Dislocation after Tri-Axial type of total elbow replacement. Note the excessive anterior and distal placement of the center of rotation.

tis.[11,28,42,43,46,53-55] This is caused in part by the frequency with which previous surgery has been done on the elbow, the presence of undetected infection, and the frequent lack of adequate bone stock in the distal humerus or humeral condyles. Our experience with 40 elbow replacements (average follow-up, seven years) revealed that 60% of the patients had severe bony deficiency (Fig. 4), 40% had supracondylar nonunions (Fig. 5), and 60% had had at least one previous operation.

Outcome was satisfactory for 75% of the patients. The average elbow retained useful motion, with an average flexion of 90 degrees in the arc from 30 to 120 degrees and pronation and supination each averaging 60 degrees.

Complications are frequent, approaching 40% in elbows with previous surgery. When infection has been noted (or suspected) previously, a two-stage reconstruction is recommended because in our series both attempts at primary exchange failed.

The Tri-Axial device is potentially inferior to the Trispherical and the custom devices in this population, because of the potential for large loads at the polyethylene interface caused by bone and soft-tissue deficiencies.

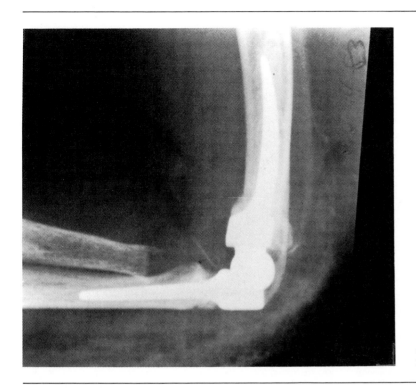

Fig. 4 Total elbow arthroplasty after complete condylar loss. Correct positioning of the elbow's center of rotation is critical in such instances.

Surgery for Complete Ankylosis of the Elbow

Ankylosis of the elbow is an infrequent indication for total elbow arthroplasty. Only sloppy-hinge devices are recommended for the management of this challenging procedure. In our experience of 19 elbows with complete ankylosis, 15 had results of good or better and three were rated as fair. Average flexion increased to 115 degrees and flexion contractures averaged 30 degrees. The average rotary arc was 95 degrees. The surgical technique is challenging. However, in selected patients, the functional improvement is dramatic and the gain in useful motion predictable.

Revision Arthroplasty

Revision of a total elbow arthroplasty presents major problems to the surgeon. The quality of the available bone is often poor, soft-tissue planes have been previously violated, and peripheral nerves are at risk. Heterotopic ossification and limited motion resulting from the previous surgery may be present.[33,43,46,51,53,55–57] Revision is most frequently performed for septic or aseptic loosening or for dislocation.

Revision for Septic Loosening

The presence of a proven infection requires a complete debridement, with the removal of all foreign material, including methylmethacrylate, implants, wear debris, and the membrane at the bone-cement interface.[51,54] As in lower-extremity implants, a mixed infection has a worse prognosis than a single organism sensitive to several antibiotics. Reimplantation may be considered after six weeks of antibiotic therapy that follows a sterile wound culture, providing that the bone and soft-tissue structures are adequate. A single-stage exchange of prosthesis for septic failure is not recommended.[46,51,54] When sepsis cannot be eradicated or if the patient's demands are not compatible with long-term success of the implant, a resection arthroplasty may be a reasonable alternative. Arthrodesis as a salvage procedure for a failed implant has not been predictably achieved (Fig. 6), and it has generally been abandoned in favor of a resection arthroplasty for this purpose.[44,58] The results of any type of revision for sepsis are generally less satisfactory than revision for other causes.[52,54] However, when the proper technical principles of reconstruction can be met, the overall results have been reported to be satisfactory in approximately 70% of cases.

Revision for Nonseptic Implant Failure

Revision surgery for aseptic failure of an implant should be approached through the medial triceps-sparing approach. When discontinuities of bone are present in the diaphysis, the stem of the proximal component must extend across the gap for a distance of at least two to three diaphyseal diameters. This usually requires fabrication of a custom prosthesis. Biologic ingrowth has been used successfully in the metaphyseal region[46,51] in both custom[46,51] and Osteonics prostheses. Allografts

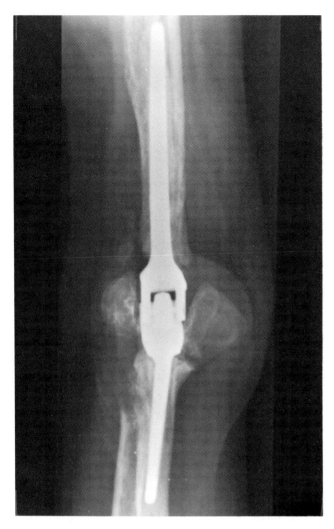

Fig. 5 Total elbow arthroplasty after supracondylar nonunion. Note that the epicondyles have been retained. Despite persistent non-union the epicondyles continue to provide resistance to varus-valgus stresses and should be retained.

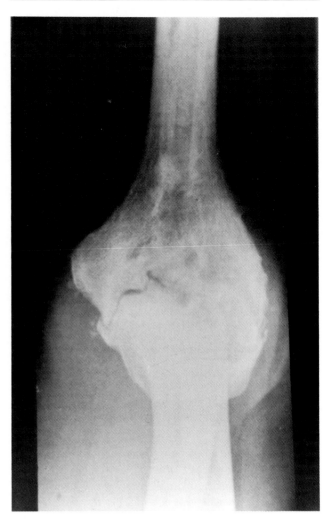

Fig. 6 Failed arthrodesis after septic failure following total elbow arthroplasty. Resection arthroplasty is preferred when the condyles are intact.

are indicated where large gaps exist in the metaphyseal bone, or where the metaphyseal bone is lost to the level of the diaphyseal junction. When the epicondyles are separated from the humeral shaft, the soft-tissue balance about the elbow has been disrupted. Reconstruction of the epicondyles at the time of surgery improves the dynamic restraints provided by the attached ligaments to varus and valgus loading. In cases in which the anteromedial ligament is incompetent, it is necessary to use a prosthesis with an inherent resistance to dislocation. Results of revision for aseptic loosening are satisfactory in approximately 70% of patients with an average follow-up of five years or longer.[8,51,53,57]

Revision for Dislocation

Dislocation of semiconstrained[8,16,42,43,49,53] implants is usually related to surgical malalignment or implant design. If the implant was initially placed in proper alignment and the implant fails by polyethylene component failure (Fig. 7), revision of the polyethylene bearing system offers a predictable and durable solution in most cases.[11,43,51,59] However, if the center of rotation was initially incorrect or has shifted to a position outside of the specified neutral range, a revision of the bearing system alone is not predictable or durable. In this instance, a revision of the malaligned component to restore a satisfactory center of rotation is usually required.

Snap-Fit Devices That Resurface the Radial Head—The ERS Device

Pritchard[47] reported on 75 elbows followed up for four months to nine years. Sixty-three total elbow replacements were in patients with rheumatoid arthritis and 12 in patients with posttraumatic arthritis.

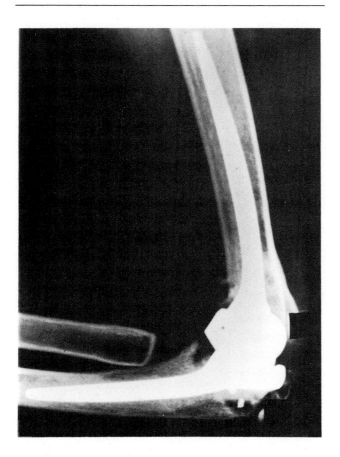

Fig. 7 Revision of polyethylene and application of a restraining spoke following polyethylene failure and dislocation.

Twenty-two of 75 elbows had a nonstemmed humeral component. Four of 22 failed by supracondylar fracture. The nonstemmed humeral component is no longer recommended.

Seven of 27 humeral components inserted without cement required revision for loosening. All components were aligned outside of a neutral alignment range. Four of 75 radial head components were revised for loosening.

The complications rate for the ERS device was 40% (31 of 75). Resurfacing of the radial head increases the complexity of the procedure. Instability was noted in more than 10% of elbows after an average follow-up of 4.5 years. Resurfacing of the radial head may prove less beneficial than originally predicted.

Cemented versus cementless fixation remains controversial. In this series, no implant aligned optimally has failed regardless of fixation (Fig. 8). Attention has been directed at increasing alignment precision to minimize the risk of instability or loosening.

The Future

Current research has been directed at several problem areas. Aseptic loosening has been a problem in

prostheses with restraints in rotation, varus, and valgus. Implant designs that allow more freedom in such planes while providing a positive block to disarticulation are currently undergoing clinical trials. In addition, these implants provide loading to the metaphyseal bone of the humerus and the ulna by the use of custom-fit metaphyseal configurations or by an anterior flange at the distal humerus. The advantage of these prostheses is that torsional loads applied to the metaphyseal bone and soft tissues about the elbow protect the relationship of the implant to the surrounding bone. Such designs have theoretically superior fatigue-lives as compared to other currently available prostheses. Early results of these prostheses have shown improved load transfer to metaphyseal bone with local bony accretion rather than stress shielding. They have provided satisfactory motion at the elbow in flexion and rotation and have not shown early failures.

In summary, recent advances regarding the understanding of elbow mechanics, optimum positioning of the implant, and load transmission, together with the benefits of custom-designed implant stems, have improved functional results during the past five years. Current research is directed at improving positioning accuracy, load transmission between implant and bone, resistance to disarticulation, and component fixation.

Summary

At this time, total elbow arthroplasty is an excellent procedure for the management of radiographic class III and IV rheumatoid arthritis. The procedure is indicated for patients who have pain, instability, and/or ankylosis. The durability of the implants in rheumatoid disease is excellent. At this time, an insidious increase in late failures caused by sepsis has been noted in all major centers. The failure rate appears to be increasing at seven to 12 years after surgery. The aseptic loosening rate remains low, however. The Tri-Axial style device becomes dislocated with time and is no longer recommended. Dislocation has not yet occurred in the Osteonics Trispherical total elbow. At present, controversies regarding fixation center less on avoidance of aseptic loosening and more on resistance to late sepsis. These controversies are not close to resolution at this time.

Surgery for posttraumatic arthritis remains difficult. Excellent results are predictably achieved in patients who have had supracondylar nonunions and no more than one previous surgical procedure. In this group, the results are predictable and approach the outcomes for rheumatoid disease. In patients who have undergone multiple procedures or who have major bony deficiencies, complication rates increase dramatically and the risk of sepsis increases. Because of the dismal experience with single-stage exchange for sepsis, we rec-

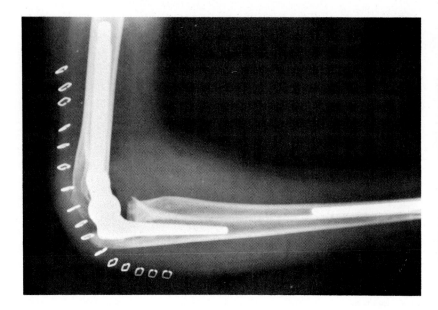

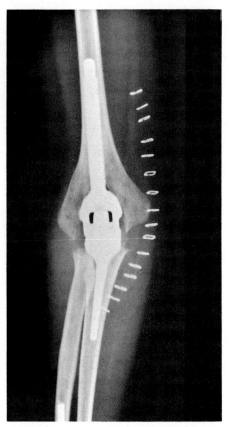

Fig. 8 A cementless total elbow replacement in satisfactory position. Note especially the filling of the metaphyseal regions by the implant. Use of hydroxyapatite as well as other enhancements may further improve fixation. The use of cementless devices remain in the investigational stages primarily for patients with a high risk for loosening or infection.

ommend a prior debridement followed by total elbow arthroplasty if there is any question of a latent or lingering septic process. Again, only hinged, semiconstrained devices are recommended for the management of posttraumatic arthritis.

Revision arthroplasty continues to be challenging. Even in the most experienced hands, only 70% achieve satisfactory outcome in a single procedure. Resection arthroplasty, if both condyles are intact, remains a reasonable alternative in the presence of severe soft-tissue deficiencies or ongoing sepsis.

Current instrumentation systems and alignment devices allow predictable management of rheumatoid disease or straightforward supracondylar nonunions by any surgeon who is experienced in elbow surgery. However, given the high complication rate and the difficulties associated with the surgery, patients with severe or massive trauma to the elbow or who require revision arthroplasty are best treated by surgeons experienced in elbow replacement.

References

1. An KN, Morrey BF: Biomechanics of the elbow, in Morrey BF (ed): *The Elbow and Its Disorders*. Philadelphia, WB Sanders, 1985, pp 43–61.

2. Nicol AC, Berme N, Paul JP: A biomechanical analysis of elbow joint function, in *Joint Replacement in the Upper Limb*. London, Mechanical Engineering Publications, 1977, pp 45–47.

3. Rosenberg GM, Turner RH: Nonconstrained total elbow arthroplasty. *Clin Orthop* 1984;187;154–162.

4. Torzilli PA: Biomechanics of the elbow, in Inglis AE (ed): American Academy of Orthopaedic Surgeons *Symposium on Total Joint Replacement of the Upper Extremity*. St. Louis, CV Mosby, 1982, pp 150–168.

5. Walker PS: *Human Joints and Their Artificial Replacements*. Springfield, Charles C Thomas, 1977, p 182–183.

6. American Academy of Orthopaedic Surgeons: *Joint Motion: Method of Measuring and Recording*. Chicago, American Academy of Orthopaedic Surgeons, 1965.

7. Morrey BF, Chao EYS: Passive motion of the elbow joint: A biomechanical analysis. *J Bone Joint Surg* 1976;58A:501–508.

8. Inglis AE: Tri-Axial total elbow replacement: Indications, surgical technique, and results, in Inglis AE (ed): American Academy of Orthopaedic Surgeons *Symposium on Total Joint Replacement of the Upper Extremity*. St. Louis, CV Mosby, 1982, pp 100–110.

9. Grant JCB: *Grant's Atlas of Anatomy*, ed 6. Baltimore, Williams & Wilkins, 1972.

10. Langman J, Woerdeman MW: *Atlas of Medical Anatomy*. Philadelphia, WB Saunders, 1978.

11. Figgie HE, Inglis AE: Current concepts in total elbow arthroplasty. *Adv Orthop* 1986;10:1–17.

12. Keats TE, Teeslink R, Diamond AE, et al: Normal axial relationships of the major joints. *Radiology* 1966;87:904–907.

13. Morrey BF: Anatomy of the elbow joint, in Morrey BF (ed): *The Elbow and Its Disorders*. Philadelphia, WB Saunders, 1985, pp 7–42.

14. London JT: Resurfacing total elbow arthroplasty. Presented at the 47th Annual Meeting of the American Academy of Orthopaedic Surgeons, Atlanta, February 1980.
15. Loomis LK: Reduction and after-treatment of posterior dislocation of the elbow, with special attention to the brachialis muscle and myositis ossificans. *Am J Surg* 1944;63:56–60.
16. Morrey BF, Askew RS: The Coonrad style total elbow replacement. Presented at the annual meeting of the American Society of Elbow and Shoulder Surgeons, New Orleans, Feb 11, 1990.
17. London JT: Kinematics of the elbow. *J Bone Joint Surg* 1981;63A:529–535.
18. Morrey BF, Askew LJ, Chao EY: A biomechanical study of normal functional elbow motion. *J Bone Joint Surg* 1981;63A:872–877.
19. Beals RK: The normal carrying angle of the elbow: A radiographic study of 422 patients. *Clin Orthop* 1976;119:194–196.
20. Schwab GH, Bennett JB, Woods GW, et al: Biomechanics of elbow instability: The role of the medial collateral ligament. *Clin Orthop* 1980;146:42–52.
21. Amis AA, Dowson D, Wright V: Muscle strengths and musculoskeletal geometry of the upper limb. *Eng Med* 1979;8:41–48.
22. Amis AA, Dawson D, Wright V: Elbow joint force predictions for some strenuous isometric actions. *J Biomech* 1980;13:765–775.
23. Amis AA, Miller JH, Dawson D, et al: Biomechanical aspects of the elbow: Joint forces related to prosthesis design. *Eng Med* 1981;10:65.
24. An KN, Hui FC, Morrey BF, et al: Muscles across the elbow joint: A biomechanical analysis. *J Biomech* 1981;14:659–669.
25. An KN, Kwak BM, Chao EY, et al: Determination of muscle and joint forces across human elbow joint. *Adv Bioeng*, 1983, pp 70–71.
26. Inglis AE: Rheumatoid arthritis, in Morrey BF (ed): *The Elbow and Its Disorders*. Philadelphia, WB Saunders, 1985, pp 638–655.
27. Friedman RJ, Ewald FC: Arthroplasty of the ipsilateral shoulder and elbow in patients who have rheumatoid arthritis. *J Bone Joint Surg* 1987;69A:661–666.
28. Figgie HE, Inglis AE, Goulet JA: Natural history and significance of heterotopic ossification about total elbow arthroplasty. *Adv Orthop* 1988;12:3–8.
29. Barr JS Eaton RG: Elbow reconstruction with a new prosthesis to replace the distal end of the humerus: A case report. *J Bone Joint Surg* 1965;47A:1408–1413.
30. Boerema I, de Waard DJ: Osteoplastische Verankerung von metallprothesen bei Pseudarthrose und bei Arthroplastik. *Acta Chir Scand* 1942;86:511–524.
31. Coonrad RW: Seven-year follow-up of Coonrad total elbow replacement, in Inglis AE (ed): American Academy of Orthopaedic Surgeons *Symposium on Total Joint Replacement of the Upper Extremity*. St. Louis, CV Mosby, 1982, pp 91–99.
32. Coonrad RW: History of total elbow arthroplasty, in Inglis AE (ed): American Academy of Orthopaedic Surgeons *Symposium on Total Joint Replacement of the Upper Extremity*. St. Louis, CV Mosby, 1982, pp 75–90.
33. Dee R: Revision surgery after failed elbow endoprosthesis, in Inglis AE (ed): American Academy of Orthopaedic Surgeons *Symposium on Total Joint Replacement of the Upper Extremity*. St. Louis, CV Mosby, 1982, pp 126–140.
34. Dee R: Total replacement arthroplasty of the elbow for rheumatoid arthritis. *J Bone Joint Surg* 1972;54B:88–95.
35. London J: Custom arthroplasty and hemiarthroplasty of the elbow, in Morrey BF (ed): *The Elbow and Its Disorders*. Philadelphia, WB Saunders, 1985, pp 540–545.
36. MacAusland WR: Replacement of the lower end of the humerus with a prosthesis: A report of four cases. *West J Surg* 1954;62:557–566.
37. Souter WA: Arthroplasty of the elbow: With particular reference to metallic hinge arthroplasty in rheumatoid patients. *Orthop Clin North Am* 1973;4:395–413.
38. Street DM, Stevens PS: A humeral replacement prosthesis for the elbow: Results in ten elbows. *J Bone Joint Surg* 1974;56A:1147–1158.
39. Swanson AB, Pericinel A, Herndon JH: Long-term follow-up of implant arthroplasty following radial head excision in rheumatoid arthritis. Presented at the 45th Annual Meeting of the American Academy of Orthopaedic Surgeons, Dallas, Feb 23–28, 1978.
40. Schlein AP: Semiconstrained total elbow arthroplasty. *Clin Orthop* 1976;121:222–229.
41. Gschwend N, Scheier H, Bahler A: GSB elbow-, wrist-, and PIP-joints, in *Joint Replacement in the Upper Limb*. London, Mechanical Engineering Publications, 1977, pp 107–116.
42. Inglis AE, Pellicci PM: Total elbow replacement. *J Bone Joint Surg* 1980;62A:1252–1258.
43. Figgie MP, Inglis AE, Mow CS, et al: Total elbow arthroplasty for complete ankylosis of the elbow. *J Bone Joint Surg* 1989;71A:513–520.
44. Evans BG, Serbousek JC, Mann RJ, et al: Comparison of mechanical design parameters in current total elbow prostheses. *Trans Orthop Res Soc* 1985;10:100.
45. Ewald FC, Scheinberg RD, Poss R, et al: Capitellocondylar total elbow arthroplasty: Two to five-year follow-up in rheumatoid arthritis. *J Bone Joint Surg* 1980;62A:1259–1263.
46. Figgie HE III, Inglis AE, Mow C: Total elbow arthroplasty in the face of significant bone stock or soft tissue losses: Preliminary results of custom-fit arthroplasty. *J Arthrop* 1986;1:71–81.
47. Pritchard RW: Results of the ERS prosthesis. Presented at the First Open Meeting of the Society of Shoulder and Elbow Surgeons, Las Vegas, 1985.
48. Bryan RS, Morrey BF: Extensive posterior exposure of the elbow: A triceps-sparing approach. *Clin Orthop* 1982;166:188–192
49. Figgie HE, Rosenberg G, Ranawat CS, et al: The results of a hinged total elbow arthroplasty for rheumatoid arthritis. Presented at the Annual Meeting of the American Shoulder and Elbow Surgeons, Atlanta, January 1988.
50. Figgie HE III, Inglis AE, Gordan NH, et al: A clinical analysis of mechanical factors correlated with bone remodeling following total elbow arthroplasty. *J Arthrop* 1986;1:175–182.
51. Figgie HE III, Iglis AE, Ranawat CS, et al: Results of total elbow arthroplasty as a salvage procedure for failed elbow reconstructive operations. *Clin Orthop* 1987;219:185–193.
52. Morrey BF, Bryan RS: Infection after total elbow arthroplasty. *J Bone Joint Surg* 1983;65A:330–338.
53. Morrey BF, Bryan RS: The results of total elbow arthroplasty in post-traumatic arthritis. Presented at the 54th Annual Meeting of the American Academy of Orthopaedic Surgeons, San Francisco, Jan 22–27, 1987.
54. Figgie MP, Inglis AE, Mow CS, et al: Reconstruction following failed total elbow replacement. Presented at the annual meeting of the American Shoulder and Elbow Surgeons, Atlanta, January 1988.
55. Morrey BF, Bryan RS: Total joint arthroplasty: The elbow. *Mayo Clin Proc* 1979;54:507–512.
56. Coventry MB, Scanlan PW: The use of radiation to discourage ectopic bone: A nine-year study in surgery about the hip. *J Bone Joint Surg* 1981;63A:201–208.
57. Inglis AE: Revision surgery following a failed total elbow arthroplasty. *Clin Orthop* 1982;170:213–218.
58. Ewald FC: Distraction arthroplasty. Presented at the annual meeting of the American Shoulder and Elbow Surgeons, Rochester, November 1983.
59. Goldberg VM, Figgie HE III, Inglis AE, et al: Total elbow arthroplasty. *J Bone Joint Surg* 1988;70A:778–783.

Capitello-Condylar Total Elbow Replacement

Mark P. Figgie, MD

Andrew J. Weiland, MD

Introduction

Rheumatoid arthritis of the elbow can severely limit function as a result of pain and loss of motion. Morrey and associates[1] reported that an arc of flexion of 100 degrees, from 30 to 130 degrees, and an arc of rotation of 100 degrees, equally divided between pronation and supination, are required for activities of daily living. Thus, loss of motion of the elbow may interfere with patients' ability to feed themselves, brush their teeth, and manage personal hygiene. Also, greater demands are placed on the elbow when there are limitations of motion of the ipsilateral shoulder and wrist. This is especially true for patients with American Rheumatism Association class III and class IV disease who have multiple joint involvement. In patients with lower-extremity involvement, who must use crutches or a walker for ambulation, the elbow may become more of a weight-bearing joint.

Treatment of the rheumatoid elbow should seek to maintain motion and provide pain relief, allowing the patient to continue to perform the activities of daily living and, thus, remain independent. In its early stages, rheumatoid disease of the elbow can be treated by splinting, therapy, and anti-inflammatory medications, including remittive agents. Cortisone injections can also help alleviate synovitis and reduce pain. Patients who are receiving optimal medical therapy and continue to have pain and dysfunction should be considered for surgical treatment.

Surgical options for the rheumatoid elbow range from synovectomy to total elbow replacement. A synovectomy can be performed either through an open approach or arthroscopically. Often it is combined with resection of the radial head. Isolated radial head replacement with a Silastic prosthesis has also been attempted. Other biologic options include fascial or interposition arthroplasty, resection arthroplasty, and arthrodesis. Total joint replacement designs include nonconstrained, semiconstrained, and fully constrained devices.

Patients with radiographic class I or class II changes are excellent candidates for synovectomy.[2-4] Results of synovectomy with stage IIIA or stage IIIB radiographic changes are less predictable, however, because pain relief is not consistent and instability can result.[5] Resection arthroplasty, with complete excision of the distal humerus, is not recommended in any circumstance because it results in a flail elbow with marked functional disability. Interpositional type arthroplasties using fascia lata, pig membrane, skin, and triceps tendon have been attempted, but in general have produced results that are no better than those of synovectomy with radial head resection.[6-9] Arthrodesis of the rheumatoid elbow is not recommended because it can be difficult to achieve and because it severely limits the patient's ability to perform the activities of daily living, especially in those patients with ipsilateral shoulder disease. Total elbow replacement should be considered when patients have marked pain and have class III or class IV radiographic changes of the joint.

Early total elbow replacement designs were metal-on-metal hinges, such as the Dee[10] and the GSB.[11] These implants initially had good results but failed rapidly because of loosening. Loosening was caused by the constraint of the prosthesis combined with wear debris secondary to the metal articulation. Semiconstrained and nonconstrained prostheses were developed to avoid these problems. The several designs of semiconstrained prostheses include the Mayo,[12] Pritchard-Walker,[13] Coonrad,[14] Volz,[15] Tri-Axial,[16] and Schlein.[17] Several designs of nonconstrained implants have been used, including the Capitello-Condylar,[18] Kudo,[19] London,[20] Souter,[21] Wadsworth,[22] ICLH,[23] Liverpool,[24] and Ishizuki.[25]

The decision as to whether to use a nonconstrained or a semiconstrained implant is based on the adequacy of the ligamentous support of the elbow, the extent of bone destruction, and the surgeon's expertise.

Indications for Nonconstrained Implants

The major indication for a nonconstrained total elbow replacement is pain that is refractory to medical treatment and associated with inflammatory arthritis and grade III or grade IV radiographic disease. In addition, the patient may find it difficult to perform such routine activities of daily living as eating without assistance, grooming, and personal hygiene. Contraindications for nonconstrained implants include recent or remote sepsis and marked joint instability with an incompetent or absent medial collateral ligament. Relative contraindications include bony ankylosis of the joint, failure of a previous arthroplasty, degenerative joint disease or posttraumatic arthritis, and marked bone loss, such as occurs in patients with supracondylar nonunions. After a period of time, supracondylar nonunions can cause arthrofibrosis of the joint and scarring of the medial collateral ligament, and in such cases it is difficult to obtain adequate motion after surgery. In addition, some patients with bony ankylosis have calcification of the medial collateral ligament. Thus, when total elbow replacement is performed, soft-tissue stability must be adequate, or a semiconstrained implant is preferable.[26] Patients in whom a previous arthroplasty has failed often have incompetent soft-tissue support and may also have large bone defects. The bone may not be adequate to support a nonconstrained implant and the ligament instability can lead to problems with soft-tissue balance. Thus, most patients who undergo revision of a failed arthroplasty will require a semiconstrained device. In addition, patients with posttraumatic or degenerative arthritis may be poor candidates for nonconstrained implants because the high demands placed across the elbow can lead to increased polyethylene wear and later dislocation. A non-prosthetic surgical option, such as a distraction arthroplasty, may be a better option for these patients.[27]

Implant Design

The Capitello-Condylar unconstrained total elbow prosthesis was designed by Dr. Frederick Ewald in Boston. It has undergone relatively few design changes since the first one was implanted in July 1974. The humeral component is a cobalt-chromium implant that mimics the natural shape of the distal humerus, having both a trochlea and capitellum. This component is supplied in both right and left configurations, and it has a medullary stem that is available in 5-, 10-, 15-, and 20-degree angles from the joint line (Fig. 1).

The ulnar component, originally a plain high-density polyethylene component, is now available in a metal-backed configuration. Initially, only two sizes were available, but now the ulnar component is available in three thicknesses with two stem sizes. The humeral and ulnar components are designed to resurface the joint and to provide stability through their matching articulations.

Although radial head replacement has been used with this prosthesis on a trial basis (F.C. Ewald, personal communication), the radial head is usually resected and not replaced at the time of surgery.

Surgical Technique

Initially, the surgical approach used for this implant was the Van Gorder approach, which involves cutting a V-shaped flap in the triceps to expose the joint. This approach was later abandoned because of problems with triceps insufficiency and with the ulnar nerve, and the extensile Kocher approach was used instead.[28,29] The procedure is performed under tourniquet control through a posterolateral incision. The incision begins approximately 8 cm above the joint line on the lateral aspect of the distal third of the humerus just posterior to the supracondylar ridge. The incision crosses the epicondylar ridge, epicondyle, and capsule; continues along the interval between the anconeus and extensor carpi ulnaris muscles; and ends medial to the subcutaneous border of the ulna approximately 6 cm distal from the joint line. The exposure is gained by elevating the triceps posteriorly along the intermuscular septum. The insertion of the triceps into the olecranon is subperiosteally elevated in a lateral-to-medial direction.

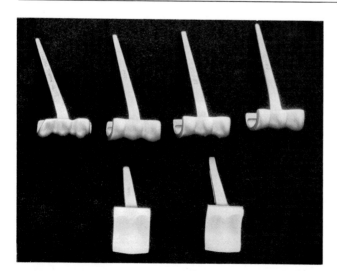 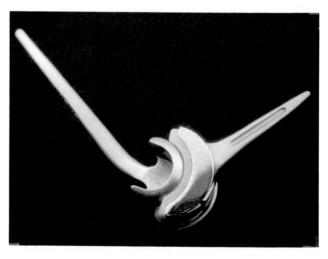

Fig. 1 **Left,** Capitello-Condylar prosthesis for the right elbow showing 20-, 15-, 10-, and 5-degree valgus stems in addition to the two ulnar components. **Right,** Lateral view of the prosthesis articulating showing the humeral and olecranon component.

The anconeus is also stripped subperiosteally in a posterior direction. Anterior exposure can be gained by elevating the extensor carpi radialis longus and extensor carpi ulnaris. The radial collateral ligament complex is subperiosteally released from its attachment to the distal humerus. The annular ligament must be spared, because its attachment to the ulna supports the proximal radius. The capsule of the elbow is detached from the humerus, and the radial head is resected just proximal to the annular ligament. Once the triceps has been reflected subperiosteally, the elbow can be dislocated, hinging along the intact medial collateral ligament. Care must be taken not to compress the ulnar nerve. If ulnar neuropathy is present before surgery, the ulnar nerve may be transposed anteriorly through a medial incision before proceeding with a lateral exposure of the elbow (Fig. 2). Preoperatively, ulnar neuropathy may often occur as marked synovitis of the rheumatoid elbow, resulting in compression of the nerve in the cubital tunnel. If the ulnar nerve is not exposed, the nerve is vulnerable to sharp instruments or saws used to cut the distal humerus and proximal ulna. In addition, care must be taken when excising the radial head, because excessive retraction or puncture can injure the posterior interosseous nerve, which courses anterior and distal to the radial head.

After the elbow has been exposed, the bone surfaces are prepared. The capitellum and trochlear notch of the humerus are shaped to accept the humeral component of the prosthesis. This is done with an oscillating saw that has a small blade and a high-speed burr. The medullary canal of the humerus is broached and is progressively reamed to accept the medullary fixation stem of the humeral component. These stems are provided in angles of 5, 10, 15, or 20 degrees depending on the configuration of the distal humerus and the relative carrying angle of the arm. In addition, different components can be selected in order to adjust the tension on the medial collateral ligament. The most commonly used components have a carrying angle of 5 to 10 degrees, but patients with marked laxity of the medial collateral ligament will require a larger carrying angle to maintain tension on the medial side.

The medullary canal of the ulna is prepared and a sharp awl is used to align the canal. The canal is offset at an angle of 15 degrees to the joint line, and care is taken not to perforate the canal. The canal is then reamed with a high-speed burr and approximately 0.5 cm of the tip of the olecranon is removed with an oscillating saw. The olecranon is then contoured with a high-speed burr to accommodate the ulnar component (Fig. 3). This component is available in three different thicknesses of plastic and in two sizes of stems. The size of the stem selected should coincide with the diameter of the canal, and the thickness of the plastic is determined by the amount of ulnar bone that has been lost

as a result of the disease process and the amount of tension required on the medial structures.

The humeral and ulnar components are then inserted and a trial reduction is carried out (Fig. 3). When the tension on the medial collateral ligament complex is tested, the component should articulate smoothly, with no tendency toward rotation or subluxation. To avoid these problems, the prosthetic components must restore the center of rotation of the joint. The normal center of rotation of the elbow is at the center of the trochlea and capitellum and is roughly 30 degrees anterior to the axis of the humerus. With the arm fully extended, the normal carrying angle of the arm should be restored within 5 to 7 degrees of valgus angulation. If there is an extension contracture, anterior capsule stripping from the distal humerus may be required to decrease the flexion contracture. After the components have been satisfactorily aligned, they are cemented in place, either with separate batches of cement or at the same time, depending on the surgeon's experience. The tourniquet can be deflated at this point and hemostasis obtained. The soft tissues are closed in layers and the soft-tissue sleeve is restored on the lateral aspect. The lateral collateral ligament complex is sutured through drill holes in the lateral epicondyle. The wound is closed over a drain, and, during closure, the triceps sleeve is restored to the lateral fascia.

After surgery, the arm is placed in a posterior splint with the elbow in 70 to 80 degrees of flexion and in neutral forearm rotation. The splint is removed five to seven days after surgery, and gentle active and passive range-of-motion exercises are begun. A resting splint with the elbow at 90 degrees of flexion is used for protection between therapy sessions. Three weeks after surgery, active range-of-motion and general soft-tissue stretching exercises are added to the regimen. At eight weeks after surgery, the protective splint is removed and active soft-tissue stretching is begun. Major ligamentous deficits or instability can require additional splinting. If there is radiographic evidence of postoperative malarticulation or dislocation during rehabilitation, the patient is treated by closed reduction and immobilization in a long arm cast for three weeks. The elbow is held in 90 degrees of flexion with neutral rotation during that time.

Results

The results of the Capitello-Condylar prosthesis for rheumatoid arthritis have been described in several studies.[18,28–31] In the initial report, in 1980, Ewald reviewed a series of 50 patients with rheumatoid arthritis who underwent 54 Capitello-Condylar total elbow replacements. The follow-up at that time ranged from two to five years, and 47 of the 54 elbows had a satisfactory result.[18] Elbows were scored on a 100-point

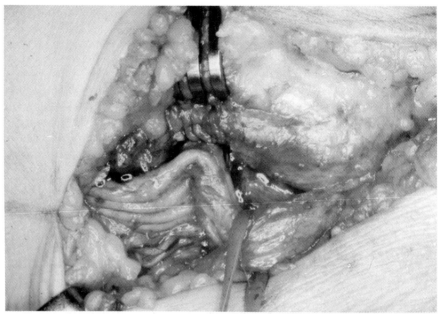

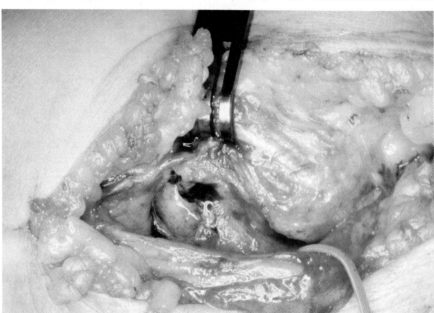

Fig. 2 Top, Intraoperative photograph of the medial aspect of the elbow with the ulnar nerve entrapped in the joint. **Bottom,** Release of the ulnar nerve with a vessel loop around the nerve proximally.

scale, with pain relief assigned 50 points, function 30 points, motion 10 points, flexion contracture 5 points, and deformity 5 points. A score of 80 to 89 points was considered a good result. Excellent results were 90 to 100 points. The average flexion improved by 14 degrees to 136 degrees, and postoperative extension remained equal to preoperative extension at 31 degrees. The average postoperative pronation and supination were 75 degrees and 53 degrees, respectively, which represented an average improvement in pronation of 23 degrees and an average loss of supination of 3.5 degrees. Postoperatively, the average flexion strength was 5.8 kg, and extension strength was 4.7 kg. Strength was not measured before surgery. Although 47 of the

54 elbows achieved good to excellent results at the two- to five-year follow-up, the complication rate in the series was 39%. In the 69 prostheses implanted, 27 complications were recorded. Fourteen patients (15 total elbow replacements) were not included in this review. Of the 14, five patients had died, three patients were lost to follow-up, and six were unable to return for follow-up. Thus, although only 54 were included in the review, the complication rate was noted as a percentage of all 69 elbows, because the complications involved problems that occurred early, during hospitalization.

Of the 27 complications, there were three deep wound infections, ulnar component loosening in one elbow, recurrent dislocation in five, five permanent and

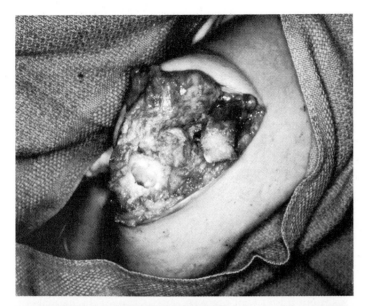

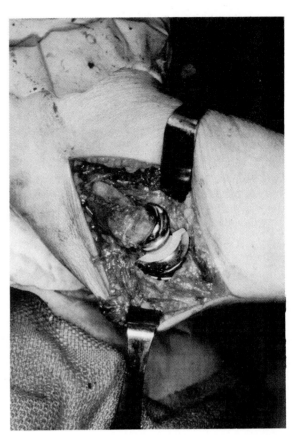

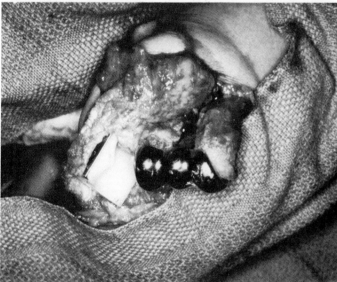

Fig. 3 **Top left,** The distal humerus and proximal ulna have been prepared for insertion of the prostheses. The medullary canal of the ulna can be seen at the left of the wound. **Bottom left,** The humeral and olecranon components have been inserted without cement for a trial reduction. **Right,** Trial reduction has been performed.

six transient ulnar nerve palsies, three postoperative fractures, three cases of skin breakdown, and one triceps rupture. Eight patients required revision surgery—four for dislocation, two for sepsis, one for loosening, and one for fracture. Of the three patients with deep sepsis, two required implant removal and one was successfully treated by debridement and antibiotic suppression.

Recurrent dislocation occurred in five elbows, with two occurring immediately after surgery. Two of these occurred in the early stages of the series, when only the 5-degree valgus stems were available. Both these patients had marked valgus deformities before surgery, and when these were corrected to 5 degrees the medial structures were still loose, causing the instability. Both

patients required implant revision. The 15-degree valgus stem was used successfully in one case; the other patient required revision to a semiconstrained prosthesis. Of the other three patients with recurrent dislocation, one had undergone fascial arthroplasty that failed and had unstable medial ligaments. An attempt to reconstruct the medial collateral ligament failed, and the patient later underwent revision surgery to a semiconstrained prosthesis. The fourth patient had anterior subluxation but remained relatively asymptomatic and did not require revision surgery. In the fifth patient, dislocation occurred months after surgery, and an attempt was made to reconstruct the medial capsule. This failed and the patient declined further reconstruction.

Ulnar nerve problems occurred in 11 elbows, with

five permanent palsies. These problems occurred during the initial phases of the series, when the posterior approach with the V-shaped triceps flap was still being used. The one patient who had loosening had received a nonmetal-backed ulnar component. The patient, who had persistent postoperative drainage, eventually required revision surgery to implant a metal-backed component.

There were no radiolucencies at the humeral bone-cement interface, but six of the 54 elbows had asymptomatic, incomplete, nonprogressive radiolucent lines at the ulnar interface. Two elbows with complete radiolucent lines wider than 2 mm at the ulnar interface were also asymptomatic.

Fractures occurred in three elbows—two at the olecranon and one at the humeral shaft. One of the fractures occurred after major trauma. One of the olecranon fractures was treated with splinting and eventually healed. The second patient required excision of the fracture fragment and repair of the triceps tendon to the remaining ulna with revision of a custom ulnar component. A third patient had an intraoperative fracture of the epicondyle, and this healed spontaneously. One triceps rupture, which occurred immediately after surgery, did not require exploration. It went on to heal spontaneously.

This initial study from the Peter Brent Brigham Hospital in Boston was followed by a combined series by Simmons and associates.[30] This series reviewed 312 Capitello-Condylar total elbow replacements performed between July 1974 and June 1987 at three centers in Buffalo, Boston, and Australia. A minimum follow-up of two years was available for 202 of the 312 implants and the mean follow-up was 69 months (range, 24 to 178 months). The predominant diagnosis was rheumatoid arthritis in 91%, with juvenile rheumatoid arthritis in 8% and posttraumatic arthritis in 1%. The average elbow score improved from 26 to 91 points, average flexion improved from 118 to 138 degrees, and average extension improved from 37 to 30 degrees. Average supination improved from 44 to 64 degrees and average pronation improved from 56 to 72 degrees. Radiolucencies were identified in eight humeral components and 23 ulnar components. Revision surgery was required for aseptic loosening in four prostheses and for instability in two. Deep infection occurred in 1.5% of the cases. Transient ulnar nerve palsy occurred in 16% of the elbows, and permanent ulnar nerve palsy occurred in 5%. The dislocation rate was 3.5%, with subluxation and malarticulation occurring in 5% of cases. Wound problems occurred in 8% of the elbows.

Two additional studies on the Capitello-Condylar total elbow replacement were performed at Johns Hopkins.[28,29] The initial series,[28] published in 1982, represented the first 30 Capitello-Condylar total elbow replacements performed at Johns Hopkins between October 1976 and June 1981. Of the 30, 28 were performed for rheumatoid arthritis and two for osteoarthritis. Of the patients with rheumatoid arthritis, 70% were steroid-dependent. The average age was 59 years. Follow-up ranged from ten to 62 months (average, 40 months). The average preoperative elbow score using the Ewald scoring system was 8 points (range, 2 to 15 points). After surgery, this improved to an average 85 points (range 55 to 95). The average range of motion before surgery was 31 degrees of extension and 121 degrees of flexion. This improved after surgery to 35 degrees and 150 degrees, respectively. Average pronation was 57 degrees and supination was 55 degrees before surgery. These improved to 79 degrees and 66 degrees, respectively. Complications included deep infections requiring prosthesis removal in two patients. Four patients had postoperative component subluxation. These elbows were treated in long arm casts and three of the four responded favorably. The fourth patient underwent open reconstruction of the medial collateral ligament and had a satisfactory result. Ulnar nerve paresthesias occurred in three patients (10%), and resolved spontaneously in two. One required neurolysis and anterior transposition of the nerve.

The follow-up study, reported in 1989, included the original 30 elbows plus an additional ten.[29] Thus, this report described 40 total elbow replacements in 35 patients with an average length of follow-up of 7.2 years (range, four to 12 years). Of the 35 patients, 32 had rheumatoid arthritis and 14 were dependent on steroids. The average Ewald elbow score before surgery, 30 points, improved to 88 points after surgery. There were 21 excellent results, ten good results, two fair results, and two poor results. Average extension and flexion improved from 42 degrees and 120 degrees before surgery to 39 degrees of extension and 133 degrees of flexion afterwards. The average pronation and supination, 56 degrees and 46 degrees before surgery, improved after surgery to 71 degrees of pronation and 67 degrees of supination (Figs. 4 to 6). Complications included two deep infections that necessitated removal of the implant. Although the infection rate was identical to that in the early series, ten elbows in this series had some degree of instability, including eight with malarticulation and two with dislocation. This represented a marked increase, because only four patients in the early series had instability. However, in six of the malarticulations in this series, the ulnar component shifted radially, and the ulna articulated with the capitellar portion of the implant.

Transient changes in the ulnar nerve occurred in seven elbows (18%); permanent ulnar nerve palsy occurred in two elbows. Again, this represents a higher rate than the earlier figure of 10%. Six elbows (15%) had superficial wound drainage. Radiolucent lines were identified in ten prostheses. Eight of these occurred at the ulna and two at the humerus. Six of the ulnar ra-

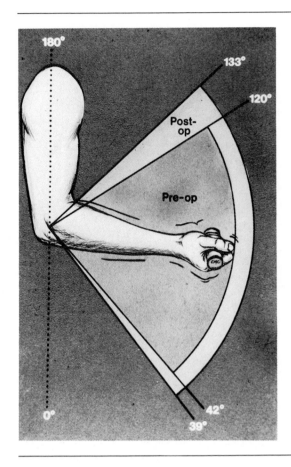

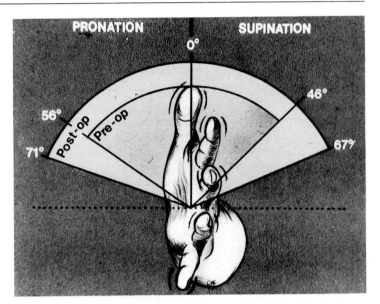

Fig. 4   Left, The improvement in flexion and extension. **Right,** The improvement in forearm rotation. (Reproduced with permission from Weiland AJ, Weiss AP, Wills RP, et al: Capitello-Condylar total elbow replacement. *J Bone Joint Surg* 1989;71A:217–222.)

diolucencies were incomplete and two were complete. Both the humeral radiolucent lines were incomplete.

A fifth study on Capitello-Condylar elbow replacement was reported by Rosenberg and Turner[31] in 1984. This series reviewed 28 Capitello-Condylar elbow replacements. Twenty-three patients with rheumatoid arthritis were examined at an average of 35 months after surgery (range, ten to 68 months). Results were satisfactory in 24 of the 28 elbows (86%). The average arc of flexion improved from 88 degrees to 101 degrees with a residual 33-degree extension contracture. The average rotation was 80 degrees of pronation and 72 degrees of supination. Three of the 28 elbows required revision surgery: one each for infection, loosening (at 53 months), and instability. A fourth patient, in whom failure was caused by loosening secondary to a fracture, chose not to have revision surgery. Of four elbows with dislocations after surgery, three responded to treatment with a long arm cast. Three patients had ulnar nerve paresthesias. There were two deep infections. One responded to debridement and antibiotic suppression; the other required removal of the prosthesis. Two patients had prolonged serous drainage, which resolved without further treatment, and one patient had a ruptured triceps tendon that required surgical repair.

One elbow had incomplete radiolucencies and another elbow had complete ulnar radiolucencies. In addition, one patient had loosening secondary to a fracture and another patient with a semiconstrained prosthesis required revision to correct clinical and radiographic loosening.

Discussion

Improvements in implant design and surgical technique, together with a heightened awareness of the importance of restoring alignment and anatomic relationships, have improved the results of total elbow replacement. Current surgical techniques and current designs of implants can achieve good to excellent results in more than 90% of total elbow replacements, using either nonconstrained or semiconstrained implants.[29,30,32] However, the decision as to whether to use a semiconstrained or a nonconstrained implant is often made on the basis of the competence of the medial collateral ligament, the quality of bone stock, and the surgeon's experience. In general, nonconstrained implants have a higher dislocation rate and semiconstrained implants have higher ultimate loosening rates. In addition, the designs of many semiconstrained implants require removal of greater amounts of humeral bone stock. Nonconstrained implants require a high level of surgical precision, because soft-tissue balancing

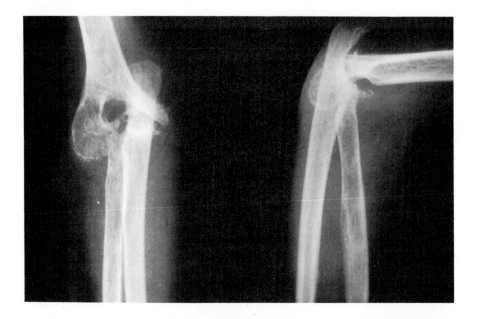

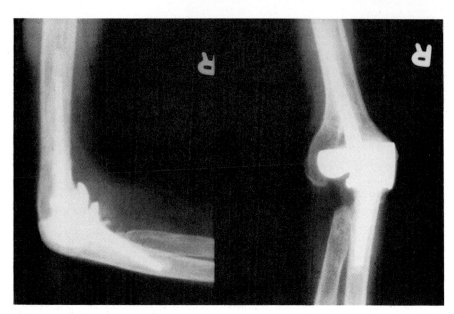

Fig. 5 Top, Anteroposterior and lateral views of the right elbow showing severe articular destruction secondary to rheumatoid arthritis. **Bottom,** Anteroposterior and lateral views of the right elbow showing Capitello-Condylar prosthesis in place.

is of utmost importance. If the medial and lateral structures are not well balanced, dislocation or malarticulation can result. In this regard, semiconstrained implants can be slightly more forgiving. In addition, nonconstrained implants have a narrower application because they require a patient with adequate bone stock and a functional and competent medial collateral ligament. In patients with medial collateral ligament insufficiency, attempts to reconstruct the ligament have not proven satisfactory. However, with proper patient selection the nonconstrained implants can give excellent results, with all series showing improvements in the average range of motion. The average arc of flexion—more than 100 degrees in each series—is within

the functional requirements as described by Morrey and associates.[1] In addition, pain relief and an improved ability to perform the activities of daily living were noted.

Although the Capitello-Condylar implant has been the one most frequently used in the United States, several other nonconstrained implant designs are available throughout Japan and Europe. Kudo and associates[19,33] presented two series on nonconstrained total elbow replacements. The Kudo nonconstrained prosthesis has undergone three modifications. The original prosthesis (type I), which had a cylindrical humeral component, was used from 1971 to 1975. In type II, the humeral component was modified to a saddle shape, with a more

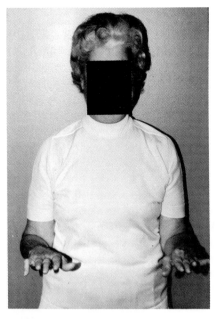 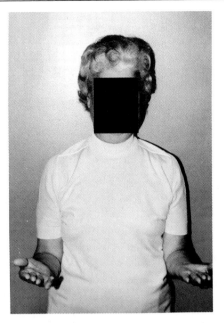 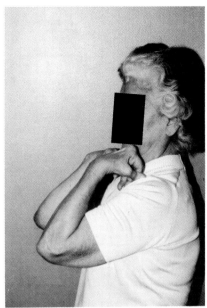

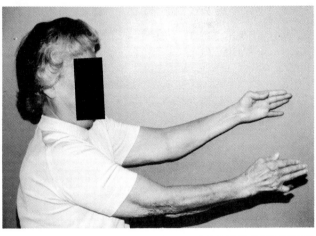

Fig. 6 **Top left,** Active flexion. **Top center,** Full pronation. **Top right,** Approximately 70 degrees of supination. **Bottom,** Active extension.

conforming articular component. In 1983, an intramedullary stem was added to the type II prosthesis, making it closer in design to the Capitello-Condylar elbow. In the follow-up series on 37 elbow replacements,[33] 30 elbows achieved a satisfactory result. Twelve type I and 25 type II prostheses were used. However, six elbows had condylar instability and four required revision surgery. Five elbows showed gross posterior displacement of the humeral component. Four patients required revision of the humeral component, and one patient required revision of the ulnar component.

The most disconcerting aspect of this study was proximal subsidence of the humeral component in 70% of the elbows. Of seven ulnar components with radiolucencies, only two showed evidence of loosening of the ulnar component. An additional elbow required revision for ulnar component loosening. Thus, on the basis of this series, loosening and progressive radiolucencies can occur even with nonconstrained implants. Because

the humeral component without a stem had a high incidence of posterior displacement, the Kudo prosthesis currently uses a stemmed humeral component and an articulation that more closely resembles normal joint surfaces. Thus, in many ways, it has become very similar to a Capitello-Condylar implant.

Most reports on other nonconstrained implants have involved small numbers of prostheses or short follow-up times. The largest series on any of these implants was the report by Soni and Cavendish[24] who reviewed the results for 80 Liverpool prostheses in 1984. The average length of follow-up in this series was 3.5 years (range, one to eight years). In 55 of these elbows, the diagnosis was rheumatoid arthritis. Sixty-six achieved a satisfactory result and 14 required revision surgery. Reasons for revision included loosening in eight, deep infection in four, dislocation in one, and ulnar component loosening in one. The complication rate, 57.5%, included six patients with ulnar nerve dysfunction, two of whom required anterior transposition of the nerve. Eight of the elbows (10%) showed some degree of instability or subluxation.

Souter[21] reported a study of 22 elbows with rheumatoid arthritis after 12 to 18 months of follow-up. Results were satisfactory in 18 of the 22, but three had instability, including frank dislocation in two and recurrent subluxation in one. Ulnar nerve dysfunction occurred in three elbows, with permanent palsy in two elbows. Tuke[23] reported a small series of ICLH prostheses implanted for rheumatoid arthritis. Of 27 elbows, 22 achieved a satisfactory result after one to three years of follow-up. However, four of the 27 required revision surgery, three requiring removal for deep infection and the fourth requiring revision for instability. The ulnar component of the nonconstrained design was modified because of a 20% rate of radiolucency. A stem was added to the humeral component for greater stability.

There have been two reports on the Wadsworth prosthesis. In the first, in 1981, Wadsworth[22] reported on 14 prostheses. In the second, in 1984, Rydholm and associates[34] reported on 19 prostheses. In the earlier series, the average follow-up was one to two years and nine of the ten elbows available for study achieved a good result. The tenth was unstable and required revision surgery. In Rydholm and associates'[34] study, follow-up ranged from 18 months to four years. Fifteen of the 19 elbows achieved a satisfactory result and two required revision surgery, one for infection and one for dislocation at 21 months. Three patients had impairment of the ulnar nerve, transient in two cases and permanent in one. However, at the most recent follow-up, ten of the 19 prostheses had evidence of loosening of the humeral components. In this small series, lower rates of loosening were associated with proper restoration of the centers of rotation.

Lowe and associates[35] reported on 47 Lowe prostheses with one to nine years of follow-up. Of 39 elbows available for follow-up, only 22 achieved satisfactory results. Fourteen elbows required revision surgery. This report evaluated 23 condylar prostheses and 16 stemmed prostheses. Of the 23 condylar prostheses, 12 were revised within two years because of loosening. Three other condylar prostheses were loose but were not revised. Two of the stemmed prostheses were revised because of loosening or instability. Of the three deep infections in this series, two were suppressed with antibiotics and one required implant removal. In addition, there were three ulnar nerve lesions. Of the three, two were transient and one was permanent. Instability occurred in eight elbows, necessitating implant removal in one case.

Roper and associates[36] reported on the Roper-Tuke elbow in 1986. In this series of 60 elbows, 36 of the 51 elbows available for study achieved satisfactory results after three to nine years of follow-up. There was a major complication rate of 27% and a minor complication rate of 23%. Of 15 elbows that required revision surgery, six were implants removed to treat deep infections that occurred within the first six months. Of the other nine revisions, seven were for ulnar loosening and two were for humeral loosening. Other complications included four transient ulnar nerve palsies, one transient posterior interosseous nerve palsy, and one triceps detachment requiring reoperation. Instability occurred in seven elbows, and there were four frank dislocations. Revision surgery was required in three of these cases.

Compared with other nonconstrained implants, the Capitello-Condylar elbow appears to have several distinct advantages. The first is the articulation, which by mimicking the natural anatomy provides greater stability to the elbow and may reduce the rate of dislocation. Other prostheses, such as that of Kudo, have undergone design modifications to improve their kinematics and thus attain greater stability through the articulation. In addition, the use of a stemmed humeral prosthesis has markedly lowered loosening rates compared with other nonconstrained implants. The latest follow-up by Kudo and Iwano[33] revealed a 70% rate of migration of the nonstemmed humeral components. Problems with nonstemmed humeral components were also reported by Tuke,[23] using the ICLH prosthesis, and by Rydholm and associates,[34] using the Wadsworth prosthesis. In the latter study, the humeral component loosening rate exceeded 50%. In addition, Lowe and associates[35] reported a revision rate for the Lowe condylar prosthesis of more than 50% within two years. The Lowe, Kudo, and ICLH prostheses have all been modified to include a stem for the humerus. However, only the Capitello-Condylar implant offers stems with different valgus orientations, which allows proper restoration of the carrying angle and improves the ability to balance the medial collateral ligament. In addition, the implant offers different ulnar stem sizes and plastic thicknesses, which also improves the ability to balance the soft tissues. Balancing of the soft tissues, by improving the kinematics of the elbow, should reduce the dislocation rate.

In summary, nonconstrained implants should be used only in patients with adequate medial collateral ligament structures. The surgical technique is demanding, and the rate of postoperative complications, including subluxation, dislocation, and ulnar nerve palsy, can be high. The extensile Kocher approach to the elbow has reduced wound complications and ultimate deep-infection rates. However, because the ulnar nerve is not exposed with this approach, it may be at higher risk. Even in the most experienced hands, complications can occur. Simmons and associates[30] reported a revision rate of 4.5%, an instability rate of 8.5%, and an ulnar nerve dysfunction rate of 20%. Weiland and associates[29] reported a revision rate of 5%, an instability rate of 25%, and an ulnar nerve dysfunction rate of 22%. However, these results included the early use of Capitello-Condylar implants, when the posterior Van Gorder surgical approach was used and the implant was not yet available in various sizes or stem alignments. Improvements in surgical technique, implant design and variability, and patient selection, along with realization of the importance of restoring the center of rotation to improve kinematics, allow a higher rate of satisfactory results in the hands of experienced surgeons.

References

1. Morrey BF, Askew LJ, Chao EY: A biomechanical study of normal functional elbow motion. *J Bone Joint Surg* 1981;63A:872–877.
2. Steinbrocker O, Traeger CH, Batterman RC: Therapeutic criteria in rheumatoid arthritis. *JAMA* 1949;140:659–662.
3. Eichenblat M, Hass A, Kessler I: Synovectomy of the elbow in rheumatoid arthritis. *J Bone Joint Surg* 1982;64A:1074–1078.
4. Inglis AE, Ranawat CS, Straub LR: Synovectomy and debridement of the elbow in rheumatoid arthritis. *J Bone Joint Surg* 1971;53:652–662.
5. Alexiades MM, Stanwyck TS, Figgie MP, et al: Elbow synovectomy for rheumatoid arthritis: Minimum ten year follow-up. Presented at the Sixth Open Meeting of the American Shoulder and Elbow Surgeons, New Orleans, Feb 1990.
6. Knight RA, Van Zandt IL: Arthroplasty of the elbow: An end-result study. *J Bone Joint Surg* 1952;34A:610–618.
7. Baer WS: Arthroplasty with the aid of animal membrane. *Am J Orthop Surg* 1918;16:1, 94, 171.
8. Froimson AI, Silva JE, Richey D: Cutis arthroplasty of the elbow joint. *J Bone Joint Surg* 1976;58A:863–865.
9. Dee R: Reconstructive surgery following total elbow endoprosthesis. *Clin Orthop* 1982;170:196–203.
10. Dee R: Total replacement arthroplasty of the elbow for rheumatoid arthritis. *J Bone Joint Surg* 1972;54B:88.
11. Garrett JC, Ewald FC, Thomas WH, et al: Loosening associated with G.S.B. hinge total elbow replacement in patients with rheumatoid arthritis. *Clin Orthop* 1977;127:170–174.
12. Morrey BF, Bryan RS, Dobyns JH, et al: Total elbow arthroplasty: A five-year experience at the Mayo Clinic. *J Bone Joint Surg* 1981;63A:1050–1063.
13. Pritchard RW: Long-term follow-up study: Semiconstrained elbow prosthesis. *Orthopedics* 1981;4:151.
14. Coonrad RW: Seven-year follow-up of Coonrad total elbow replacement, in Inglis AE (ed): American Academy of Orthopaedic Surgeons *Symposium on Total Joint Replacement of the Upper Extremity.* St. Louis, CV Mosby, 1982, pp 91–99.
15. Volz RG: Development and clinical analysis of a new semiconstrained total elbow prosthesis, in Inglis AE (ed): American Academy of Orthopaedic Surgeons *Symposium on Total Joint Replacement of the Upper Extremity.* St. Louis, CV Mosby, 1982, pp 111–125.
16. Inglis AE, Pellicci PM: Total elbow replacement. *J Bone Joint Surg* 1980;62A:1252–1258.
17. Schlein AP: Semiconstrained total elbow arthroplasty. *Clin Orthop* 1976;121:222–229.
18. Ewald FC, Scheinberg RD, Poss R, et al: Capitellocondylar total elbow arthroplasty: Two to five-year follow-up in rheumatoid arthritis. *J Bone Joint Surg* 1980;62A:1259–1263.
19. Kudo H, Iwano K, Watanabe S: Total replacement of the rheumatoid elbow with a hingeless prosthesis. *J Bone Joint Surg* 1980;62A:277–285.
20. London JT: Resurfacing total elbow arthroplasty. *Orthop Trans* 1978;2:217.
21. Souter WA: A new approach to elbow arthroplasty. *Eng Med* 1981;10(2):59.
22. Wadsworth TG: A new technique of total elbow replacement. *Eng Med* 1981;10(2):69.
23. Tuke MA: The ICLH elbow. *Eng Med* 1981;10(2):75.
24. Soni RK, Cavendish ME: A review of the Liverpool elbow prosthesis from 1974 to 1982. *J Bone Joint Surg* 1984;66B:248–253.
25. Ishizuki M, Nagatsuka Y, Arai T, et al: Preliminary experiences with hingeless total elbow arthroplasty. *Ryumachi* 1977;17:403–408.
26. Figgie MP, Inglis AE, Mow CS, et al: Total elbow arthroplasty for complete ankylosis of the elbow. *J Bone Joint Surg* 1989;71A:513–520.
27. Morrey BF: Post-traumatic contracture of the elbow operative treatment including distraction arthroplasty. *J Bone Joint Surg* 1990;72A:601.
28. Davis RF, Weiland AJ, Hungerford DS, et al: Nonconstrained total elbow arthroplasty. *Clin Orthop* 1982;171:156–160.
29. Weiland AJ, Weiss AP, Wills RP, et al: Capitellocondylar total elbow replacement: A long-term follow-up study. *J Bone Joint Surg* 1989;71A:217–222.
30. Simmons ED, Sullivan JA, Ewald FC: Long-term review of the capitello-condylar total elbow replacement. Presented at the Sixth Open Meeting of the American Shoulder and Elbow Surgeons, New Orleans, Feb 1989.
31. Rosenberg GM, Turner RH: Nonconstrained total elbow arthroplasty. *Clin Orthop* 1984;187:154–162.
32. Inglis AE, Figgie MP, Figgie HE III, et al: Semi-constrained total elbow arthroplasty in rheumatoid arthritis. Presented at the 57th Annual Meeting of the American Academy of Orthopaedic Surgeons, New Orleans, Feb 13, 1990.
33. Kudo H, Iwano K: Total elbow arthroplasty with a non-constrained surface-replacement prosthesis in patients who have rheumatoid arthritis: A long-term follow-up study. *J Bone Joint Surg* 1990;72A:355–362.
34. Rydholm U, Tjörnstrand B, Pettersson H, et al: Surface replacement of the elbow in rheumatoid arthritis: Early results with the Wadsworth prosthesis. *J Bone Joint Surg* 1984;66B:737–741.
35. Lowe LW, Miller AJ, Allum RL, et al: The development of an unconstrained elbow arthroplasty: A clinical review. *J Bone Joint Surg* 1984;66B:243–247.
36. Roper BA, Tuke M, O'Riordan SM, et al: A new unconstrained elbow: A prospective review of 60 replacements. *J Bone Joint Surg* 1986;68B:566–569.

Semiconstrained Total Elbow Arthroplasty

Bernard F. Morrey, MD

The results of total elbow arthroplasty are directly correlated to surgical experience, patient selection, and implant design. With improvements in surgical expertise and technique, the spectrum of pathology potentially treated by joint replacement arthroplasty has increased and become largely dependent on the implant design. This chapter discusses the experience with semiconstrained implants used at the Mayo Clinic from 1976 to the present.

Surgical Technique

The surgical approach to joint replacement arthroplasty used by the Mayo Clinic has been described previously.[1] Essential elements of the technique include careful bone resection to avoid stress risers that might allow condylar fractures to occur, careful cleansing and drying in the intramedullary canal, and, most importantly, the use of injection systems to provide an adequate prosthesis-cement-bone interface (Fig. 1). The high incidence of infection prompted the addition of antibiotics to the powdered cement. These elements have markedly improved the radiographic appearance of the total elbow arthroplasty immediately after surgery (Fig. 2).

Extension strength has been shown to be adversely influenced by the various triceps exposures.[2] As a result of this study, an improved technique of reattaching the triceps mechanism has been developed, but it is too early to know whether this will result in significant improvement of extension function (Fig. 3).

Postoperative Management

There have been no dramatic changes regarding postoperative care in recent years. The elbow is routinely splinted in full extension with a plaster splint placed anteriorly away from the incision. The arm is elevated for about three days, and then motion is begun. Physical therapy is not used nor is continuous passive motion unless the elbow is markedly stiff before surgery.

The patient is told not to repetitively lift more than 1 to 2 lb or more than 5 to 10 lb at any single time to preserve the longevity of the implant.

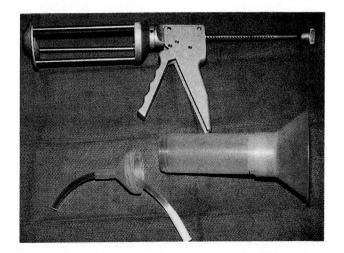

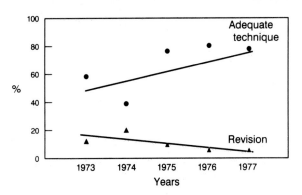

Fig. 1 Top, Cement is injected down the medullary canal with flexible tubes and standard injection systems. **Bottom,** This has provided markedly improved cement technique, which should lessen the incidence of revision. (Reproduced with permission of the Mayo Foundation.)

The Pritchard-Walker Implant

The first experience with a semiconstrained implant was with the Pritchard-Walker implant first used at the Mayo Clinic in 1976. Since then, 47 of the semiconstrained implants have been used (Fig. 4). Only 48% of these patients had rheumatoid arthritis; the remainder either were treated for posttraumatic arthritis or received the implant as a revision procedure.

In function, this experience resulted in an arc of motion of 30 to 135 degrees of flexion and extension, 60 degrees of pronation, and 65 degrees of supination.

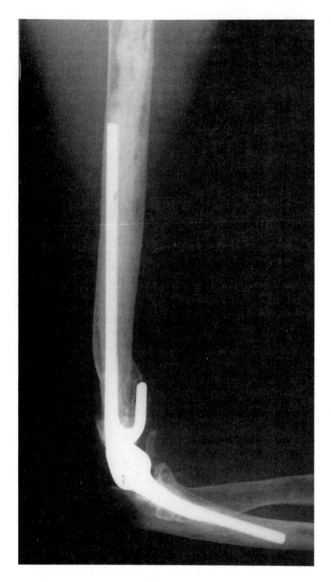

Fig. 2   Improved cement technique has been associated with a lessened incidence of revision surgery and improved bone-cement interface. (Reproduced with permission of the Mayo Foundation.)

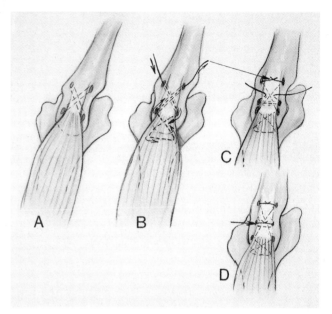

Fig. 3   Current technique used to reattach the triceps to the olecranon. (Reproduced with permission of the Mayo Foundation.)

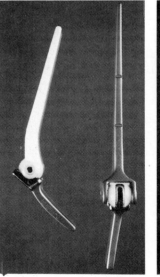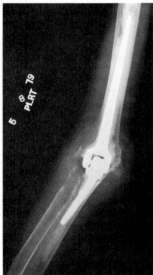

Fig. 4   **Left,** The semiconstrained Pritchard-Walker implant. **Right,** After implantation in a patient with rheumatoid arthritis.

Pain relief was obtained in 90%. The complication rate was 32%; the major complication in this particular subset was infection (14%). Only 4% of the patients had mechanical loosening.

The importance of this particular experience is the expansion of indications for joint replacement, as more than half of the patients were treated for nonrheumatoid conditions. The Kaplan-Meier survival curve of the Pritchard-Walker implant, excluding cases involving infection, is demonstrated in Figure 5.

The Coonrad Implant

In 1978 the rigid or constrained Coonrad hinge implant was modified to allow about 8 to 10 degrees of varus-valgus tolerance or play. After this modification, a plasma spray and a flange were added in 1981 to enhance fixation (Fig. 6). Since that time, 236 Mayo-modified Coonrad implants have been inserted at the Mayo Clinic for a spectrum of problems.

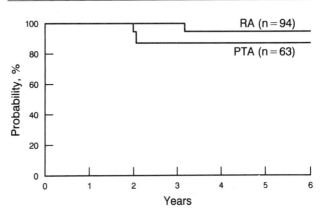

Fig. 5 Kaplan-Meier survival curve for Pritchard and Mayo-modified semiconstrained Coonrad devices.

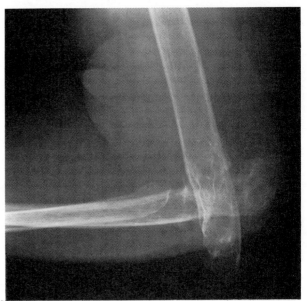

Fig. 7 Kaplan-Meier survival for rheumatoid and posttraumatic cases. (Reproduced with permission of the Mayo Foundation.)

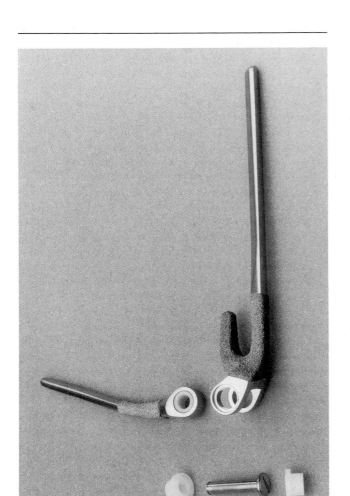

Fig. 6 Mayo-modified flanged, semiconstrained Coonrad implant. (Reproduced with permission of the Mayo Foundation.)

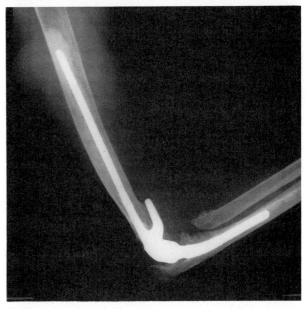

Fig. 8 **Top,** Nonunion of the distal humerus. **Bottom,** Nonunion treated with the modified Coonrad device is asymptomatic at five years.

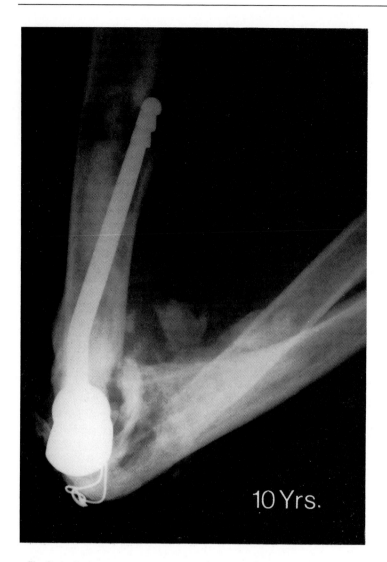
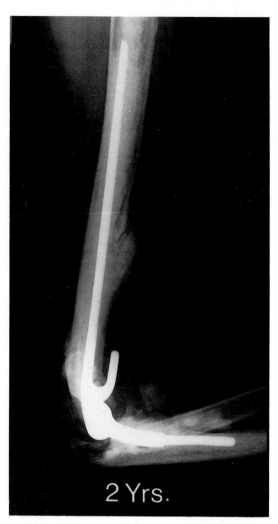

Fig. 9 **Left,** Failed Mayo implant at ten years. **Right,** After treatment with an 8-inch, stemmed modified Coonrad implant, the revision is asymptomatic at two years.

Table 1
Results of semiconstrained joint replacement in 509 replacements

Author	Implant	No.	% With Rheumatoid Arthritis	Follow-up (yr)	Extension and Flexion	Pronation and Supination	Pain Relief (%)	Complications (%)	Revised Loose	Satisfactory (%)
Inglis & Pellicci[7]	Triaxial	44	64	3.5	—	—	89	36	2	—
Pritchard[8]	Pritchard II	92	60	2.5	—	—	98	15	2	85
Bayley[5]	Stanmore	30	90	3.5	107-degree arc	107-degree arc	67	67	—	87
Rosenfeld[9]	Pritchard I & II	14	100	2.6	—	—	100	53	—	94
Bell et al[6]	GSB III	45	82	2.6	29 & 137	65 & 60	96	25	5	87
Morrey et al[3]	Pritchard II	47	48	>5	30 & 135	60 & 65	90	32	4	80
Morrey et al[2]	Coonrad-Morrey	237	40	>5	26 & 132	64 & 62	92	15	2	88
Total or mean		509	54	>3	29 & 135	63 & 63	90	24	3	88

Indications

In this patient population, 41% received implants for rheumatoid arthritis and 29% for posttraumatic conditions. Revisions of prior total elbow arthroplasty constituted 23% of this population. The implant typically has a 6-inch humeral stem; however, for revisions and in cases in which there is distal humeral bone loss, an 8-inch stem is used. Conversely, if the shoulder has been replaced or if it is anticipated that the shoulder will be replaced, a 4-inch humeral stem is employed.

Results

Functionally, patients have done quite well after this joint replacement. The arc of motion averages 26 to 136 degrees of flexion, 64 degrees of pronation, and 60 degrees of supination. Pain relief has been reported in 92% of the overall population.

Complications

Even in this difficult patient population, only a 15% incidence of complications was reported, markedly less than the 45% previously reported.[3] Three percent had mechanical loosening, 1.7% because of particulate synovitis caused by the titanium plasma spray. This problem has been eliminated in the current design, which uses sintered beads. Other complications have been dramatically reduced, with infections in 3%, intraoperative fractures in 4%, and triceps rupture, implant failure, and ulnar neuropathy in 1% each. Overall, the five-year survival for reoperation of any kind excluding infection was 95% (Fig. 5).

Specific Diagnoses

Rheumatoid Arthritis

This particular semiconstrained implant (modified Coonrad) was used for severe rheumatoid involvement in 94 instances. Under these circumstances, the results have been 100% at two years and 97% at five years (Fig. 7).

Posttraumatic Arthritis

This condition is significantly more complex (Fig. 8). Before implantation, 15% of the patients had less than 50 degrees of motion and 15% had had flail elbows for at least two years. Four of 26 patients had nonprogressive lucent lines, two underwent revision because of infection and one because of metallic synovitis. Overall, a survival rate of 100% was observed at two years and 90% at ten years.

Revision Surgery

Since 1981, the modified Coonrad device has been employed in 42 instances of revision replacement arthroplasty (Fig. 9). There have been no infections and no revisions.

Summary and Conclusions

In summary, experience with semiconstrained joint replacement is dramatically and significantly improved compared with that with earlier devices.[4] Improved results have also been reported with other semiconstrained devices, both in this country and in Europe (Table 1).[5-9] Results have improved for a variety of designs using different articulations. Research has demonstrated that the semiconstrained devices do tend to function through an arc of flexion that does not stress the bone-cement interface.

Overall, the semiconstrained implants provide a significant enhancement of the options and broaden the spectrum for which joint replacement arthroplasty may be considered. The Mayo Clinic continues to reserve the implant for individuals less than 65 years old for posttraumatic conditions, but there is no age restriction for those with rheumatoid arthritis. In our experience, reliability in rheumatoid arthritis is comparable to that obtained with resurfacing devices. Additional time must pass before the full impact of these studies can be known, but current data allow cautious optimism regarding the use of semiconstrained total elbow arthroplasty for an increasing variety of conditions.

References

1. Bryan RS, Morrey BF: Extensive posterior exposure of the elbow: A triceps-sparing approach. *Clin Orthop* 1982;166:188–192.
2. Morrey BF, Askew LJ, An KN: Strength function after elbow arthroplasty. *Clin Orthop* 1988;234:43–50.
3. Morrey BF, Bryan RS, Dobyns JH, et al: Total elbow arthroplasty: A five-year experience at the Mayo Clinic. *J Bone Joint Surg* 1981; 63A:1050–1063.
4. Morrey BF (ed): *The Elbow and Its Disorders.* Philadelphia, WB Saunders, 1985.
5. Bayley JI: Elbow replacement in rheumatoid arthritis. *Reconstr Surg Traumatol* 1981;18:70–83.
6. Bell S, Gschwend N, Steiger U: Arthroplasty of the elbow: Experience with the Mark III GSB prosthesis. *Aust NZ J Surg* 1986; 56:823–827.
7. Inglis AE, Pellicci PM: Total elbow replacement. *J Bone Joint Surg* 1980;62A:1252–1258.
8. Pritchard RW: Long-term follow-up study: Semi-constrained elbow prosthesis. *Orthopedics* 1981;4:151.
9. Rosenfeld SR, Ansel SH: Evaluation of the Pritchard total elbow arthroplasty. *Orthopedics* 1982;5:713.

Advances in Implant-Bone Interface

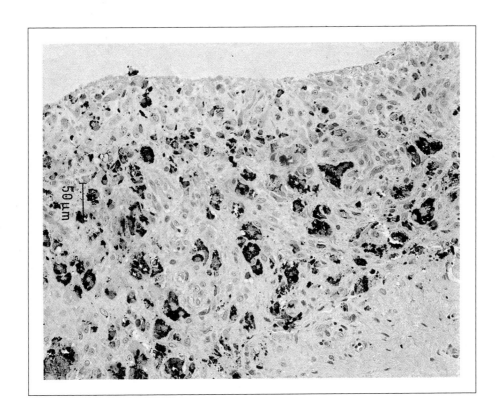

Biologic Ingrowth of Porous-Coated Knee Prostheses

John P. Collier, DE

Michael B. Mayor, MD

Victor A. Surprenant, BA

Les A. Dauphinais

Helene P. Surprenant

Robert E. Jensen, MS

Introduction

The use of porous coatings to permit ingrowth of bone into orthopaedic prostheses was first demonstrated to be clinically efficacious in femoral hip applications. Early clinical studies in the United States began in 1977 with a porous-coated Moore-type endoprosthesis. The success of porous coatings in regard to tissue fixation was demonstrated when retrieved specimens were examined in the late 1970s and early 1980s.[1-6] These early prostheses had a porous coating with a very small pore and were developed using sintering techniques and a fine cobalt-chromium powder. In Europe, a femoral hip prosthesis developed by Gerald Lord, using a lost-wax casting technique, had a pore size of nearly 1 mm. The early retrievals of Lord and associates[7] also demonstrated the presence of tissue ingrowth. Immediately after the early successes of the porous-coated femoral hip prostheses, the use of porous-coated acetabular components and total knee components was initiated.

The first porous-coated knee prosthesis made available in the United States was a cobalt-alloy prosthesis with a sintered, large-pore, beaded porous coating. Soon other manufacturers began providing prostheses that used either cobalt-alloy beads in a variety of pore sizes or wire-mesh titanium coatings. This prompted a series of studies to determine optimal pore size, whether cobalt alloy was superior or inferior to titanium alloy, and whether a fiber-mesh surface was more or less conducive to bone ingrowth than a beaded surface. Early reports on retrieved knee prostheses indicated that ingrowth of femoral knee prostheses was more reliable than ingrowth of either patellar or tibial prostheses.[8,9] Subsequently, manufacturers have modified the designs of all three components in an effort to increase the opportunity for bone ingrowth.

This chapter documents the results with 500 retrieved knee components with the goals of determining if there is a difference between the appearance or frequency of bone ingrowth of titanium versus cobalt-alloy prostheses, large versus small pores, and beaded versus wire-mesh systems. The relative reliability of ingrowth of femoral, patellar, and tibial components is also discussed.

Methods

Sent to the laboratory in a 10% buffered formalin solution, each prosthesis was photographed on receipt and, by means of microscopic and mechanical techniques, was examined for areas of bone and fibrous tissue adherence and ingrowth. Typically, a map of the prosthesis was developed and areas of tissue ingrowth were typed and their locations indicated. The prosthesis was then dried in a series of alcohol and acetone solutions, was embedded in ethyl methacrylate, and was sectioned on a diamond wheel or carbide wheel cut-off saw. Each section, 0.5 mm thick, was polished on one side, glued to a glass microscope slide with its orientation relative to the original prosthesis noted, and ground to a thickness of 10 μ to 40 μ. After being polished, stained, and covered with glass, the sections were examined and photographed with a photomicroscope. Microscopic examination documented bone and fibrous tissue ingrowth, the extent of ingrowth, and the presence or absence of osteoclastic activity, wear debris, and soft-tissue inflammatory reaction. This information, together with an examination of the postoperative and preretrieval radiographs and all patient data, made up the case reports. Additionally, patellar and tibial polyethylene articular surfaces were examined for the degree of wear and creep using the process developed by Hood and associates.[10]

Results and Discussion

Bone ingrowth of femoral knee prostheses was seen with relative frequency, independent of type, when compared with other total knee components (Tables 1 and 2). It was unusual for a femoral knee component to be revised because of fixation failure. The vast majority of these components were made available to us because of breakdown of the tibial or patellar ingrowth interfaces or separation or wear of the polyethylene articulating surfaces. Nearly 35% of the femoral knee prostheses examined demonstrated bone ingrowth. In no case, however, was 100% of the available porous surface ingrown by bone. Rather, the appearance of bone ingrowth was patchy (Fig. 1) and was inconsistent

Table 1
Bone ingrowth of total knee components

Component	No.	Bone Ingrowth	
		No.	%
Femoral	144	49	34.0
Tibial	209	51	24.4
Patellar	147	48	32.7
Total	500	148	29.6

Table 2
Bone ingrowth of femoral components by type

Component	No.	Bone Ingrowth	
		No.	%
PCA	30	16	53.3
Synatomic	28	10	35.7
LCS	41	12	29.3
Ortholoc	16	6	37.5
Miller-Galanté	8	3	37.5
AMK	3	2	66.6
Other	18	0	0.0
Total	144	49	34.0

from one prosthesis to another even within a given prosthesis type. In some cases, ingrowth occurred only in the anterior and posterior flanges of the component or within either the medial or lateral compartment. However, evidence of osteoclastic activity representative of resorption was relatively unusual and, in the vast majority of these prostheses, the interfaces between host and prosthesis appeared to be healthy and well-maintained. Bone ingrowth of large-pore prostheses represented by the PCA and Ortholoc devices (Fig. 2) and the small-pore components represented by the Synatomic and LCS prostheses (Fig. 3) was seen with similar frequency. The appearance of bone ingrowth of the beaded cobalt-alloy prostheses (LCS, Synatomic, Ortholoc, PCA) and the titanium wire-mesh prostheses (Miller-Galante, Fig. 4) was similar in all respects.

Bone ingrowth occurred in the patellar prostheses about as frequently as in the femoral knee prostheses (Table 3). Of 147 patellar prostheses examined, 48 (32.7%) presented regions of bone ingrowth. A high percentage of these prostheses were retrieved for pain, for wear of the polyethylene surface, or for separation of the polyethylene from the metal backing. Histologic examination of the interfaces of patellar components demonstrated the presence of polyethylene wear debris and osteoclastic activity at the margins of the porous coating more frequently than was seen in femoral components. Bone ingrowth of large-pore and small-pore prostheses appeared to be similar, as did that of cobalt-alloy and titanium wire-mesh systems. However, fixation of patellar prostheses appeared to be more difficult and less reliable than fixation of femoral knee prostheses. The polyethylene articulating surface frequently underwent severe wear, and its proximity to the porous-coated surface resulted in a high proportion of these prostheses demonstrating significant amounts of wear debris at the tissue-ingrowth interface.

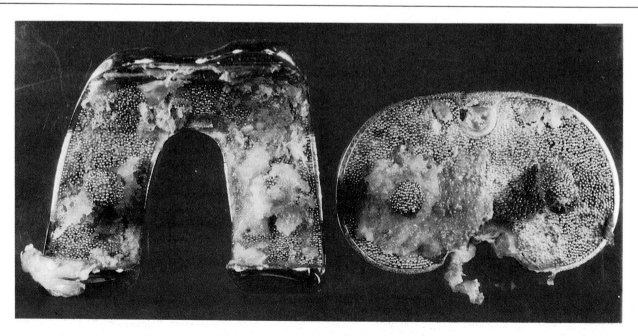

Fig. 1 Appearance of uncemented, porous-coated knee components retrieved one year postoperatively because of pain. Note patchy nature of bone and fibrous tissue adherence.

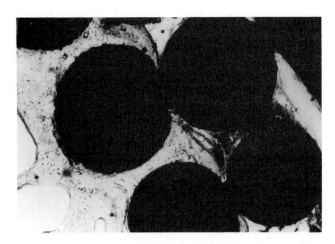

Fig. 2   Bone ingrowth of large-pore (>400 μ) cobalt-alloy porous coating.

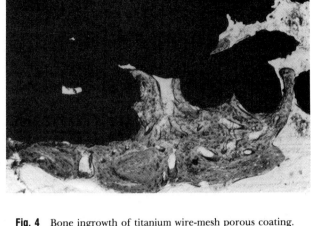

Fig. 4   Bone ingrowth of titanium wire-mesh porous coating.

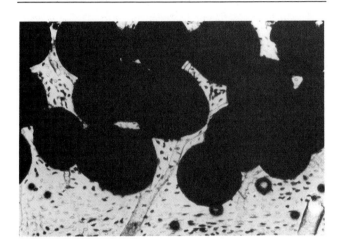

Fig. 3   Bone ingrowth of small-pore (<400 μ) cobalt-alloy porous coating.

Table 3
Bone ingrowth of patellar components by type

Component	No.	Bone Ingrowth	
		No.	%
PCA	33	8	24.2
Synatomic	48	19	39.6
LCS	27	12	44.4
Ortholoc & Ortholoc II	17	7	41.2
Miller-Galanté	8	1	12.5
AMK	2	1	50.0
Natural Knee	0	—	—
Freeman-Samuelson	3	—	—
Microloc	0	—	—
Other	9	—	—
Total	147	48	32.7

Table 4
Bone ingrowth of tibial components by type

Component	No.	Bone Ingrowth	
		No.	%
PCA	62	14	22.6
Synatomic	39	5	12.8
LCS	55	13	23.6
LCS-RP	17	5	29.4
Ortholoc	18	4	22.2
Ortholoc II	2	1	50.0
Miller-Galanté	8	6	75.0
AMK	4	3	75.0
Other	4	0	—
Total	209	51	24.4

Bone ingrowth of tibial knee prostheses was seen less frequently than in either of the other two knee components (Table 4). Biomechanical analysis of the components indicated that the interface between the bone and tibial prosthesis is subjected to considerable rocking forces and that if it is not securely fixed to the tibial plateau, the rocking between component and bone will inhibit bone ingrowth. Those prostheses with little mechanical interlock between themselves and the bone generally demonstrated little evidence of bone ingrowth (Fig. 5). Titanium tibial prostheses provided with four-screw fixation fared better, demonstrating ingrowth in 75% of the cases. The appearance of bone ingrowth of the wire-mesh (Fig. 4) and beaded systems of titanium (Fig. 6) were quite similar. Bone resorption and evidence of wear debris were frequently seen at the ingrowth interfaces of prostheses that were not bone ingrown or that were ingrown in only one small portion of the plateau (Fig. 7).

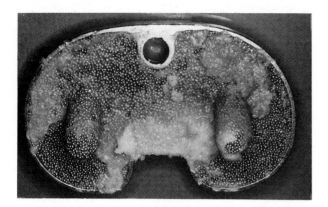

Fig. 5 Appearance of a tibial component fixed only by loose fibrous tissue.

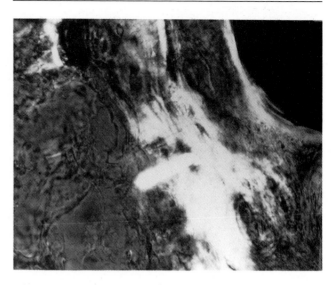

Fig. 7 Wear debris (bright white object in center of photograph) found in fibrous tissue adjacent to porous coating of a prosthesis retrieved because of polyethylene wear.

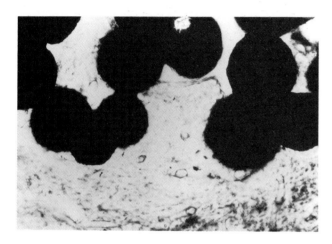

Fig. 6 Bone ingrowth of small-pore (<400 μ) titanium beaded porous coating.

Conclusions

The geometry of the femoral knee prosthesis provides sufficient fixation and resistance to micromotion that ingrowth of the large variety of porous surfaces appears reliable. Well-fixed patellar prostheses also demonstrate bone ingrowth, but their ingrowth interfaces appear to be at early risk of breaking down because of the presence of polyethylene wear debris generally associated with the metal-backed polyethylene design. Tibial prostheses evidently present a much more difficult fixation problem. The quality of bone in the proximal tibia often varies widely between medial and lateral compartments and the loads rock the prostheses in both the medial-lateral plane and the anterior-posterior plane. The most common appearance of tissue ingrowth of these prostheses is that of a fibrous interdigitation of varying quality. Plateaus that were poorly

anchored to the bone generally present the appearance of a fibrous membrane and osteoclastic activity in the adjacent bone. Prostheses that were better anchored, either by screws or central pegs, characteristically present the appearance of well-interdigitated fibrous tissue, which may lack any osteoclastic activity. Only devices with very firm mechanical fixation and contact with bone of good quality demonstrated bony ingrowth.

The polyethylene of the tibial insert was frequently severely worn, and the resulting wear debris was often found at the interface between metal backing and tibia. Long-term fixation of these prostheses by either bone or well-interdigitated fibrous tissue appears to be at risk because of the factors released by wear debris. The work by Willert[11] and Howie[12] indicates that in the presence of wear debris, the host can be expected to release prostaglandins and collagenase, which may well break down the interface of even well-fixed prostheses.

In the range of pore sizes currently available, bone ingrowth of knee prostheses occurs independent of pore size. Also, it appears to make little difference in the appearance of bone ingrowth whether the porous coating is composed of cobalt alloy or titanium. Both beaded and wire-mesh systems demonstrated the ability to permit bony fixation. Bone ingrowth of titanium tibial prostheses with multiple-screw fixation was seen with greatest frequency, but it was not determined whether this was more a function of the material used or of the type of fixation. On the basis of experience with other orthopaedic prostheses, it seems reasonable to assume that mechanical fixation is the dominant variable in these systems. Therefore, our concerns need to be focused both on better fixation mechanisms for the tibial component and on better articulation mechanisms, which will eliminate the high wear rates currently found in most designs.

References

1. Cameron HU, Pilliar RM, MacNab I: The effect of movement on the bonding of porous metal to bone. *J Biomed Mater Res* 1973;7:301–311.
2. Cameron HU, Pilliar RM, MacNab I: The rate of bone ingrowth into porous metal. *J Biomed Mater Res* 1976;10:295–302.
3. Cameron HU: Six-year results with a microporous-coated metal hip prosthesis. *Clin Orthop* 1986;208:81–83.
4. Collier JP, Colligan GA, Brown SA: Bone ingrowth into dynamically loaded porous-coated intramedullary nails. *J Biomed Mater Res* 1976;10:485–492.
5. Collier J, Mayor MB, Engh CA, et al: Bone ingrowth of porous-coated Moore prostheses. *Biomater Trans* 1984;7:113.
6. Collier JP, Mayor MB, Bobyn JD, et al: The histology of tissue ingrowth into porous-metal coated femoral hip prostheses in five humans. *Trans Soc Biomater* 1983;6:79.
7. Lord G, Marotte JH, Blanchard JP, et al: Etude experimentale de l'ancrage des arthroplasties totales madreporiques de hanche [The fixation of madreporic total hip prosthesis: An experimental study]. *Rev Chir Orthop* 1978;64(6):459–470.
8. Collier JP, Mayor MB, Townley CO, et al: Histology of retrieved porous-coated knee prosthesis. Presented at the 53rd Annual Meeting of the American Academy of Orthopaedic Surgeons, New Orleans, Feb 21, 1986.
9. Haddad RJ, Cook SD, Thomas KA, e al: Histologic and microradiographic analysis of noncemented retrieved PCA knee components. Presented at the 53rd Annual Meeting of the American Academy of Orthopaedic Surgeons, New Orleans, Feb 21, 1986.
10. Hood RW, Wright TM, Burstein AH: Retrieval analysis of total knee prostheses: A method and its application to 48 total condylar prostheses. *J Biomed Mater Res* 1983;17:829–842.
11. Willert HG: Reactions of the articular capsule to wear products of artificial joint prostheses. *J Biomed Mater Res* 1977;11:157–164.
12. Howie DW, Vernon-Roberts B: A rat model of resorption of bone at the cement-bone interface in the presence of polyethylene wear particles. *J Bone Joint Surg* 1988;70B:257–263.

Macroscopic and Microscopic Evidence of Prosthetic Fixation With Porous-Coated Materials

John P. Collier, DE

Michael B. Mayor, MD

John C. Chae, MD

Victor A. Surprenant, BA

Helene P. Surprenant

Les A. Dauphinais

The use of porous metal coatings to permit bone ingrowth as a mechanism for fixation of orthopaedic prostheses was first evaluated in animals in the early 1970s by a number of researchers.[1-4] Experience with cobalt-chromium alloy implants in rabbits and dogs indicated that, under specific conditions, bone would grow into the pores of the coating and provide fixation to the bone. Galanté and associates[5,6] studied the ingrowth of bone into fully porous prostheses made of titanium wire and implanted into baboons. These early experiments provided valuable information about the proper pore size, pore geometry, and biocompatibility of materials for use in animals. These studies also highlighted the importance of proper fit and the elimination of micromotion as critical for the ingrowth of bone rather than fibrous tissue into the porous surfaces.

In the ten years since the introduction of porous-coated prostheses for clinical use, the scope of available configurations and applications has expanded enormously. Many of these devices are designated for use with cement, but it is evident that a significant proportion of them are implanted without cement, with the goal being to provide fixation by bone ingrowth.

The use of uncemented, porous-coated prostheses has proliferated because of the expectation by surgeons that ingrowth will occur in humans with the same regularity demonstrated in laboratory animals. To date, however, there has been little scientific evidence, other than clinical data and radiographic analysis, to support this view. Therefore, a histologic evaluation of significant numbers of specimens of retrieved, porous-coated, uncemented prostheses appears warranted.

This paper is based on the gross examination of 226 retrieved, uncemented, porous-coated hip prostheses provided by 115 surgeons. Of these prostheses, 162 were selected for detailed macroscopic and histologic examination, and the two largest categories of devices (AML and PCA stems) were subjected to statistical analysis to determine whether the differences in geometry and amount or type of porous coating would result in statistically different amounts of bone adherence.

Objectives

The objectives of the study were (1) to determine the efficacy of porous coatings in permitting bone and/or fibrous tissue ingrowth as a mechanism for long-term implant fixation; (2) to determine the role of such porous-coating characteristics as composition and geometry in the performance of the prostheses; (3) to assess the amount of available porous-coating ingrown by bone and/or dense fibrous tissue; and (4) to determine whether any generalization about the amount or location of ingrowth could be made.

Methods

All of the retrieved, porous-coated prostheses were fixed in formalin and were shipped wet to the laboratory. There they were photographed for documentation, catalogued, and put in fresh formalin solution. The type of ingrowth, whether fibrous tissue, bone, or a combination of the two, was assessed, and a rough map of the adherent tissue was produced. Because of the time required to section the prostheses, only specific areas of interest were selected for evaluation. Of the 226 prostheses, 64 were not included in the statistics; the majority of these were eliminated as being too few of a specific type to provide viable information. Only when five or more of a specific prosthesis type were available were the results included.

Over a two-week period each prosthesis was immersed sequentially in containers of increasing concentrations of alcohol, followed by immersion in acetone for a week. Once the implants were fully dried, they were embedded in ethyl methacrylate. The mold containing the specimen and liquid ethyl methacrylate was placed into a dessicating jar and put under vacuum for a period of about an hour to remove as much entrapped air as possible. Once bubbling ceased, the mold was put into a high-pressure bomb at a pressure of 100 lb/in^2. This pressure was maintained while the ethyl methacrylate cured. This inhibited bubble formation, resulting in a very clear, bubble-free, embedded sample. The embedded specimens were then sawed into sections 0.5 mm thick. Each section was hand polished on one side and glued to a microscope slide with epoxy. The slides were mounted in a petrographic slide holder, ground by hand to a thickness of approximately 40 to 60 μ, polished, stained with hematoxylin and eosin, and covered with glass. Histologic examination of the specimens was carried out with a photomicroscope. Photographic slides of the sections were made available to the participating surgeons.

Of the 162 prostheses examined histologically for this study, 104 were femoral hip prostheses and 58 were acetabular components. Prostheses that clearly demonstrated only loose fibrous tissue by extensive macroexamination were not sectioned and are included in the results as "fibrous tissue only" along with the reason for retrieval. An effort was made to assess the amount and extent of bone ingrowth of the AML and PCA stems by mapping the bone adherent to the stems, verifying the presence of bone ingrowth by examination of histologic sections, and extrapolating the presence or absence of bone in the regions between the sections. This data was then subjected to statistical analysis using the two-tailed t-test.

Results

Sixteen of 70 AML femoral components were found to be ingrown by bone. Five of 16 PCA components demonstrated bone ingrowth. Of the 12 Trilock retrievals, four presented evidence of bone ingrowth; of these, two were postmortem retrievals done more than one year after implantation. Three of six Harris-Galanté stems showed bone ingrowth; of the three, two were retrieved because of symptoms of pain and looseness.

Four of the eight Harris-Galanté cups showed some evidence of bone ingrowth and one of 12 PCA cups demonstrated bone ingrowth. Four of 38 AML cups demonstrated bone ingrowth; of these, three were retrieved because of malposition. It should be noted that in most cases the prostheses had been implanted for so short a time that bone ingrowth could not be expected. The average postoperative preretrieval period was four months for the AML cup, ten months for the PCA, and nine months for Harris-Galanté.

The femoral stems were revised after longer postoperative periods ranging from ten to 20 months. Overall, 28 of 104 femoral stems and nine of 58 acetabular components demonstrated some bone ingrowth.

Discussion

This study was subject to a large number of limitations, including nonuniformity of surgical technique; a variety of implant types, sizes, and fits; and variations in bone quality, patient age, weight, sex, and disease process. A further limitation is that only a limited number of sections of each prosthesis could be prepared because of the large number of retrieved devices. Because of this, considerable extrapolation of the amount of bone and fibrous tissue adherence was required. Additionally, because the prostheses were retrieved for a variety of reasons, generalizations from this examination of components, many of which must be considered failures, is difficult.

Histologic examination confirmed that at the time of implantation surgery, the bone is traumatized by the cutting, reaming, and broaching and responds by attempting to replace the removed material with new bone. If a porous surface has been implanted tightly against this front of new bone, an opportunity for fixation is provided through growth into the pores. The ingrowth of bone into the porous coating, however, is not guaranteed and, in fact, appears to depend on a number of factors. Among the most important of these factors is sufficient stability to eliminate relative motion between the prosthesis and surrounding bone. Prostheses that are undersized, fixed against structures of poor quality, inadequately press-fitted, or implanted in patients who overload the bone-implant interface in the early postoperative period are commonly ingrown only with fibrous tissue, an event that may be likened to a nonunion.

When a properly designed and implanted porous-coated prosthesis is well-fitted to bleeding bone, there is an initial fracture healing response that results in bone ingrowth after approximately four to six weeks. This initial period is followed by a remodeling phase that lasts at least a year and can last considerably longer. There is only very rare evidence of endochondral ossification. Cartilage does not appear to be a precursor to bone ingrowth; rather, primary bone ingrowth occurs in the early phases, with bone remodeling resulting in additional ingrowth and bone maturation in the later phases. Complete bone ingrowth of all of the available porous coating area of any of these retrieved prostheses was not seen. The geometry of the prosthesis profoundly influences its early stability and may be a factor in the amount of bone ingrowth necessary for long-term stability.

Well-stabilized prostheses that are partially porous-coated typically demonstrate interdigitation of bone or fibrous tissue with the porous coating and fibrous encapsulation of the uncoated portion of the stem. Thus, there is a profoundly different response of the body to the two regions of these devices.

Bone ingrowth was demonstrated in more than 25% (28 of 104) of the femoral hip components retrieved for all reasons. Prostheses retrieved for pain showed a somewhat higher incidence of bone ingrowth (seven of 21) than did those retrieved for all other reasons (21 of 85), indicating that bone ingrowth alone is not sufficient to guarantee relief from pain.

A significant proportion of all retrieved femoral hip prostheses demonstrated burnishing of the smooth portion of the stem, evidence of relative motion between the stem and bone. The polished areas were generally present on the lateral, distal margins of the straight-stemmed prostheses and at the anterior tip of the bowed PCA stems.

The analysis of femoral stems retrieved after short implantation periods indicates that the first region to be ingrown is generally the lateral aspect of prostheses that are porous-coated in that region and in the lateral margins of the anterior and posterior surfaces of all femoral devices.

The amount of porous coating of AML and PCA femoral prostheses demonstrating bone adherence was found to be statistically different (P<.05). Approximately 16% of the porous surface of the AML and 31% of the surface of the PCA were commonly adhered to by bone. However, when the amount of available coating of the two prostheses was normalized, no significant difference in the amount of bone adherence was demonstrated.

Histologically, bone ingrowth of coatings with the largest and smallest pore sizes appeared similar in every respect. Bone ingrowth of the pure titanium fiber-mesh pads was indistinguishable from the ingrowth of the beaded cobalt-alloy coatings. Very little direct bone apposition to the uncoated portions of any of the femoral prostheses was found and this occurred only in the closest possible proximity to the porous-coated regions. The frequency of apposition of bone to smooth titanium and cobalt-alloy surfaces and the appearance of a direct bone-metal contact with no discernible fibrous tissue interposed were in all ways similar for the two systems.

Bone ingrowth was seen in approximately 16% (nine of 58) of the acetabular components retrieved for all reasons. The majority of the cups removed for pain were found to be ingrown only with fibrous tissue. It appears that stabilization of these components is less frequently achieved than is the case with femoral components. The histologic appearance of the tissue surrounding loose or painful prostheses typically consists of a thick layer of highly organized, load-bearing fibrous tissue. This tissue separates the prosthesis from bone, which often demonstrates evidence of osteoclastic activity. Those prostheses that are grossly loose are encapsulated with loose, fibrous tissue, and, in these cases, there is often evidence of osteoclastic activity in the adjacent bone.

Conclusions

The host response to porous-coated prostheses appears favorable, and there is little evidence of any adverse tissue response or significant osteoclastic activity except in grossly loose specimens. Femoral hip prostheses are most likely to demonstrate bone ingrowth along the lateral quadrant of their porous coating. The frequency of bone ingrowth of femoral components was nearly twice that of retrieved acetabular devices. Pore size, geometry, and porous-coating composition did not appear to influence the appearance of bone and fibrous tissue ingrowth. Direct bonding of bone to the uncoated portion of the prostheses was rarely seen and occurred only within several millimeters of the porous-coated regions.

Indications of pain and looseness are evidence that fibrous tissue ingrowth alone is not always sufficient to assure stability. Additionally, some prostheses with bone ingrowth were retrieved because of pain, which leads to the conclusion that local bone ingrowth cannot assure a general freedom from pain, especially with partially coated prostheses. The bone and fibrous tissue response to the porous coatings is generally through interdigitation, whereas the response to the uncoated regions is fibrous tissue encapsulation. Burnishing of the distal tips of many of the partially coated femoral prostheses is an indication of relative motion in that region, which is a potential source of pain.

References

1. Pilliar RM, Cameron HU, MacNab I: Porous surface layered prosthetic devices. *J Biomed Eng* 1975;10:126–131.
2. Cameron HU, Pilliar RM, MacNab I: The effect of movement on the bonding of porous metal to bone. *J Biomed Mater Res* 1973;7:301–311.
3. Cameron HU, Pilliar RM, MacNab I: The rate of bone ingrowth into porous metal. *J Biomed Mater Res* 1976;10:295–302.
4. Collier JP, Colligan GA, Brown SA: Bone ingrowth into dynamically loaded porous coated intramedullary nails. *J Biomed Mater Res* 1976;10:485–492.
5. Galanté J, Rostoker W: Fiber metal composites in the fixation of skeletal prosthesis. *J Biomed Mater Res* 1973;7:43–61.
6. Galanté J, Rostoker W, Lueck R, et al: Sintered fiber metal composites as a basis for attachment of implants to bone. *J Bone Joint Surg* 1971;53A:101–114.

Advances in Our Understanding of the Implant-Bone Interface: Factors Affecting Formation and Degeneration

Myron Spector, PhD

Sonya Shortkroff, MS

Clement B. Sledge, MD

Thomas S. Thornhill, MD

Overview

Important issues related to the formation and degeneration of the implant-bone interface are embodied in the following questions: (1) What are the chemical and topographic features of an implant that best facilitate its incorporation into host bone? (2) How do the chemistry and geometry of materials contribute to the activation of certain cells to cause the degeneration of bone and other tissues around prostheses? The formation of the interface has its biologic basis in the cellular and biomechanical processes involved in wound healing. The degeneration of the interface is related to the activation of macrophages and other cells to produce cytokines, eicosanoids, and enzymes that are capable of stimulating and facilitating bone resorption.

Answers to the two questions posed above will make possible more rational development and implementation of materials that will facilitate the incorporation of the prosthesis into the musculoskeletal system and, at the same time, limit the degenerative processes if some failure in the prostheses should cause production of particulate debris.

Formation of the Implant-Bone Interface

Wound Healing

The tissue that forms around implants is the result of the influence of the device on (1) the wound-healing response initiated by the surgical trauma of implantation (Fig. 1) and (2) subsequent tissue remodeling.[1] Implantation of a medical device sets into motion a sequence of cellular and biochemical processes that leads to healing by second intention. This type of healing, which initially involves formation of granulation tissue within a defect, differs from healing by first intention, of which the healing of an incision is an example. The first phase of healing is inflammation.[2] This is followed by a reparative phase, during which dead or damaged cells are replaced by healthy cells. The pathway that the reparative process takes depends on the regenerative capability of the cells that make up the injured tissue, that is, the tissue or organ into which the implant has been placed. Cells can be distinguished as labile, stable,

or permanent on the basis of their capacity to regenerate.[2] Labile cells continue to proliferate throughout life, replacing cells that are continually being destroyed. Epithelial and blood cells are examples of labile cells. Cells of splenic, lymphoid, and hematopoietic tissues are also labile cells. Stable cells retain the capacity for proliferation, although they do not normally replicate. These cells can undergo rapid division in response to a variety of stimuli and are capable of reconstituting the tissue of origin. Stable cells include the parenchymal cells of all of the glandular organs of the body, including the liver, kidney, and pancreas; mesenchymal derivatives such as fibroblasts, smooth muscle cells, osteoblasts, and chondroblasts; and vascular endothelial cells. Permanent cells are cells, such as nerve cells, that cannot reproduce themselves.

Tissue made up of labile and stable cells can regenerate itself after surgical trauma (Fig. 1). Injured tissue is replaced by parenchymal cells of the same type, often leaving no residual trace of injury. However, tissues constituted of permanent cells are repaired by the production of fibrocollagenous scar. Scar will also form in tissues with the capability for regeneration if the tissue stroma that remains after injury or is constructed during the healing process is destroyed (Fig. 1).[2] The biologic response to materials thereby depends on the influence of the material on the inflammatory and reparative stages of wound healing. Does the material yield leachables or corrosion products that interfere with the normal reparative processes initiated by the surgical trauma? Does the presence of the material interfere with the stroma required for the regeneration of tissue at the implant site? These are the types of questions that must be addressed when assessing the biocompatibility of materials.

A number of systemic and local factors influence the inflammatory-reparative response. Systemic influences include age, nutrition, hematologic and metabolic derangements, hormones, and steroids. Although the general impression is that the elderly heal more slowly than the young, there are few human data or animal experiments to support this notion.[2] However, recent observations of the decreased cellularity and regenerative capability of bone[3] and impaired bone ingrowth[4] with aging in dogs suggest that care must be taken in

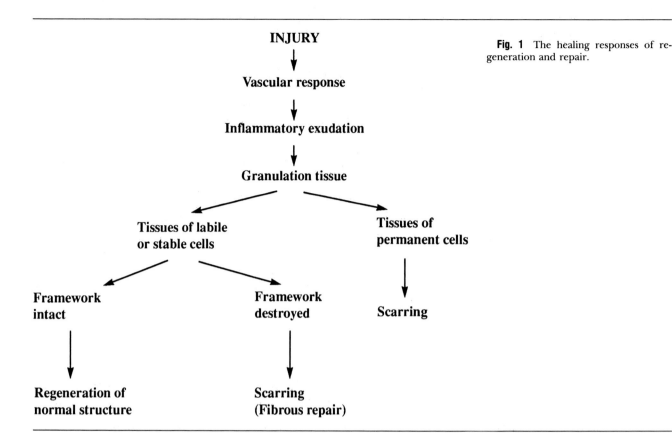

INJURY

↓

Vascular response

↓

Inflammatory exudation

↓

Granulation tissue

**Tissues of labile
or stable cells**

**Tissues of
permanent cells**

**Framework
intact**

**Framework
destroyed**

Scarring

**Regeneration of
normal structure**

**Scarring
(Fibrous repair)**

Fig. 1 The healing responses of regeneration and repair.

recommending the use of biologically fixed implants in the elderly. Nutrition can also profoundly affect the healing of wounds. Prolonged protein starvation can inhibit collagen formation, while high-protein diets can enhance the rate of tensile strength gained during wound healing.[2] Local influences that can affect wound healing include infection, an inadequate blood supply, and the presence of a foreign body.

Osseointegration, Bone Ingrowth, and Bone Bonding

Wound healing governs the makeup of the tissue that forms around implants. Because it is capable of regeneration, bone can be expected to appose cemented and noncemented orthopaedic prostheses and to form within the pore spaces of porous coatings. Is this bone bonded in any way to the implant? Bonding of a prosthesis to bone enhances its stability by limiting the relative motion between the implant and bone. In addition, bonding can provide a more favorable distribution of stress to surrounding osseous tissue.

Bone can bond to an implant by either mechanical or chemical means. Interdigitation of bone with bone cement or with irregularities in implant topography and bone ingrowth into porous surfaces can yield interfaces capable of supporting shear and tensile as well as compressive forces. These types of mechanical bonding have been extensively investigated and are reasonably well understood.[5-11] Chemical bonding of bone to ma-

terials results from molecular (for example, protein) adsorption and bonding to surfaces with subsequent attachment of osteoblasts. This phenomenon has undergone intensive investigation in recent years but is not yet as well understood as mechanical bonding.

The term "osseointegration" has been used to describe the presence of bone on the surface of an implant with no histologically demonstrable intervening fibrous or other nonosseous tissue. All cemented and noncemented orthopaedic implants should become osseointegrated unless the bone regeneration process is inhibited. Initially it was suggested that chemical bonding of bone to the implant surface was a prerequisite for osseointegration[12-15] and that osseointegration occurred with commercially pure titanium, but not with titanium alloyed with aluminum, vanadium, or other metals; this has never been conclusively proven. Observations indicate that implants fabricated from any of the orthopaedic metals, as well as polymers and ceramics, can become osseointegrated. With respect to the osseointegration of bone cement, Charnley[16] noted that "in load-bearing areas no tissue of any kind intervenes between the cement surface and the caps of changing bone on the ends of the load-bearing trabeculae." The question remains as to whether chemical bonding of bone to any of these orthopaedic biomaterials, including commercially pure titanium, occurs. Results of mechanical tests of the strength of attach-

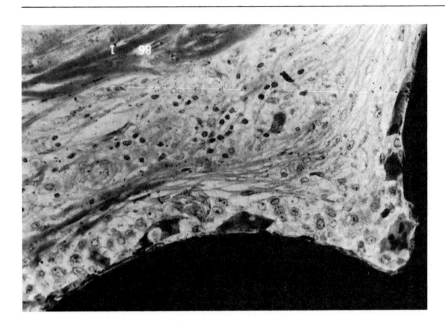

Fig. 2 Histology of tissue in the pore of a porous cobalt-chromium alloy tibial plateau prosthesis retrieved at revision arthroplasty for reasons other than loosening from a patient more than one year after implantation. Note the multiple layers of macrophages on the cobalt-chromium microsphere. A few multinucleated foreign body giant cells can also be seen on the implant surface. One of these cells is in the process of phagocytosing material. Undecalcified ground section is stained with paragon.

ment of implants of these materials to bone suggest that it does not.

Although there are few data that demonstrate chemical bonding of bone to the current orthopaedic biomaterials, previous investigations have provided evidence of bone bonding to calcium containing bioactive glasses[17-20] and to many different types of calcium phosphate.[21-24] Chemical bonding was evidenced by the high strength of the implant-bone interface that could not be explained by a mechanical interlocking bond alone. In addition, transmission electron microscopy has shown that there is no identifiable border between these calcium-containing implants and adjacent bone.

Many recent studies have investigated the bonding of bone to one particular calcium phosphate mineral, hydroxyapatite. Although hydroxyapatite was chosen because it was considered to be the primary mineral constituent of bone, natural bone mineral is actually calcium-deficient carbonate apatite. Experiments have been performed on both hydroxyapatite-coated metallic implants[23] and on particulate and block forms of the mineral employed as bone substitute materials.[25-29] Histologic specimens from animals[23] and retrieved from human subjects[30] show that a layer of new bone approximately 100 μ in thickness covers most of the hydroxyapatite surface within a few weeks of implantation.

In studying the mechanism of bone bonding, researchers have found that, within days of implantation, biologic apatite precipitates from body fluid onto the surface of implants made of hydroxyapatite and bioactive glass.[31-37] This biologic apatite is carbonate apatite, comparable to natural bone mineral. Proteins probably adsorb to this biologic mineral layer, thereby facilitating

bone-cell attachment and the production of osteoid directly onto the implant. The bone cell responds to the biologic apatite layer that has formed on the implant and not directly to the implant itself. Recent studies have shown that this biologic apatite layer can form on many different calcium phosphate substances, which explains why bone-bonding behavior has been reported for a variety of calcium phosphate materials. Of course, the clinical value of this phenomenon depends, in part, on how well these substances can be bonded to orthopaedic implants. However, the finding that bone can become chemically bonded to certain biomaterials is a significant advance in our understanding of the implant-bone interface.

Fibrous Interface

The features of the tissue around prostheses that are not osseointegrated vary widely. At one end of the spectrum are the narrow radiolucent lines, parallel to the implant surface, that are found in clinical radiographs of asymptomatic patients. These are considered to reflect stable, fibrous interfaces[9] that might function successfully for an indefinite period. However, there have been no systematic investigations of the mechanical properties of this fibrous tissue to validate its suitability as a support vehicle for a prosthesis. At the other end of the spectrum are interface zones around loose prostheses characterized by widening, divergent radiolucent, fibrous seams and aggressive osteolytic lesions.

Histologic examination of fibrous capsules around noncemented and cemented implants in bone often reveals macrophages on the biomaterial and bone-cement surfaces (Fig. 2). These cells are attracted to the pros-

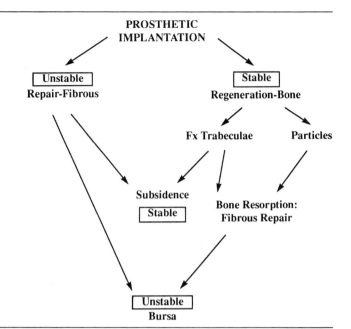

Fig. 3 Paradigm for stability/instability of implanted prostheses.

thesis as they are to a dead space, presumably because of such microenvironmental conditions as low oxygen and high lactate levels.[1] In this regard, it is not clear why macrophages are absent from the surface of osseointegrated implants. Perhaps stromal and osteoblast precursor cells migrate to the implant surface and begin forming new osseous tissue before macrophages have an opportunity to infiltrate.

In light of the above, the stability of these fibrous interfaces is questionable because they contain cellular elements such as macrophages that could be activated at some later time (by motion, particles, or metal ions) to release bone-resorbing agents that would promote loosening and cause pain.

Factors Affecting Degeneration of the Interface

As noted earlier, it is the wound-healing response that initially establishes the tissue characteristics of the implant-tissue interface. Several agents can initiate degenerative changes in the interface tissue. Others probably promote the production of pro-inflammatory mediators that stimulate bone resorption, leading to prosthesis loosening. Two factors that affect the implant-bone interface—motion of the prosthetic component and particulate debris—are of particular importance, because they are clearly present in most specimens retrieved at revision arthroplasty. However, it is difficult to determine the causal relationships between these factors and implant failure from study of end-stage tissue alone. Other histopathologic findings and laboratory studies indicate that metal ions and immune reactions may play roles in the degenerative pro-

cesses leading to prosthesis loosening in certain patients. Systemic diseases, and the drugs used to treat them, could also contribute to the breakdown of the implant-bone interface. Finally, there might be interindividual differences in genetically determined cellular responses that could explain why prostheses fail in some patients for whom the mechanical risk factor for failure is low.

A Paradigm for Loosening

The paradigm for loosening shown in Figures 3 and 4 can serve as a framework for considering the factors that influence the degeneration of the implant-bone interface and loosening.

The surgical trauma of implantation initiates the wound-healing response that should lead to the regeneration of osseous tissue in the surgically prepared implant site (Fig. 3). In the case of a stable prosthesis, bone envelopes the device, resulting in its osseointegration. Motion of a mechanically unstable implant during the initial stage of wound healing can disrupt the regenerating osseous stroma and lead to fibrous repair and encapsulation of the device. Depending on its design, subsidence of the fibrous-encapsulated prosthesis can stabilize it to the extent that it may become adequately supported by bone; the interposed fibrous tissue may persist indefinitely as a fibrous, stable interface.

In late loosening, fibrous tissue replaces bone around previously stable, osseointegrated devices either because of fracture of apposed bone (a mechanical factor) or because of a bone-resorption response (a biologic factor) associated with particulate debris and/or metal ions acting on joint synovium, infiltrating the implant-

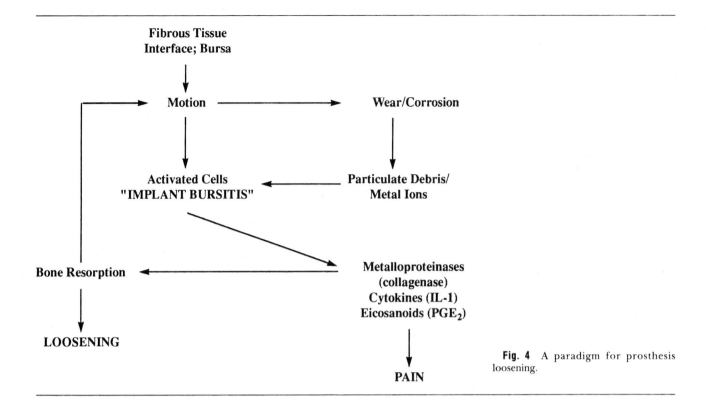

Fibrous Tissue
Interface; Bursa

Motion ————→ Wear/Corrosion

Activated Cells
"IMPLANT BURSITIS" ←———— Particulate Debris/
Metal Ions

Bone Resorption ←————

Metalloproteinases
(collagenase)
Cytokines (IL-1)
Eicosanoids (PGE$_2$)

LOOSENING

PAIN

Fig. 4 A paradigm for prosthesis loosening.

bone interface from the joint space, or appearing in localized lesions around the device.

Fibrous tissue formation around the prosthesis (Fig. 3), regardless of the cause, is accompanied by accretion of macrophages that eventually migrate to the surface of the implant,[1] probably attracted by the microenvironment associated with the dead space.[38] Some macrophages on or near the implant surface fuse to form multinucleated foreign body giant cells. This giant cell formation is probably influenced by the topography of the surface[39-42] and other, as yet unidentified, factors. Histologically, the nonosseous tissue around the prosthesis is made up of a layer of macrophage- and fibroblast-like cells supported by fibrous tissue, a formation characteristic of a synovial membrane. This has led to the use of the term "pseudomembrane." Because this synovium-like tissue contains a defect—the implant site—and experiences friction caused by implant micromotion, its histologic characteristics are similar to those of a bursa (Figs. 2 to 4).

Motion of the prosthesis (Figs. 4 and 5) can affect the cells around the implant in two ways. The motion can act directly by activating macrophages to produce certain cytokines, eicosanoids, and metalloproteinases. The motion can also create conditions that promote wear and corrosion, yielding metallic and polymeric particulate debris and metal ions. The debris and ions can activate the bursal cells to elaborate pro-inflammatory mediators and enzymes. The inflammatory process involving the cells at the interface of the prosthesis

could be referred to as "implant bursitis." Previously this condition has been referred to as "prosthetic synovitis."

Agents such as interleukin-1, prostaglandin E$_2$, and collagenase are known to stimulate bone resorption.[43-46] Bone loss can contribute to further motion, aggravating the inflammatory condition at the implant-tissue interface. These and other mediators of inflammation produced by the activated cells of the interface are probably responsible, at least in part, for the pain experienced by the patient (Fig. 4).

Motion

As noted earlier, motion can interfere with the wound-healing response of bone regeneration by destroying the regenerating osseous stroma. Fibrous, scar-like tissue results. Another important effect of motion is the formation of a bursa within connective tissue in which shearing and tensile movement have disrupted tissue continuity, forming a void space or sack lined by synovium-like cells. It is to be expected, then, that tissue around prosthetic components removed because of loosening might display features of synovium-like tissue. The presence of synovial cells (macrophage- and fibroblast-like cells) is important because they can be activated by other agents, such as particulate debris, to produce pro-inflammatory molecules (Fig. 4). The process of activation of this tissue may be similar to that which occurs in inflammatory joint synovium or bursitis.

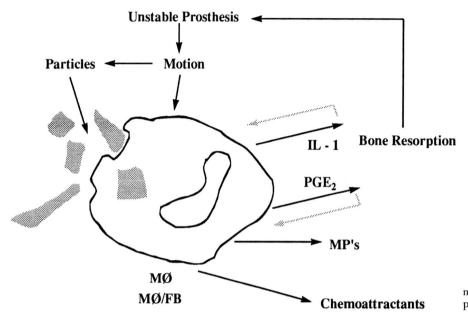

Unstable Prosthesis

Particles ← **Motion**

IL - 1 **Bone Resorption**

PGE$_2$

MP's

MØ
MØ/FB **Chemoattractants**

Fig. 5 Schema of the response of a macrophage-fibroblast to motion and particulate debris.

An explanation of how prosthetic motion leads to the formation of synovium-like tissue can be found in previous studies such as that by Edwards and associates[47] that has shown that a "synovial lining is simply an accretion of macrophages and fibroblasts stimulated by mechanical cavitation of connective tissue." This finding is based on experiments in which the mechanical disruption of connective tissue was produced by injecting air and/or fluid into the subcutaneous space of animals.[48,49] The resulting sack was initially described as a "granuloma pouch."[48] After demonstrating that the membrane lining the pouch displayed the characteristics of synovium, Edwards and associates[47] referred to this tissue as "facsimile synovium."

Prosthetic motion can also contribute to wear of the prosthetic component abrading against the bone-cement sheath or surrounding bone, thereby generating increased amounts of particulate debris that may contribute to activation of the macrophages and synovium-like cells at the implant-tissue interface (Figs. 3 and 4).

Particulate Debris

Particulate debris can be generated by wear occurring at the articulating surfaces of total joint replacement prostheses and by abrasion of the components against fragments of the bone-cement sheath or against surrounding bone. This particulate debris can induce changes in the joint synovium and in the tissue around the prosthetic components. Adverse responses have been found to both metallic and polymeric particles. The biologic reactions to particles are related to particle size, quantity, chemistry, topography, and shape. Although it is not clear what role each of these factors plays in the biologic response, particle size appears to be particularly important. Particles small enough to be phagocytosed (smaller than 10 μ) elicit a more adverse cellular response than larger particles.

Recent investigations[50] have shown that intra-articular injection of laboratory-prepared particulate cobalt-chromium alloy particles induced rapid proliferation of macrophages and focal degeneration of synovial tissues in rats. This reaction resembles changes seen in the articular tissue around loose total joint prostheses in human subjects. Because previous animal investigations and histopathologic studies of tissues retrieved from human subjects have suggested that titanium alloy is more biocompatible than cobalt-chromium alloys, it has been assumed that titanium particulate debris causes fewer problems than particles of cobalt-chromium alloy. Histologic studies of pigmented tissue surrounding titanium implants have generally revealed considerably fewer macrophages and multinucleated foreign body giant cells than are seen around cobalt-chromium alloy particles and polymeric particulate debris. However, a recent study of titanium alloy particles generated by the abrasion of femoral stems against bone cement in human subjects revealed histiocytic and lymphoplasmacytic reactions to the metallic particles.[51] In another recent investigation, titanium particles were found to cause fibroblasts in culture to produce elevated levels of prostaglandin E_2.[52] These findings indicate that the biologic response to titanium particles is not as benign as was initially believed.

Many investigations evaluating the histologic response to polyethylene and polymethylmethacrylate particles in animals and in tissue recovered from revision surgery have revealed the histiocytic response to these polymeric particles. It has been shown that this macrophage response can lead to bone resorption, causing loosening. The ability of polymeric particles to promote the destruction of the implant-bone interface and infiltrate the resulting fibrous membrane has been demonstrated in a recent animal investigation.[53] Injection of polyethylene particles into the knee joint of rats induced resorption of bone and the formation of a membrane at the interface of a nonweightbearing plug of bone cement implanted through the knee joint into the distal part of the femur. Polyethylene particles infiltrated the fibrous tissue around the acrylic plug. Results of this experiment could explain why such particles are found at distal sites around femoral stems.

The effect of calcium-containing ceramic particles on synovial cells has also been investigated.[54] Local leukocyte influx and levels of proteinase, prostaglandin E_2, and tumor necrosis factor increased after injection of three calcium-containing ceramic materials into the "air pouch model" described above.[54] This reaction shows that substances with surface chemistries that elicit a beneficial tissue response, such as bone bonding, when implanted in bulk form can cause destructive cellular reactions when present in particulate form.

Investigations indicate that all the orthopaedic biomaterials, when present as particles small enough to be phagocytosed (less than 10 μ), can elicit a biologic response that can cause the bone resorption that initiates and promotes the loosening process. This degenerative process has been referred to as small particle disease.

Recent studies have added to our knowledge of the fundamental response of cells to biomaterial chemistry and topography. One recent investigation,[55] carried out in vitro, assayed the bone-resorption activity of the medium conditioned by macrophages exposed to orthopaedic biomaterials in culture. Bone-resorption activity was greater in medium conditioned with macrophages on hydrophilic and rough surfaces than in that conditioned with cells on hydrophobic and smooth surfaces. Using this experimental method, high-density polyethylene elicited approximately 20% more bone resorption than did polymethylmethacrylate. Although

research of this type is advancing our understanding of the implant-bone interface, its clinical importance is not yet clear.

Metal Ions

Animal and human investigations have revealed increased levels of metal ions in serum and urine and peri-implant tissues in subjects with joint replacement prostheses and other types of implants. Our knowledge is still incomplete regarding the mechanisms of metal-ion release. Results are often variable with respect to the concentration of specific metal ions in tissues and fluids. The fact that metal in ionic form cannot always be distinguished from that present as particles further confounds interpretation of results.

One recent investigation of 14 patients undergoing conventional cemented cobalt-chromium alloy hip replacement revealed postoperative increases in serum and urinary chromium levels.[56] However, an attempt to determine the valency of chromium as either $+3$ or $+6$ from the concentration of metal ions in blood clot was not successful. This experiment was based on the fact that erythrocytes display a unidirectional uptake of $+6$ chromium while effectively excluding $+3$ chromium. Identification of the valency of chromium is important because $+6$ chromium is much more biologically active than $+3$ chromium.

Unfortunately, our knowledge of the local and systemic biologic and clinical sequelae of metal-ion release has not advanced significantly during the last several years. One recent study explored the effect of metal ions on cells in culture.[57] Addition of cobalt ions in the form of cobalt fluoride solutions to the media of lapine or human synovial cells stimulated their production of neutral proteinases and collagenase. Production of prostaglandin E_2 by lapine cells was enhanced 30% to 40% by cobalt solutions that slightly depressed the production of prostaglandin E_2 by human cells. Lapine synovial cells stimulated by cobaltous chloride also produced a substance that provoked synthesis of collagenase, gelatinase, caseinase, and prostaglandin E_2 by monolayers of articular chondrocytes. It has been suggested that these findings may be relevant to aseptic loosening of joint prostheses, in that metal ions could activate synovial cells, located in the joint capsule and in the pseudomembrane at the implant-bone interface, to produce agents that promote osteolysis.

Diseases and Drugs

There has been little work correlating the failure of orthopaedic prostheses with disease states and drugs employed to treat the disorders. Most investigations in this area have studied the role of anti-inflammatory drugs[58-62] and other agents employed to prevent heterotopic ossification, on the bone ingrowth into noncemented, porous-coated prostheses. Generally, these results have shown that these anti-inflammatory agents,

Table 1
Biochemistry of pseudomembrane tissue (human)

Patient No.	Interleukin-1β (pg/ml)	Prostaglandin E$_2$ (ng/ml)	Prosthesis
1	3440	82.5	Uncemented total knee replacement (Co-Cr)
2	6240	384.6	Cemented total hip replacement (Co-Cr)
3	730	910.0	Uncemented total knee replacement (Ti alloy)

as well as certain anticancer drugs,[63] reduce the amount of bone ingrowth in the early stages of wound healing after implantation. There have been almost no studies of the role of these and other agents on the remodeling and degeneration of the implant-bone interface after longer periods of implantation.

The role of disease in the formation, remodeling, and degeneration of the implant-bone interface is still unclear. One investigation[64] employed estrogen deficiency in a canine model to determine the effect that postmenopausal osteoporosis might have on bone ingrowth. The results, which were not definitive, suggested that this condition might be expected to yield greater amounts of fibrous tissue ingrowth into porous-coated prostheses.

Unfortunately, there have been no studies investigating the role of selected diseases on the longer-term remodeling and degeneration of the implant-bone interface.

Immune Reactions and Genetic Determinants

It is not uncommon for two patients matched for sex, age, weight, activity level, and other factors that might be expected to affect the performance of the prosthesis to have very different outcomes. This suggests that in some patients immune reactions or genetically determined responses may play a role in the failure of prostheses.

Immune responses include antibody- and cell-mediated reactions and activation of the complement system. Metal ions behave as haptens, which, when complexed with serum proteins, can trigger an immune response. However, the lymphocytes and plasma cells that might be expected to occur at sites of antibody- and cell-mediated reactions are not often found in tissue retrieved during revision surgery. In one recent report,[51] a lymphoplasmacytic infiltrate was found in pseudomembrane tissue containing titanium alloy particulate debris. However, this finding, and the observation of occasional lymphocytic infiltrates in the pseudomembrane tissue, does not presently provide enough information to determine the role of immune reactions in implant loosening.

Several studies[65-67] have demonstrated that many biomaterials can activate (cleave) certain molecules (C3 and C5) in the complement system. It has been suggested that complement activation by biomaterials may play a role in adverse reactions to certain devices. However, additional studies are required.

One form of cell-mediated immune reaction associated with implants is the delayed hypersensitivity response. "Metal allergy" has been seen to cause failure in certain patients.[68-70] However, results obtained to date are not definitive.

> The incidence of metal sensitivity in the normal population is high, with up to 15% of the population sensitive to nickel and perhaps up to 25% sensitive to at least one of the common sensitizers Ni, Co, and Cr. The incidence of metal sensitivity reactions requiring premature removal of an orthopedic device is probably small (less than the incidence of infection). Clearly there are factors not yet understood that cause one patient but not another to react.[68]

A similar situation exists with respect to sensitivity reactions to bone cement (polymethylmethacrylate, PMMA). The monomer of polymethylmethacrylate is a strong skin sensitizer.[71] However, failure of cemented devices has not yet been correlated with a hypersensitivity response in patients.

The fact that in some patients there is no clear cause for prosthesis loosening, whereas in others, with multiple risk factors for failure, the prosthesis functions well suggests that there may be genetic determinants for loosening.

A recent investigation[72] has shown interindividual differences in the in vitro cytokine and prostaglandin E$_2$ production by macrophages stimulated with lipopolysaccharide. Individuals who were HLA-DR2-positive and their first-degree relatives were found to be low-responders. Studies of this type suggest that in certain individuals genetic determination may play a role in the degree to which cells in the tissue around prostheses can be activated to produce pro-inflammatory agents that stimulate bone resorption. Additional studies of this type could be of value in identifying patients who might be high-responders to prosthetic motion and particulate debris, putting them at high risk for prosthesis failure.

Carcinogenicity

Chromium and nickel are known carcinogens, and cobalt is a suspected carcinogen. Therefore, it is understandable that there is some concern about the release of these metal ions into the human body from orthopaedic prostheses. Fortunately, there have been

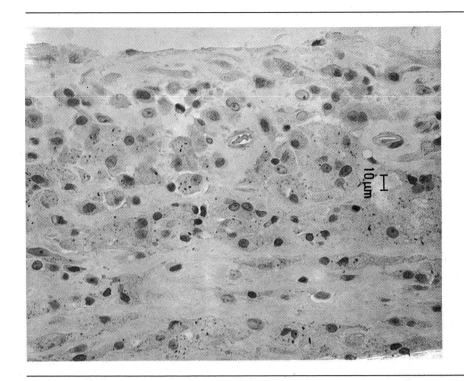

Fig. 6 Patient 2. Histology of tissue around a loose cemented cobalt-chromium total hip prosthesis showing small metallic particles in macrophages, multinucleated giant cells, and, occasionally, fibroblast-like cells.

few reports of neoplasms around orthopaedic implants. Although no causal relationship has been demonstrated, there is a high enough index of suspicion to warrant serious investigation of this matter through epidemiologic and other studies. The use of noncemented, porous-coated metallic stems (with large surface area) in younger patients has increased concern about the long-term clinical consequences of metal-ion release because of the prolonged exposure of such patients to metal ions.

Recent publications have reviewed the relationship between metal-ion release and oncogenesis,[73] and reports of neoplasms found around orthopaedic implants have recently been reviewed.[74] Differences in tumor types, times to appearance, and types of prostheses confound attempts to associate neoplasms with implant materials and products of degradation.

In a recent epidemiologic investigation conducted in New Zealand,[75] more than 1,300 patients who underwent total joint replacement were followed up to determine the incidence of remote-site tumors. In the decade after arthroplasty, incidences of tumors of the lymphatic and hemopoietic systems were found to be significantly greater than expected. It is important to note that the incidences of cancer of the breast, colon, and rectum were significantly less than expected. The investigators acknowledged that although the association might result, in part, from an effect of the prosthetic implants, other mechanisms, particularly drug therapy, must also be considered. Somewhat similar results were obtained from another recent study[76] of can-

cer incidence in 443 patients who underwent total hip replacement between 1967 and 1973 and who were followed up through 1981. The risk of leukemias and lymphomas increased, whereas the risk of breast cancer decreased. The authors concluded that the local occurrence of cancer associated with prostheses made of cobalt-chromium-molybdenum as reported in the literature indicates some connection between the two.

Histology and Biochemistry of Tissue Around Loose Prostheses

Biochemical studies of pseudomembrane tissue retrieved with loose prostheses have revealed the presence of molecules, such as prostaglandin E_2, interleukin-1, and collagenase, that are known to contribute to bone resorption. Goldring and associates[77] provided the first report of the cellular and biochemical features of the pseudomembrane around aseptic loose cemented femoral stems. They found a synovium-like lining adjacent to the cement sheath, and increased levels of prostaglandin E_2 and collagenase. Moreover, tissue culture medium, conditioned by exposure to cells from the pseudomembranes, demonstrated bone resorption activity in vitro. In a later study this group found no increase in prostaglandin E_2 in fibrous tissue around rigid (stable) implants.[78] More recently, Goldring and associates[79] reported a difference in the histologic features of pseudomembranes obtained from patients with rheumatoid arthritis and those with os-

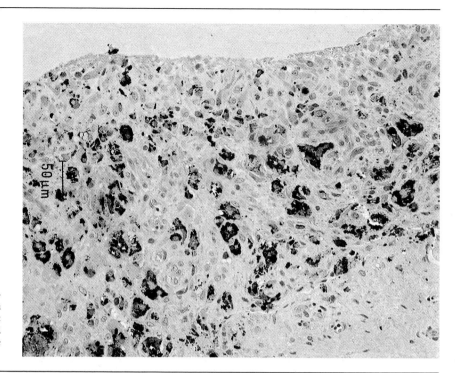

Fig. 7   Patient 3. Synovium-like tissue retrieved with a loose noncemented titanium alloy total knee prosthesis showing metallic particles in macrophages and giant cells, and occasionally in cells consistent in appearance with fibroblasts.

teoarthritis. Tissue from patients with rheumatoid arthritis displayed "marked papillary transformation with nodular lymphocytic infiltration. Surface fibrin, lining layer hyperplasia, and proliferation of vascular elements characteristic of rheumatoid synovium are also seen."

Interleukin-1-like activity, determined by the mouse thymocyte co-mitogenesis assay, has also been found in pseudomembranes.[80] However, immunoassay determination of interleukin-1β, while yielding positive findings in one study,[81] produced negative results in another.[82]

The pro-inflammatory cellular elements and molecules found in pseudomembrane tissue are responsible for the bone resorption that promotes loosening and the associated pain. However, the roles played by specific cells and molecules in this process are still unclear.

Correlation of histologic with biochemical characteristics of interface tissue in selected cases can be of value in determining the role of certain cells in the degenerative response and comparing the response to different types of particulate debris. In a recent study,[83] pseudomembrane tissues obtained from patients at revision surgery were analyzed for interleukin-1β and prostaglandin E_2, and the results were correlated with histologic findings. Although all the interface tissues retrieved from three selected patients with different types of prostheses displayed synovium-like features characteristic of a pseudomembrane, there were variations in interleukin-1β and prostaglandin E_2 levels (Table 1). There was no correlation between the levels of interleukin-1β and prostaglandin E_2. Polyethylene

debris was predominant in the histologic sections from two of the patients (Patient 1 and Patient 2). Smaller polymeric particles were found within macrophages; the large particles were interstitial and surrounded by multinucleated foreign body giant cells. Large amounts of cobalt-chromium and titanium alloy particulate debris (of comparable size distribution) were found in Patient 2 (Fig. 6) and Patient 3 (Fig. 7), respectively. Both types of metallic particles were found in macrophages and giant cells. The titanium particles appeared to be aggregated to a greater extent than were the cobalt-chromium particles, perhaps because there were more titanium particles. The tissue with the greatest amount of cobalt-chromium alloy contained the most interleukin-1β and the tissue with a large amount of titanium alloy debris had the most prostaglandin E_2. These findings highlight the need for additional studies to determine how the chemistry of particulate material influences the biologic response.

Many of the cells constituting the pseudomembrane did not have the morphologic features of macrophages. These cells were more consistent in appearance with fibroblasts. Histopathologically, cells of this type have been referred to by some as fibrohistiocytes, reflecting the proposition that certain mesenchymal cells can reversibly express the phenotypes of fibroblasts and histiocytes. Moreover, it has not been possible to distinguish monocyte-derived, mobile macrophages from tissue-fixed histiocytes. Resolution of issues about the lineage and phenotype of cells in the tissue around prostheses will deepen our understanding of mechanisms underlying the degeneration of the implant-bone interface.

Rationale for Nonsurgical Treatment of Loose Prostheses

As noted in the paradigm for loosening shown in Figures 3 and 4, certain eicosanoids (prostaglandin E_2), cytokines (interleukin-1), and metalloproteinases (collagenase) can serve as agents to initiate and promote the resorption of bone at the implant interface, thereby causing loosening. The question is raised as to whether drugs or other treatments, such as electrical stimulation, might help stabilize the response, thereby delaying or, possibly, avoiding revision. Can a patient who has pain and radiographic evidence of an ongoing osteolytic process be treated in a way such that the symptoms will disappear and the radiographic changes cease? It is unlikely that any treatment will be effective for advanced loosening because of mechanical instability and the necessity of ameliorating the inflammatory and bone resorption processes and also replacing the fibrous tissue with new bone. The prosthetic component would probably have to be stabilized mechanically while new bone formed, and it is not clear how this could be accomplished.

The increased levels of prostaglandin E_2 in tissue retrieved from loose prostheses have suggested that nonsteroidal anti-inflammatory drugs (NSAIDs) might be of value in reducing one of the inflammatory components of the tissue around loose prostheses. Specific NSAIDs might be of particular value in reducing levels of cyclo-oxygenase, which is responsible for converting arachidonic acid to prostaglandins. There have been no controlled prospective studies performed as yet to determine the efficacy of NSAIDs in reducing the inflammatory component of tissue around loose prostheses. In many cases, patients who have undergone total joint replacement are already taking NSAIDs for the arthritic condition of other joints. However, it is difficult to determine from this patient population the effectiveness of this class of drugs in treating prosthesis loosening.

Recent studies have shown the effectiveness of an NSAID, flurbiprofen, in reducing the resorption of alveolar bone in naturally occurring chronic destructive periodontal disease in dogs.[84] In another study, ibuprofen was also shown to be effective.[85] The inflammatory tissue in periodontal disease shares many characteristics with the tissue around loose prostheses, particularly increased levels of prostaglandin E_2.

Interleukin-1 and collagenase probably also play important roles in the bone destruction associated with the loosening process. In the future, interleukin-1 inhibitors may be identified for investigation of this application. It is possible that retinoids or analogs of tissue inhibitors of metalloproteinases may also be of value in the treatment at certain stages of loosening of patients who have undergone total joint replacement. A recent study has suggested the potential value of chelators for reducing the activity of metalloproteinases in arthritic joint tissues.[86]

The complex interrelationships between agents that can contribute to inflammation and bone destruction around joint replacement prostheses make it difficult to determine the effectiveness of drugs and other treatments for loose prostheses through human trials alone. This highlights the importance of establishing animal models to gain a better understanding of the loosening process and to evaluate modes of treatment.

Summary

Many factors influence the formation, remodeling, and degeneration of the tissue around implants. Because of its capability for regeneration, bone should be expected to appose prostheses, thereby leading to their osseointegration. However, early postoperative motion can destroy regenerating osseous stroma and thereby lead to fibrous (scar) encapsulation of an orthopaedic prosthesis. Replacement of bone with fibrous tissue around previously osseointegrated devices may result from fracture of bone trabeculae or cement at the implant-bone interface or from the biologic response to particulate debris or metal ions. Continued motion of fibrous-encapsulated prostheses can disrupt the fibrous tissue, leading to the formation of a synovium-like structure (bursa) at the implant-tissue interface. Particulate debris (and perhaps metal ions) can further activate cells in the pseudomembrane to produce cytokines, eicosanoids, and metalloproteinases that can result in additional bone resorption and pain. Any orthopaedic biomaterial, when present in particulate form of a size that can be phagocytosed (smaller than 10μ), can provoke an inflammatory response. This includes materials such as calcium phosphates, which in bulk form display "biocompatible" (bone-bonding) behavior.

Advances in our understanding of the formation and degeneration of the implant-bone interface will facilitate the rational development and implementation of materials for the fabrication of joint replacement prostheses.

References

1. Spector M, Cease C, Xia T-L: The local tissue response to biomaterials. *CRC Crit Rev Biocompat* 1989;5:269–295.
2. Robbins SL, Cotran RS: *Pathologic Basis of Disease*, ed 2. Philadelphia, WB Saunders, 1979.
3. Kelly PJ, Williams EA, Pinto MR, et al: The effects of age and

bony ingrowth, in Fitzgerald RH Jr (ed): *Non-Cemented Total Hip Arthroplasty.* New York, Raven Press, 1988, pp 111–117.

4. Magee FP, Longo JA, Hedley AK: The effect of age on the interface strength between porous coated implants and bone. *Trans Soc Biomater* 1989;12:85.

5. Spector M: Bone ingrowth into porous metals, in Williams DF (ed): *Biocompatibility of Orthopedic Implants.* Boca Raton, CRC Press, 1982, pp 89–128.

6. Spector M: Bone ingrowth into porous polymers, in Williams DF (ed): *Biocompatibility of Orthopedic Implants.* Boca Raton, CRC Press, 1982, pp 55–88.

7. Spector M: Historical review of porous-coated implants, *J Arthrop* 1987;2:163–177.

8. Spector M: Current concepts of bone ingrowth and remodeling, Fitzgerald RH Jr (ed): *Non-Cemented Total Hip Arthroplasty.* New York, Raven Press, 1988, pp 69–85.

9. Engh CA, Bobyn JD, Glassman AH: Porous-coated hip replacement: The factors governing bone ingrowth, stress shielding, and clinical results. *J Bone Joint Surg* 1987;69B:45–55.

10. Engh CA, Bobyn JD, Glassman AH: Theory and practice of cementless revision total hip arthroplasty, in Brand RA (ed): *The Hip.* St. Louis, CV Mosby, 1987, pp 271–317.

11. Bobyn JD, Engh CA: Biologic fixation of hip prostheses: Review of the clinical status and current concepts. *Adv Orthop Surg* 1983; 7:137.

12. Albrektsson T: Direct bone anchorage of dental implants. *J Prosthet Dent* 1983;50:255–261.

13. Brånemark PI, Adell R, Albrektsson T, et al: Osseointegrated titanium fixtures in the treatment of edentulousness. *Biomaterials* 1983;4:25–28.

14. Linder L, Albrektsson T, Brånemark PI, et al: Electron microscopic analysis of the bone-titanium interface. *Acta Orthop Scand* 1983;54:45–52.

15. Albrektsson T, Brånemark PI, Hansson H-A, et al: The interface zone of inorganic implants in vivo: Titanium implants in bone. *Ann Biomed Eng* 1983;11:1–27.

16. Charnley J: *Low Friction Arthroplasty of the Hip: Theory and Practice.* Berlin, Springer-Verlag, 1979.

17. Hench LL, Splinter RJ, Allen WC, et al: Bonding mechanisms at the interface of ceramic prosthetic materials. *J Biomed Mater Res Symp* 1971;2:117–141.

18. Hench LL, Wilson J: Surface-active biomaterials. *Science* 1984; 226:630–636.

19. Gross U, Brandes J, Strunz V, et al: The ultrastructure of the interface between a glass ceramic and bone. *J Biomed Mater Res* 1981:15:291–305.

20. Gross U, Strunz V: The interface of various glasses and glass ceramics with a bony implantation bed. *J Biomed Mater Res* 1985; 19:251–271.

21. de Groot K: *Bioceramics of Calcium Phosphate.* Boca Raton, CRC Press, 1983.

22. Klein CP, de Groot K, Driessen AA, et al: A comparative study of different beta-whitlockite ceramics in rabbit cortical bone with regard to their biodegradation behaviour. *Biomaterials* 1986;7: 144–146.

23. Geesink RG, de Groot K, Klein CP: Chemical implant fixation using hydroxyl-apatite coatings: The development of a human total hip prosthesis for chemical fixation to bone using hydroxyl-apatite coatings on titanium substrates. *Clin Orthop* 1987;255: 147–170.

24. Geesink RG, de Groot K, Klein CP: Bonding of bone to apatite-coated implants. *J Bone Joint Surg* 1988;70B:17–22.

25. Bucholz RW, Carlton A, Holmes RE: Hydroxyapatite and tricalcium phosphate bone graft substitutes. *Orthop Clin North Am* 1987;18:323–334.

26. Holmes RE, Bucholz RW, Mooney V: Porous hydroxyapatite as a bone-graft substitute in metaphyseal defects: A histometric study. *J Bone Joint Surg* 1986;68A:904–911.

27. Martin RB, Chapman MW, Holmes RE, et al: Effects of bone ingrowth on the strength and non-invasive assessment of a coralline hydroxyapatite material. *Biomaterials* 1989;10:481–488.

28. Fitzgerald RH Jr, Chao EYS, McDonald DJ, et al: A comparison of autografts, allografts, and tricalcium phosphate hydroxyapatite crystals, in Fitzgerald RH Jr (ed): *Non-Cemented Total Hip Arthroplasty.* New York, Raven Press, 1988, pp 159–174.

29. Russotti GM, Okada Y, Fitzgerald RH, et al: Efficacy of using a bone graft substitute to enhance biological fixation of a porous metal femoral component, in Brand RA (ed): *The Hip.* St. Louis, CV Mosby, 1987, pp 120–154.

30. Osborn JF: Bonding osteogenesis under loaded conditions-the histological evaluation of a human autopsy specimen of a hydroxyapatite ceramic coated stem of a titanium hip prosthesis, in Oonishi H, Aoki H, Sawai K (eds): *Bioceramics.* St. Louis, Ishiyaku Euro America Inc, 1989, pp 388–399.

31. Heughebaert M, LeGeros RZ, Gineste M, et al: Physiochemical characterization of deposits associated with HA ceramics implanted in nonosseous sites. *J Biomed Mater Res* 1988;22(suppl 3):257–268.

32. Daculsi G, Passuti N, Martin S, et al: A comparative study of bioactive calcium phosphate ceramics after implantation in cancellous bone in the dog. *Fr J Orthop Surg* 1989;3:43–48.

33. Passuti N, Daculsi G, Rogez JM, et al: Macroporous calcium phosphate ceramic performance in human spine fusion. *Clin Orthop* 1989;248:169–176.

34. Daculsi G, Passuti N, Hamel L, et al: Biointegration of HAP coating titanium implant: Structural, ultrastructural and electron microprobe studies, in Oonishi H, Aoki H, Sawai K, (eds): *Bioceramics.* St. Louis, Ishiyaku Euro America Inc, 1989, pp 375–381.

35. Kokubo T, Kushitani Y, Ebisawa Y, et al: Apatite formation on bioactive ceramics in body environment, in Oonishi H, Aoki H, Sawaik (eds): *Bioceramics.* St. Louis, Schiyaku EuroAmerica, 1989, p 157.

36. Kitsugi T, Yamamuro T, Nakamura T, et al: Bonding behavior between two bioactive ceramics in vivo. *J Biomed Mater Res* 1987; 21:1109–1123.

37. Kokubo T, Ito S, Huang ZT, et al: Ca,P-rich layer formed on high-strength bioactive glass-ceramic A-W. *J Biomed Mater Res* 1990;24:331–343.

38. Silver IA: The physiology of wound healing, in Hunt TK (ed): *Wound Healing and Wound Infection: Theory and Surgical Practice.* New York, Appleton-Century-Crofts, 1980, pp 11–28.

39. Behling CA, Spector M: Quantitative characterization of cells at the interface of long-term implants of selected polymers. *J Biomed Mater Res* 1986;20:653–666.

40. Rich A, Harris AK: Anomalous preferences of cultured macrophages for hydrophobic and roughened substrata. *J Cell Sci* 1981;50:1–7.

41. Mariano M, Spector WG: The formation and properties of macrophage polykaryons (inflammatory giant cells). *J Pathol* 1974; 113:1–19.

42. Taylor SR, Gibbons DF: Effect of surface texture on the soft tissue response to polymer implants. *J Biomed Mater Res* 1983; 17:205–227.

43. Dinarello CA: Interleukin-1. *Dig Dis Sci* 1988;33(suppl 3):25S–35S.

44. Galasko CS, Bennett A: Relationship of bone destruction in skeletal metastases to osteoclast activation and prostaglandins. *Nature* 1976;263:508–510.

45. Garrett IR, Mundy GR: Relationship between interleukin-1 and prostaglandins in resorbing neonatal calvaria. *J Bone Miner Res* 1989;4:789–794.

46. Klein DC, Raisz LG: Prostaglandins: Stimulation of bone resorption in tissue culture. *Endocrinology* 1970;86:1436–1440.

47. Edwards JC, Sedgwick AD, Willoughby DA: The formation of a structure with the features of synovial lining by subcutaneous

injection of air: An in vivo tissue culture system. *J Pathol* 1981; 134:147–156.

48. Selye H: Use of "granuloma pouch" technic in the study of antiphlogistic corticoids. *Proc Soc Exp Biol Med* 1953;82:328–333.

49. Selye H: On the mechanism through which hydrocortisone affects the resistance of tissues to injury: An experimental study with the granuloma pouch technique. *JAMA* 1953;152:1207–1213.

50. Howie DW, Vernon-Roberts B: The synovial response to intraarticular cobalt-chrome wear particles. *Clin Orthop* 1988;232:244–254.

51. Agins HJ, Alcock NW, Bansal M, et al: Metallic wear in failed titanium-alloy total hip replacements: A histological and quantitative analysis. *J Bone Joint Surg* 1988;70A:347–356.

52. Goldring SR, Kroop SF, Petrison KK, et al: Metal particles stimulate prostaglandin E$_2$ (PGE$_2$) release and collagen synthesis in cultured cells. *Trans Orthop Res Soc* 1990;15:444.

53. Howie DW, Vernon-Roberts B, Oakeshott R, et al: A rat model of resorption of bone at the cement-bone interface in the presence of polyethylene wear particles. *J Bone Joint Surg* 1988;70A:257–263.

54. Nagase M, Baker DG, Schumacher HR Jr: Prolonged inflammatory reactions induced by artificial ceramics in the rat air pouch model. *J Rheumatol* 1988;15:1334–1338.

55. Murray DW, Rae T, Rushton N: The influence of the surface energy and roughness of implants on bone resorption. *J Bone Joint Surg* 1989;71B:632–637.

56. Bartolozzi A, Black J: Chromium concentrations in serum, blood clot and urine from patients following total hip arthoplasty. *Biomaterials* 1985;6:2–8.

57. Ferguson GM, Watanabe S, Georgescu HI, et al: The synovial production of collagenase and chondrocyte activating factors in response to cobalt. *J Orthop Res* 1988;6:525–530.

58. Ahrengart L, Lindgren U, Reinholt FP: Comparative study of the effects of radiation, indomethacin, prednisolone, and ethane-1-hydroxy-1, 1-diphosphonate (EHDP) in the prevention of ectopic bone formation. *Clin Orthop* 1988;229:265–273.

59. Keller JC, Trancik TM, Young FA, et al: Effects of indomethacin on bone ingrowth. *J Orthop Res* 1989;7:28–34.

60. Longo JA, Hedley AK, Weinstein AM: Comparative effect of EHDP, radiation, indomethacin, on bone growth in a porous ingrowth model in rabbits. *Trans Eur Soc Biomater* 1985;5:195.

61. Longo JA, Magee FP, Hedley AK, et al: The effect of chronic indomethacin on fixation of porous implants to bone. Presented at the 15th Annual Meeting of the Society for Biomaterials, Lake Buena Vista, Florida, 1989.

62. Trancik T, Mills W, Vinson N, et al: The effect of several therapeutic agents on bone ingrowth into a porous coated implant. *Trans Soc Biomater* 1989;12:87.

63. Barth E, Roenningen H, Solheim LF, et al: Influence of cis-platinum on bone ingrowth into porous fiber titanium, mechanical and biochemical correlations. *Trans Soc Biomater* 1986;9:170.

64. Martin RB, Paul HA, Bargar WL, et al: Effects of estrogen deficiency on the growth of tissue into porous titanium implants. *J Bone Joint Surg* 1988;70A:540–547.

65. Anderson JM, Miller KM: Biomaterial biocompatibility and the macrophage. *Biomaterials* 1984;5:5–10.

66. Kazatchkine MD, Carreno MP: Activation of the complement system at the interface between blood and artificial surfaces. *Biomaterials* 1988;9:30–35.

67. Ward CA, Koheil A, Johnson WR, et al: Reduction in complement activation from biomaterials by removal of air nuclei from the surface roughness. *J Biomed Mater Res* 1984;18:255–269.

68. Merritt K, Brown SA: Biological effects of corrosion products from metals, in Fraker A (ed): *Corrosion and Degradation of Implant Material*. Philadelphia, ASTM STP 859, 1985, pp 195–207.

69. Merritt K, Brown SA: Hypersensitivity of metallic biomaterials, in Williams DF (ed): *Systemic Aspects of Biomaterials*. Boca Raton, CRC Press, 1980, pp 33–48.

70. Brown SA, Devine SD, Merritt K: Metal allergy, metal implants and fracture healing. *Biomater Med Devices Artif Organs* 1983;11:73–81.

71. Merritt K: Role of medical materials, both in implant and surface applications, in immune response and in resistance to infection. *Biomaterials* 1984;5:47–53.

72. Molvig J, Baek L, Christensen P, et al: Endotoxin-stimulated human monocyte secretion of interleukin 1, tumour necrosis factor alpha, and prostaglandin E$_2$ shows stable interindividual differences. *Scand J Immunol* 1988;27:705–716.

73. Black J: Metallic ion release and its relationship to oncogenesis, in Fitzgerald RH Jr (ed): *The Hip*. St. Louis, CV Mosby, 1985, pp 199–213.

74. Martin A, Bauer TW, Manley MT, et al: Osteosarcoma at the site of total hip replacement: A case report. *J Bone Joint Surg* 1988;70A:1561–1567.

75. Gillespie WJ, Frampton CM, Henderson RJ, et al: The incidence of cancer following total hip replacement. *J Bone Joint Surg* 1988;70B:539–542.

76. Visuri T, Koskenvuo M: Cancer risk after McKee-Farrar total hip replacement, abstract. *Acta Orthop Scand* 1989;60(suppl 231):25.

77. Goldring SR, Schiller AL, Roelke M, et al: The synovial-like membrane at the bone-cement interface in loose total hip replacements and its proposed role in bone lysis. *J Bone Joint Surg* 1983; 65A:575–584.

78. Jasty M, Goldring SR, Harris WH: Comparison of bone cement membrane around rigidly fixed versus loose total hip implants. *Trans Orthop Res Soc* 1984;9:125.

79. Goldring SR, Wojno WC, Schiller AL, et al: In patients with rheumatoid arthritis the tissue reaction associated with loosened total knee replacements exhibits features of a rheumatoid synovium. *J Orthop Rheumatol* 1988;1:9–21.

80. Appel AM, Sowder WG, Hopson CN, et al: Production of mediators of bone resorption by prosthesis associated pseudomembranes. *Trans Orthop Res Soc* 1988;13:362.

81. Mather SE, Magee FP, Emmanual J, et al: Interleukin and prostaglandin E$_2$ in failed total hip arthroplasty. Presented at the Symposium on Retrieval and Analysis of Surgical Implants and Biomaterials, Snowbird, Utah, 1988.

82. Goodman SB, Chin RC, Chiou SS, et al: A clinical-pathologic-biochemical study of the membrane surrounding loosened and nonloosened total hip arthroplasties. *Clin Orthop* 1989;244:182–187.

83. Thornhill TS, Ozuna RM, Shortkroff S, et al: Biochemical and histological evaluation of the synovial-like tissue around failed (loose) total joint replacement prostheses in human subjects and a canine model. *Biomaterials* 1990;11:69–72.

84. Williams RC, Jeffcoat MK, Kaplan ML, et al: Flurbiprofen: A potent inhibitor of alveolar bone resorption in beagles. *Science* 1985;227:640–642.

85. Williams RC, Jeffcoat MK, Howell TH, et al: Ibuprofen: An inhibitor of alveolar bone resorption in beagles. *J Periodont Res* 1988;23:225–229.

86. Ehrlich MG, Armstrong AL, Treadwell BV, et al: Degradative enzyme systems in cartilage. *Clin Orthop* 1986;213:62–68.

Advances in Total Hip Reconstruction

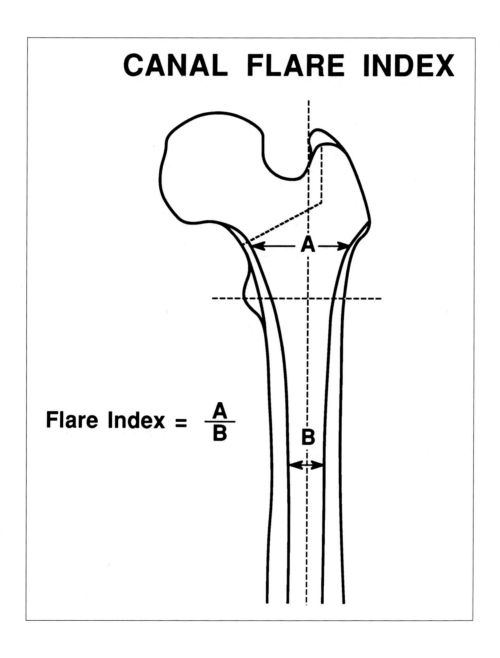

CANAL FLARE INDEX

Flare Index = $\dfrac{A}{B}$

Results and Experiences With Uncemented and Hybrid Primary Total Hip Replacements

John J. Callaghan, MD

Uncemented Total Hip Replacement

Our understanding of uncemented total hip replacement is in an evolutionary state. The following chapter updates the clinical and scientific data available today concerning uncemented replacement. Although the majority of surgeons and manufacturers have elected to achieve microlock fixation with porous surfaces for bony ingrowth, the other option is to omit porous surfaces and obtain macrolock with press-fit fixation. Advocates of this method believe that press-fit fixation provides more uniform stress transfer to proximal bone than is possible with porous surfaces.[1] On the other hand, those favoring porous-surface devices question the long-term stability and durability of press-fit fixation. This discussion focuses on porous-surface devices, the type currently used by most surgeons.

Type of Ingrowth Surfaces Available

Two common forms of manufactured porous surfaces use either sintered bead or fiber mesh technology. Attaching either of these surfaces to the device requires that the material be sintered to the underlying substrate. The high temperatures involved in sintering increase the grain size of the substrate and weaken the material. Fiber mesh attachment is currently accomplished with lower temperatures, with the addition of high pressure. These lower temperatures reduce the risk of weakening the prosthesis. Because titanium is more notch-sensitive than cobalt-chromium, the mesh is usually reduced in area or excluded on the tension (lateral) surfaces of titanium devices to avoid weakening them. The breakage of noncemented implants has not yet been reported, however, and this issue may not be clinically important.

With either type of porous surface, bone ingrowth appears to occur satisfactorily. Bobyn and associates[2] demonstrated in an animal model that prostheses coated with chrome cobalt sintered beads with pore sizes of 50 μ to 400 μ allow bony ingrowth with stability at six to eight weeks after implantation. Galanté and associates[3] demonstrated bony ingrowth into titanium fiber mesh. In comparing the two in a canine model, Turner and associates[4] reported relatively minor differences in bony ingrowth between stems with cobalt-chromium sintered beads (23.3%) and those with titanium mesh (37.3%). Retrieved specimens from human patients have also demonstrated bony ingrowth into both types of surface.[5,6] The potential for wear debris

and biocompatibility problems caused by ion release need continued clinical and basic investigation with both technologies. More recently, the potential of enhancing bony ingrowth by applying ceramics (most notably hydroxyapatite) to the porous surfaces has been investigated. These studies require further follow-up to determine the merit of this technology.

Uncemented Femoral Component Considerations

Femoral Stem Designs The stems of uncemented hip replacements are designed in two basic shapes, straight and curved. When straight stems are used, the femur is machined to accept the prosthesis. Hence, a straight reamer is used to machine a tight isthmus fit and a broach is used to shape a triangle proximally. The largest prosthesis that will fit tightly into the isthmus of the femur is the size used. With curved stems, the prosthesis is machined to fit the femur. Stems of this design are curved to fit the bow of the femur. Other design concepts that are presently undergoing evaluation include modular systems, in which proximal and distal fit are independently sized, and custom designs, which provide optimal fill of the femur for each patient by using a computed tomographic scan of the patient's femur to manufacture the prosthesis. Bargar[7] and Stulberg and associates[8] have reported better early results with custom devices than with off-the-shelf devices. Although modular designs may provide a custom design for each patient with an off-the-shelf device, more research into the potential fretting of metal at the interlock of the modular components is necessary. Table 1 depicts results, after a minimum of two years, of various investigators using the designs discussed above. In general, the clinical hip ratings are good or excellent for all devices. Some patients have persistent thigh pain or limp, and there is a small percentage of early femoral side failures (J. Galanté, personal communication; W.N. Capello, personal communication; L.D. Dorr, personal communication).[9–12]

Extent of Porous Coating The more extensive the porous coating (for example, if the device is fully coated rather than one-third coated), the larger the area available for bony ingrowth. However, increasing the extent of porous surfacing creates three potential problems. Most obvious is the extensive bone resorption demonstrated in animal models along the entire area of porous coating.[4] In addition to the evidence from the animal models, Engh and associates[9,13] reported more exten-

Table 1
Results of primary uncemented total hip replacement

Authors	Design	Stem Type	Hips (No.)	Average Age (yr)	Follow-up (yr)	Rating	Pain (%)	Limp (%)	Revisions (%)
Engh et al[9]	AML	Straight	307	—	Minimum 2	5.8 pain 5.6 walking	14%*	21	0
Galanté	Harris-Galanté	Straight	122	51	Minimum 4	95	25%*	4.2†	2.6‡
Capello	Omnifit	Straight	91	46	Average 4	—	12%	0†	0
Gustilo[10]	BIAS	Curved	69	43	Minimum 5	92	6%*	4†	2.9‡
Hedley et al[11]	PCA	Curved	118	51	Minimum 2	90	4%*	5	1.7‡
Dorr	APR	Curved	100	56	Minimum 2	94	16%*	14	2‡
Callaghan et al[12]	PCA	Curved	100	58	Minimum 4	92	26%*	9†	0
Capello	Omniflex	Modular	61	48	Average 22 mos.	—	12%	2	0

*Thigh.
†Moderate limp.
‡Femoral.

sive loss of femoral bone density in humans with the more extensively coated prostheses. However, coating only the proximal area can lead to secure fixation proximally with increased micromotion distally, a possible explanation for the thigh pain reported in approximately one fifth of the patients. Engh and associates[9,13] reported less thigh pain with a more extensively coated prosthesis. Other potential problems with more extensive coating include the risk of greater ion release from the additional surface area and increased difficulty of retrieval.

Material and Diameter of the Stem Theoretically, a more flexible stem (for example, one made of titanium rather than cobalt-chromium) transfers more load to the proximal femur than does a stem of higher material stiffness. However, the larger stems used to obtain a tight femoral fit have structural rigidity whether the material is stiff or not, because the stem's rigidity increases in increments to the fourth power of its diameter. Clinically, Engh and Bobyn[13] observed greater loss of femoral cortical bone (presumably because of stress shielding) when stems larger than 13.5 mm in diameter were used. Loss of proximal density occurred in two thirds of our cases during the first two years, with minimal progressive loss of density over the next three years.[12]

Uncemented Acetabular Component Considerations

Except for screw-in sockets, all reported uncemented acetabular components demonstrated stable radiographic interfaces by two to four years after implantation. The primary differences in uncemented acetabular designs today relate to the type of supplementary fixation. Spikes, lugs, and screws have all been used. Lachiewicz and associates[14] demonstrated better fixation with three screws than with lugs and spikes. However, it is imperative to appreciate the relationship of the intrapelvic vasculature to the acetabulum if screws are used. The anterior acetabulum should be avoided

to prevent injury to the external iliac vessels (superiorly) and obturator vessels (inferiorly). Surgeons are also attempting to increase cup stability by underreaming the acetabulum 1 or 2 mm (interference fit), rather than reaming to the size of the cup selected (on-line fit). Interference fits provide better initial stability, but it is not clear that this stability enhances bone ingrowth or long-term durability. Additionally, substantial underreaming can result in acetabular fractures at the time of insertion and can prevent medial wall contact.

Hybrid Total Hip Arthroplasty

Theory

As other authors have noted, excellent long-term results can be achieved with cemented total hip replacements. However, animal,[15] human retrieval,[16] and long-term follow-up studies[17-19] have demonstrated differences at the femoral and acetabular interfaces in the fixation achieved between bone and cement. Paul and Bargar[15] demonstrated in an animal model that at the acetabular interface a fibrous layer always occurred between bone and cement, whereas at the femoral bone-cement interface, cement and bone interlocked with no interposed fibrous layer. Malcolm,[16] in a retrieval analysis of Charnley's cases, demonstrated similar findings—mechanical interlock with no interposed fibrous layer between bone and cement at the femoral interface, but with a fibrous layer interposed between cement and bone at the acetabular interface in patients who were asymptomatic and had no bone-cement interface lucencies on radiographs. Wroblewski,[17] in a 15- to 21-year follow-up of the Charnley total hip prosthesis, demonstrated acetabular migration in 22.5% and complete acetabular radiolucencies in 35% of cases. In addition, the ten-year cemented results reported by Sutherland and associates[18] and Stauffer[19] demonstrated a marked increase in acetabular loosening with time and

Outline 1
Harris and Maloney hybrid results

No. of hips, 126
Average age, 63 years
Average follow-up, 3.6 years
Average hip rating, 93
Mild pain, 6%
Thigh pain, 0%
Mild limp, 6%
Revisions, 0%

leveling off of femoral loosening at five years using noncontemporary techniques. Using contemporary techniques and designs, Mulroy and Harris,[20] reported 42% acetabular loosening and only 3% femoral loosening at ten years. These data, along with previously mentioned excellent early results with uncemented acetabular components and the potential for improving cement by decreasing porosity (either by centrifugation or vacuum mixing), provide the theoretical rationale for "hybrid" total hip arthroplasty with uncemented acetabular fixation and cemented femoral fixation.

Early Results

The reported early results of hybrid total hip replacement are encouraging. The results of Harris and Maloney[21] (Outline 1) demonstrated secure acetabular and femoral interfaces with excellent hip ratings and no thigh pain at two to four years. My early (minimum follow-up, two years) results in 28 hips were similar, with no evidence of femoral or acetabular loosening and no thigh pain. In women physiologically older than 60 years and men physiologically older than 65 years, this is the form of fixation I presently use.

References

1. Poss R, Robertson DD, Walker PS, et al: Anatomic stem design for press-fit and cemented application, in Fitzgerald RH Jr (ed): *Non-Cemented Total Hip Arthroplasty.* New York, Raven Press, 1988, pp 343–363.
2. Bobyn JD, Pilliar RM, Cameron HU, et al: The optimum pore size for the fixation of porous-surfaced metal implants by the ingrowth of bone. *Clin Orthop* 1980;150:263–270.
3. Galanté J, Rostoker W, Lueck R, et al: Sintered fiber metal composites as a basis for attachment of implants to bone. *J Bone Joint Surg* 1971;53A:101–114.
4. Turner TM, Sumner DR, Urban RM, et al: A comparative study of porous coatings in a weight-bearing total hip-arthroplasty model. *J Bone Joint Surg* 1986;68A:1396–1409.
5. Cook SD, Barrack RL, Thomas KA, et al: Quantitative analysis of tissue growth into human porous total hip components. *J Arthrop* 1988;3:249–262.
6. Collier JP, Mayor MB, Townley CO, et al: Histology of retrieved porous-coated knee prosthesis. Presented at the 53rd Annual Meeting of the American Academy of Orthopaedic Surgeons, New Orleans, Feb 20–25, 1986.
7. Bargar WL: Shape the implant to the patient: A rationale for the use of custom-fit cementless total hip implants. *Clin Orthop* 1989;249:73–78.
8. Stulberg SD, Stulberg BN, Wixson RL: The rationale, design characteristics, and preliminary results of a primary custom total hip prosthesis. *Clin Orthop* 1989;249:79–96.
9. Engh CA, Bobyn JD, Glassman AH: Porous-coated hip replacement: The factors governing bone ingrowth, stress shielding, and clinical results. *J Bone Joint Surg* 1987;69B:45–55.
10. Gustilo RB, Bechtold JE, Giacchetto J, et al: Rationale, experience, and results of long-stem femoral prosthesis. *Clin Orthop* 1989;249:159–168.
11. Hedley AK, Gruen TA, Borde LS, et al: Two year followup of the PCA noncemented total hip replacement, in Brand RA (ed): *The Hip.* St. Louis, CV Mosby, 1989.
12. Callaghan JJ, Dysart SH, Savory CG: The uncemented porous-coated anatomic total hip prosthesis: Two-year results of a prospective consecutive series. *J Bone Joint Sug* 1988;70A;337–346.
13. Engh CA, Bobyn JD: The influence of stem size and extent of porous coating on femoral bone resorption after primary cementless hip arthropasty. *Clin Orthop* 1988;231:7–28.
14. Lachiewicz PF, Suh PB, Gilbert JA: In vitro initial fixation of porous-coated acetabular total hip components: A biomechanical comparative study. *J Arthrop* 1989;4:201–205.
15. Paul HA, Bargar WL: Histologic changes in the dog acetabulum following total hip replacement with current cementing techniques. *J Arthrop* 1987;2:71–76.
16. Malcolm A: Retrieval analysis of asymptomatic Charnley total hip arthroplasty. Presented at the Closed Meeting of the Hip Society, Montreal, Canada, 1988.
17. Wroblewski BM: 15–21-year results of the Charnley low-friction arthroplasty. *Clin Orthop* 1986;211:30–35.
18. Sutherland CJ, Wilde AH, Borden LS, et al: A ten-year follow-up of one hundred consecutive Müller curved-stem total hip replacement arthroplasties. *J Bone Joint Surg* 1982;64A:970–982.
19. Stauffer RN: Ten-year follow-up study of total hip replacement: With particular reference to roentgenographic loosening of the components. *J Bone Joint Surg* 1982;64A:983–990.
20. Harris WH, Mulroy RD Jr: Cemented femoral total hip replacement: Eleven-year loosening-rate of three percent. Presented at the 57th Annual Meeting of the American Academy of Orthopaedic Surgeons, New Orleans, Feb 8–13, 1990.
21. Harris WH, Maloney WJ: Hybrid total hip arthroplasty. *Clin Orthop* 1989;249:21–29.

Cemented Total Hip Replacement: Long-Term Results and Future Outlook

Eduardo A. Salvati, MD

Michael H. Huo, MD

Robert L. Buly, MD

Introduction

In the 30 years since Sir John Charnley[1] first reported his new operation, total hip arthroplasty has become one of the most frequently performed reconstructive procedures in orthopaedic surgery. Mechanical failure of prosthetic fixation remains the leading long-term problem in patients with cemented total hip replacements.

Much of the current debate over cemented versus cementless total hip replacement focuses on theoretical projections of the longevity of both types of fixation. Concern over the long-term failure of cemented total hip replacements has led many orthopaedic surgeons to favor the newer cementless prostheses (Table 1). However, a careful review of reported results in several large series of well-performed primary total hip arthroplasties, using proper designs and adequate surgical and cementing techniques, demonstrates a very good prognosis in more than 90% of these patients (Fig. 1). Analysis of these data also shows the long-term prognosis for cemented total hip prostheses to be less favorable for young, active, obese individuals, for patients with osteonecrosis (particularly if secondary to sickle cell disease, steroids, or alcoholism), and for those undergoing revision surgery, especially if they have poor bone stock.

This chapter summarizes the published long-term follow-up data in primary, cemented total hip replacements. Characteristics of stable and failed bone-cement interfaces, polyethylene and metal wear, improvements in cement preparation and delivery, acetabular metal-backing, modular heads, and improvements in the articulating surfaces, implant design, and biomaterials are discussed. Finally, it summarizes the recent results of total hip arthroplasty using newer cementing and surgical techniques.

Long-Term Results With Cemented Total Hip Replacements

Charnley and Cupic[2] were the first to report the nine- to ten-year results of low-friction arthroplasty of the hip. Among 106 hips evaluated, there were only three failures caused by mechanical loosening (two cups and one stem). Wroblewski[3] reported the clinical outcome in 32 hips from Charnley's original group of patients at 15 to 21 years after surgery. Pain relief was good to excellent in 96.5%. Radiographic evidence of loosening was seen in 29% of the femoral stems, and 22.5% of the sockets showed signs of migration. The true revision rate, however, was not specified. Older[4] reported a ten- to 12-year follow-up of 153 hips operated on by Charnley, with a revision rate of 5.25% for mechanical loosening and stem fracture.

McCoy and associates[5] reported that the rate for revision because of aseptic loosening was 4% in the first 100 Charnley total hip arthroplasties performed at The Hospital for Special Surgery. These patients were followed up for a minimum of 15 years. Survivorship analysis depicted 91% survival of the prostheses at 15 years. Acetabular components required removal or revision half as frequently as did the femoral components. The survival probability for the sockets was 96% at 15 years. With the two infections excluded, the survival rates were 93% and 98% for the stem and the socket, respectively. At final follow-up, 87.5% of the patients had good or excellent results.

Fowler and associates[6] reported a 5.5% aseptic failure rate in 426 arthroplasties using the Exeter design at a mean follow-up of 13.4 years. Clinically, there was no deterioration between the five- to ten-year review and the 11- to 16-year review in the surviving patients. Amstutz and associates[7] reported an overall aseptic revision rate of 17% for primary total hip arthroplasties using the T-28 prostheses at 12 to 14 years of follow-up. However, among patients older than 65 years of age, the revision rate was only 5.5% at 12 years.

Sarmiento and associates[8] noted progressive loosening in 8.5% of Charnley total hip replacements 11 years after surgery. The survival rate for the straight-stem design using low-modulus titanium alloy was 96.4% at 11 years. Even though the designs had been used in separate time periods, the surgeons' surgical and cementing techniques were unchanged. Clinical success was seen in more than 90% of the patients evaluated at follow-up, regardless of the prosthesis used.

Table 1
Percentages of cemented, porous, and hybrid primary total hip replacements performed at The Hospital for Special Surgery

Type	1985	1986	1987	1988	1989
Cement	97.5%	95%	81%	72%	54%
Porous	1.5%	4%	13%	13%	20%
Hybrid	1%	1%	6%	15%	26%
Total number	813	909	912	976	1,011*

*Revision excluded.

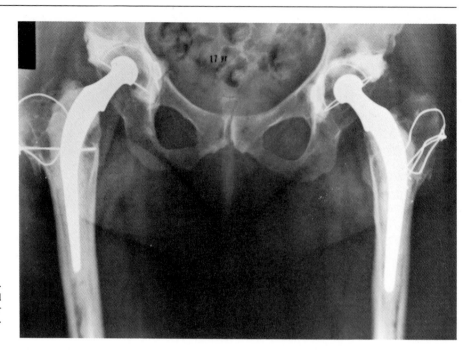

Fig. 1 Bilateral cemented Charnley total hip replacements in a 52-year-old woman with osteoarthritis, 17 years after surgery. The clinical and radiographic result is excellent.

Collis[9] reported a 7% revision rate for mechanical failure at ten years, for procedures performed by a single surgeon using a variety of prosthetic designs.

Kavanagh and associates[10] recently reported the survivorship analysis of 166 Charnley total hip replacements followed up for a minimum of 15 years. The failure rate was 12.7% at 15 years, and 80% of these patients were free of pain at follow-up. Furthermore, these authors did not find that the rate of failure increased as the length of follow-up increased. The overall rate of revision was approximately 1% per year. It should be emphasized that all these studies reflect the long-term experience with early prosthetic designs and metallurgy, implanted with early surgical and cementing techniques.

Bone-Cement Interface

The mechanically stable bone-cement interface has been well documented by Draenert[11] in an elaborate animal model. The cement mantle was surrounded by viable bone with active osteoblasts, and there was no evidence of fibrous tissue. Linder and Hansson,[12] using electron microscopy, found only a thin layer of proteoglycan between bone and cement. Calcium deposition in the collagen was evident. Ulmansky and associates[13] confirmed hydroxyapatite formation in the bone-cement interface in an animal model.

Most recently, in separate studies of human retrieval specimens after successful long-term implantation,

Malcolm[14] and Jasty and associates[15] demonstrated that on the femoral side the host bone was in intimate contact with the cement mantle, with no evidence of an intervening biologically active fibrous membrane. Long-term bone remodeling around well-fixed cemented stems forms a neocortex that encircles the prosthetic composite, providing continued stable fixation and no adverse biologic reactions to the cement, even after ten to 20 years of successful in vivo function. On the acetabular side, however, a fibrous membrane of variable thickness is usually present between cement and bone with plastic particulate debris, particularly in the periphery.

The histologic characteristics of the bone-cement interface in failed cemented total hip replacements have been well characterized.[16,17] A layer of fibrous connective tissue containing predominantly macrophages and foreign body giant cells is uniformly present. These cells may contribute to bone resorption mediated through prostaglandins and collagenase. Proliferation of these reactive cells may also create a space-occupying mass, leading to prosthetic fixation failure. Plastic, acrylic, and metal wear debris from the articular surfaces and the prosthesis-bone interface has been detected within the macrophages in the tissues surrounding loose implants.[17-20] Increasing numbers of wear particles have also been associated with increases in histiocytic response and necrosis. Additionally, wear debris may have metabolic, immunogenic, and oncogenic effects.[21,22]

Polyethylene Wear

Improved methods of fixation have increased the longevity of total hip prostheses, making wear an increasingly important issue to consider, particularly as the indications have been extended to younger patients. Much attention has been focused on the mechanical properties and wear characteristics of polyethylene that has an ultrahigh molecular weight.[2,5,23,24] Charnley and Cupic[2] estimated that polyethylene wear averaged 1.2 mm after ten years of use. Wroblewski[24] determined that the rate of socket wear was 0.19 mm per year (0.017 to 0.52 mm) in 22 acetabular components retrieved at the time of revision surgery. The radiographic estimates correlated well with actual measurements. He later reported a wear rate of 0.096 mm per year in a clinical review of patients with successful results after 15 to 21 years of follow-up.[3] The wear rate of the socket is greater in young and active patients. Body weight has not been a significant factor. More recently, McCoy and associates[5] reported an average wear rate of 1.2 mm after 15 years of use in 40 hips (average, 0.08 mm per year). The wear rate was higher in men.

Livermore and associates[25] concluded that wear correlated significantly with head size, with 32-mm heads having the greatest volumetric wear and 22-mm heads showing the most linear wear (Figs. 2 and 3). Because of this, use of an intermediate head size (26 or 28 mm) is recommended, to minimize penetration and volumetric wear.

Isaac and associates[26] examined three-body wear and the articulating prosthetic head counterface. Their studies indicate that polymethylmethacrylate and its predominant radiographic contrast medium, barium sulfate, can scratch the prosthetic head. Barium sulfate has a hardness similar to that of stainless steel. We have documented by atomic absorption spectrophotometry the consistent presence of barium in synovial fluid obtained by hip aspiration of well-fixed cemented total hip replacements (mean, 19 μg/L; range, 1 to 51 μg/L). In loose prostheses, the mean synovial barium level was 16-fold greater (mean, 302 μg/L; range, 30 to 8,856 μg/L). This observation explains in part the increased wear of plastic cups in failed total hip prostheses compared with well-fixed cups.

The homogeneous distribution of barium sulfate in the cement is essential to avoid clumps that, if liberated from the cement and entrapped among the articulating surfaces, could scratch the prosthetic head, causing increased wear on the plastic cup. Interestingly, Isaac and associates[27] recently reported minimal plastic wear in eight cases in which no cement was used for acetabular fixation. They postulated that the cement debris contributing to the wear probably came from the acetabular side of the joint, in cases in which both components were fixed by cement.

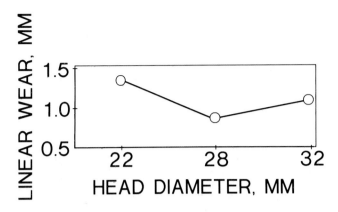

Fig. 2 Mean linear wear rate (per year) of polyethylene as a function of head diameter. (Modified with permission from Livermore J, Ilstrup D, Morrey B: Effect of femoral head size on wear of the polyethylene acetabular component. *J Bone Joint Surg* 1990;72A:518–528.)

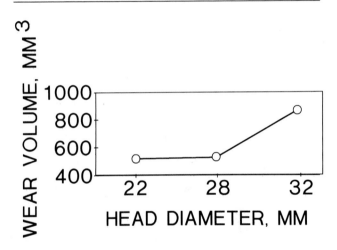

Fig. 3 Mean wear volume of polyethylene as a function of head diameter. (Modified with permission from Livermore J, Ilstrup D, Morrey B: Effect of femoral head size on wear of the polyethylene acetabular component. *J Bone Joint Surg* 1990;72A:518–528.)

As plastic wear progresses, an associated problem, in addition to the increased production of particulate debris, is the penetration of the prosthetic head into the cup. Advancing penetration decreases the hip's range of motion because of earlier impingement between the cup margin and the prosthetic neck, especially with the 22-mm heads. This impingement also increases impact stresses on the prosthetic-bone interface, challenging the fixation. A statistically significant correlation between cup wear, head penetration, and cup loosening has been demonstrated by Wroblewski.[28]

Plastic wear debris has been associated with calcar, acetabular, and endocortical bone resorption (Fig. 4).[5,16,17] Recently, Howie and associates[29] demonstrated in an animal model that injected, intra-articular polyethylene debris can produce bone resorption at the bone-cement interface.

Metallic Wear Debris

In addition to polymeric and methylmethacrylate particles, increasing evidence supports the potential synergistic role of metallic wear particles in aseptic loosening of cemented total hip prostheses.[18,20,30-32] Michel and associates[30] found significantly increased levels of cobalt, chromium, and nickel in the pericapsular tissues of 36 patients with failed cemented total hip prostheses. Pazzaglia and associates[31] found intracellular metallic debris in macrophages present in the bone-cement granulation tissue in four failed total hip reconstructions.

Agins and associates[18] reported on nine cases of failed all-titanium femoral implants (eight cemented). Excessively high tissue levels of titanium, aluminum, and vanadium were found in all cases. Most importantly, the mean duration from implantation to failure of these prostheses was only 33 months. Robinson and associates,[33] after a mean follow-up of only three years, reported a 49% incidence of bone cement femoral radiolucency, 23% subsidence, and 4.3% revision among 47 hips in which the all-titanium DF-80 femoral component was used. Martell and associates[34] reported 3.5% revision and 27.1% loosening rates, at a mean follow-up time of seven years, in 137 hips with the all-titanium SixTi-28/32 femoral component. Lombardi and associates[20] recently reported two cases of failed titanium prostheses caused by metallosis. One of these cases was entirely cementless. Buchert and associates[32] also reported two cementless implants with excessive metal release that led to early loosening. Obviously, in these three cementless implants, cement particles could not have been implicated in the failure.

We recently obtained tissues from the area surrounding the screw holes of four mechanically well-fixed cementless sockets that required reoperation (three for recurrent dislocation, one for infection). The mean titanium level, measured by atomic absorption spectrophotometry, was 4,653 μg/g of dry tissue (range, 99 to 11,900 μg/g). The high titanium levels probably resulted from fretting corrosion between the screws and the holes in the socket. Even higher levels would be expected in loose cups.

We studied 71 all-titanium femoral components retrieved at revision surgery. Fifty patients (51 hips) underwent revision of a primary total hip arthroplasty, eight patients (eight hips) underwent rerevision, and 11 patients (12 hips) underwent removal for infection. Radiographs were evaluated for endosteal scalloping, and bone loss was quantified. Retrieved components were examined for head and stem abrasion. Areas of head burnishing were mapped and quantified with a computerized digitizer.

Early postoperative radiographs in most cases showed a properly cemented prosthesis by current standards, yet the mean time to failure was only 4.5 years (Fig. 5). Prerevision radiographs showed that endosteal scalloping of the femur was present in 90% of the cases. Acetabular scalloping was seen in only 5.9%. The prosthetic femoral heads showed consistent abrasion and burnishing, with an average area of 49.5% and a range from 2% (in one hip revised at two weeks) to 96% (Fig. 6). Stem burnishing was present in 70% of the stems with aseptic loosening, and in none of the infected cases in which the stem was well fixed. Polyethylene wear averaged 0.22 mm per year (range, 0.02 to 0.60 mm per year).

The intraoperative observation of the periprosthetic tissues showed variable degrees of gray staining and, in several instances, marked black staining (Fig. 7). Histologic specimens demonstrated an intense histiocytic reaction at the site of metallic debris, which was present in 85.9% (Fig. 8). The tissue metal levels, measured by atomic absorption spectrophotometry, were approximately 100 times greater in titanium alloy failure than those observed in a comparable series of failed cemented cobalt-chromium femoral components (Table 2).

The short duration of service and degree of femoral bone loss suggest accelerated loosening and failure. The amount of polyethylene wear was higher than that reported in other series, including those with revisions. Bone scalloping and granuloma formation were probably caused by increased plastic and metal debris generated from the articulating surfaces, as evidenced by the abraded heads and the increased rate of polyethylene wear. The pattern of failure and high metallic levels in the tissues do not support the use of titanium alloys for bearing surfaces in total hip replacement. Its use for the stem is also questioned, because increased metallic debris will be liberated when it loosens, as the stem abrades with the fragmented cement. Nitrogen ion implantation has been proposed[20] to increase the hardness and wear resistance of the titanium-alloy prosthetic surface. However, the depth of the ion implantation is only 0.2 μ, at best. This thin layer can be easily scratched and eroded if acrylic fragments or metallic beads become entrapped, producing three-body wear.

High levels of titanium, aluminum, and vanadium debris liberated to the tissues can produce a toxic effect on the local bone metabolism that may contribute to the early failure. Increasing evidence supports this observation. Rae[35] demonstrated that particulate vanadium from titanium-based alloys can damage human synovial fibroblasts in cell cultures. In addition, titanium and vanadium can adversely affect hydroxyapatite nucleation and growth.[36] Intracellular debris particles

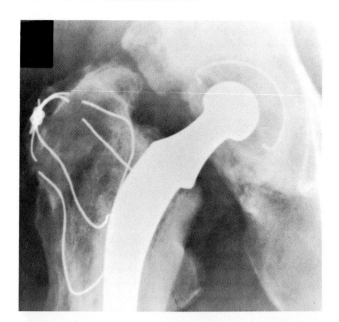

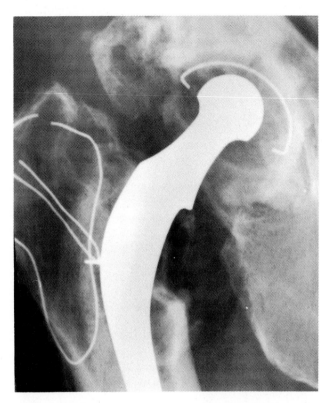

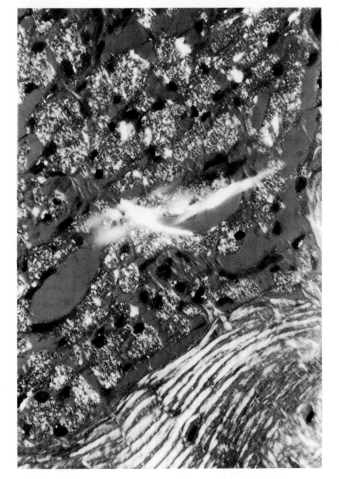

Fig. 4 A 62-year-old man with osteoarthritis. **Top left,** A radiograph taken immediately after surgery. **Top right,** Fourteen years after surgery, significant calcar resorption is seen. **Bottom left,** Photomicrograph showing intracellular polyethylene wear debris in the histiocytes. The needle-like material is larger particulate debris of polyethylene. (Reproduced with permission from Johanson NA, Callaghan JJ, Salvati EA, et al: 14-year follow-up study of a patient with massive calcar resorption: A case report. *Clin Orthop* 1986;213: 189–196.)

may lead to cell death of the macrophages, in turn contributing to the release of lysosomal enzymes. Resultant bone resorption can cause the prosthesis to fail.

On the basis of this information, we prefer to use cobalt-chromium alloy for the cemented femoral component.

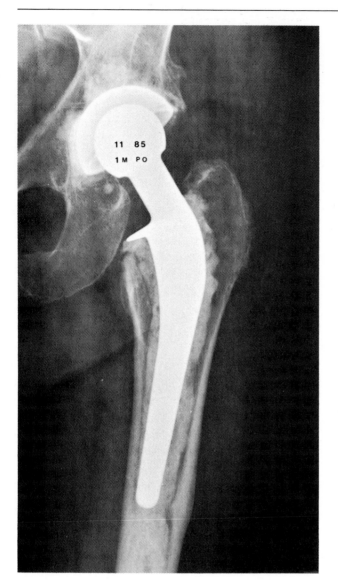
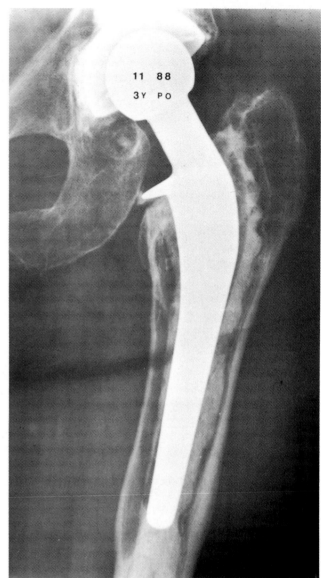

Fig. 5 **Left,** Radiograph taken one month after surgery shows an adequately cemented titanium-alloy total hip arthroplasty. **Right,** Radiograph three years after surgery shows significant osteolysis and mechanical failure.

Improved Polymethylmethacrylate Preparation and Delivery

The primary cause of aseptic loosening of cemented total hip prostheses is loss of acrylic fixation to bone,[10] which probably starts with a fatigue fracture of the cement mantle.[15] Porosity within the polymethylmethacrylate can contribute to failure under repetitive loads. Pores decrease the cross-sectional area and increase stress concentration.[37-39] Lindén[40] demonstrated that manual mixing lacked reliability, producing cement with mean porosity of nearly 30% per volume. Improvement of the mechanical properties of poly-

methylmethacrylate by centrifugation and vacuum mixing has been advocated by several investigators.[37,41,42]

Burke and associates[37] demonstrated, with Simplex P cement, that centrifugation at 4,000 rpm could significantly reduce porosity and improve the cement's mechanical properties. After centrifugation, only small pores (200 to 400 μ) were present, in comparison with much larger voids (up to 5,000 μ) seen in the manually mixed specimens. The ultimate tensile strength was improved by 24%, and the fracture strain was increased by 54%. Mean fatigue life was increased 136%. In addition, the centrifuged specimens showed more uniform testing data, reflected in the smaller standard de-

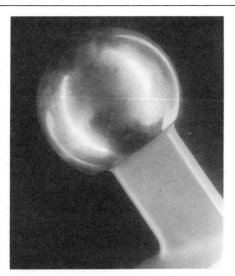

Fig. 6   Burnishing of a titanium-alloy femoral head.

viations from specimen to specimen. Continuing centrifugation for longer than 30 seconds did not improve these parameters significantly. Davies and associates[41] further demonstrated that centrifugation significantly reduced crack initiation, even in the presence of such impurities as air and bone debris.

Wixson and associates[42] demonstrated that vacuum mixing also improved polymethylmethacrylate, reducing porosity to less than 1% compared with 9.4% in manually mixed specimens. Vacuum mixing also increased compressive and tensile strength by 24% and 44%, respectively. In this study, all biomechanical parameters proved superior to those seen in centrifuged

specimens. More recently, Lindén and Gillquist[43] confirmed that vacuum mixing produced less porosity than did manual mixing or centrifugation.

In contrast, Rimnac and associates[38] reported that centrifugation had no significant effect on the fracture toughness tested by cyclic loading of four commercially available polymethylmethacrylate products. Resistance to fatigue crack propagation was not affected by centrifugation. They concluded that acrylic surface imperfections, such as those present at the sites of interdigitation between cement and cancellous bone, would constitute greater stress risers, and that these, rather than the porosity within the cement, would be more likely to lead to fatigue failure. Recently, Chin and associates[44] reported that in an in vitro total hip arthroplasty model, centrifuged cement had greater static strength than hand-mixed cement. Under low-cycle fatigue tests, however, there was no significant difference. The authors concluded that centrifugation cannot be currently justified. These in vitro testing results underline the need for a prospective, randomized clinical study to evaluate the clinical relevance of centrifugation or vacuum mixing in total hip reconstruction.

Oh and associates,[45] using in vitro experiments, demonstrated the advantage of a distal femoral plug for cement pressurization. In addition, cleansing of the bone bed with jet lavage and brushing, using hypotensive anesthesia to minimize bleeding, and retrograde injection of cement under pressure have all contributed to improvements in cement fixation in recent years.

Metal-Backed Acetabular Component

Contact between the metallic head and the polyethylene causes complex stress distributions on the sur-

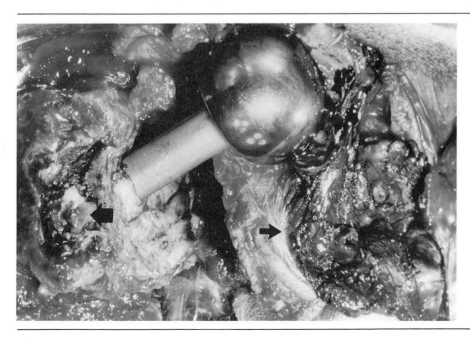

Fig. 7   Intraoperative photograph obtained at the time of revision surgery of a grossly loose titanium femoral component. Severe black staining of the tissues is observed around the burnished prosthetic head, under the osteotomized greater trochanter (right small arrow) and within the intramedullary canal (left large arrow).

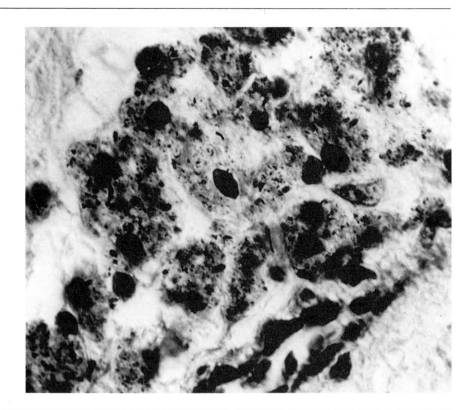

Fig. 8 Photomicrograph showing marked metallic debris (1 to 3 μ in size) within the histiocytes (hematoxylin-eosin, $\times$ 800).

face, within the plastic, and in the underlying trabecular bone. Cyclic tensile and compressive stresses acting tangentially to the surface encourage propagation of subsurface cracks, generally associated with shear stresses (Figs. 9 and 10).[23] Magnitude and direction of the contact stresses vary according to the change in conformity of the surfaces throughout the normal arc of hip motion and upon loading during gait.

Metal-backing has the theoretical advantage of distributing surface forces evenly to the underlying cement and bone.[23] Encouraging clinical results were reported initially,[46] but late fixation failure is a persistent problem. A 12.5% revision rate and a 19% migration rate of metal-backed cups were reported by Harris and Penenberg[47] after a minimum follow-up of ten years. Ritter and associates[48] reported that the incidence of radiographic loosening, migration, and revision was significantly higher in patients with 138 metal-backed acetabular components than in a similar group of patients with 100 all-plastic cups. After a mean follow-up of nearly four years, the incidence of radiolucency was 39% in the metal-backed group and only 23% in the polyethylene group (P<.001). We have compared our own experience in a consecutive series of total hip replacements, performed by Salvati. At a mean follow-up of 3.5 years of 69 metal-backed and 55 plastic cups articulating with 22-mm heads, no difference was observed in radiographic loosening (none), migration (none), and radiolucent lines.

If the outer dimension of the cup is maintained, the polyethylene must be thinner with larger head sizes and with metal-backing. When the thickness of the plastic is reduced, the contact stress increases significantly (Fig. 11).[23] A minimum thickness of 8-mm is essential for long-term success. Ritter and associates[49] reported a significantly higher incidence of cup failure among the Muller prostheses with 32-mm head components than were seen with 22-mm Charnley components. Morrey and Ilstrup[50] also reported that the cumulative acetabular revision rate was 1% for both the 22-mm and the 28-mm heads at ten years, as compared with a 3.5% revision rate for the 32-mm heads.

Modular Head

Modular heads require less inventory and allow more flexibility at surgery to adjust leg length and offset and to select head size. If acetabular revision is necessary later and the stem is well fixed, the modular head can be removed, allowing increased exposure. Three and four neck lengths are possible for 28-mm and 32-mm heads, respectively. Modular 22-mm heads offer the option of only two neck lengths because of the space limitations of the Morse taper.

The potential problems of disassociation in recurrent dislocation (Fig. 12), prosthetic neck fracture, and fretting and crevice corrosion at the Morse taper remain

Table 2
Mean tissue levels of metals

Tissue Levels (μ/g)			
Titanium Revisions (No. = 12)		Cobalt-Chromium Revisions (No. = 19)	
Titanium	4171.3	Cobalt	14.07
Aluminum	198.2	Chromium	19.95
Vanadium	100.8	Nickel	8.31
		Molybdenum	2.88
Range	110 to 24,314*		5 to 248

*The highest value was measured in a patient with very severe metallosis, as shown in Figure 7. The urine output of titanium in this patient was 20 μg/day and the serum level was 45 μg/L.

to be fully studied.[51] Another disadvantage of modular systems is the variation in offset simultaneously with changes in length. It would be preferable if these two parameters could be varied independently.

Improvements in the Articulating Surfaces

Many factors can affect the performance of ultrahigh-molecular-weight polyethylene. Enhanced or ex-tended-chain ultrahigh-molecular-weight polyethylene has been developed and its use in orthopaedic implants is currently being studied. This material has been demonstrated to have three times less creep on loading and a twofold increase in tensile and flexural strength, with no change in the coefficient of friction as compared with regular ultrahigh-molecular-weight polyethylene.

Ceramic represents a broad class of materials. The most common biostable ceramic, aluminum oxide, has excellent biocompatibility and resistance to corrosion. Ceramics produced with present technology have very hard and highly polished surfaces. The flexural fatigue and impact strengths of present ceramics are adequate for the mechanical requirements of artificial joints. Ceramic also has the lowest wetting coefficient, which makes the tribology of the ceramic-on-polyethylene articulation superior to that of the metal-on-polyethylene.[52] Ceramic-on-ceramic articulation has been discouraged because of possible impact crack initiation, especially in smaller-diameter 22-mm heads. Further development in total hip designs, applying extended-chain polyethylene articulating with a ceramic femoral head, may improve wear resistance and reduce the

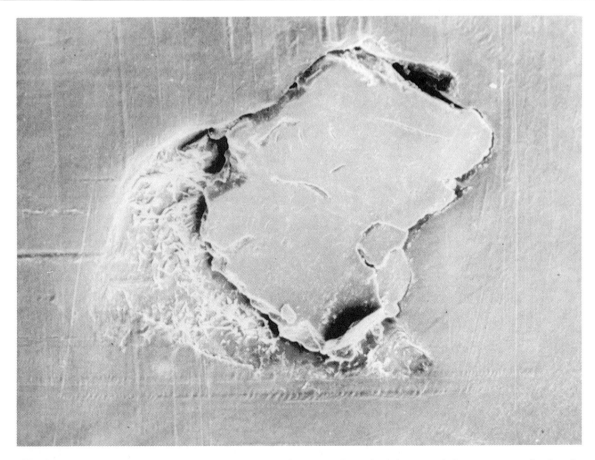

Fig. 9 Scanning electron micrograph of the articulating surface of a polyethylene acetabular component showing the development of a pit with the eventual release of a large plastic fragment.

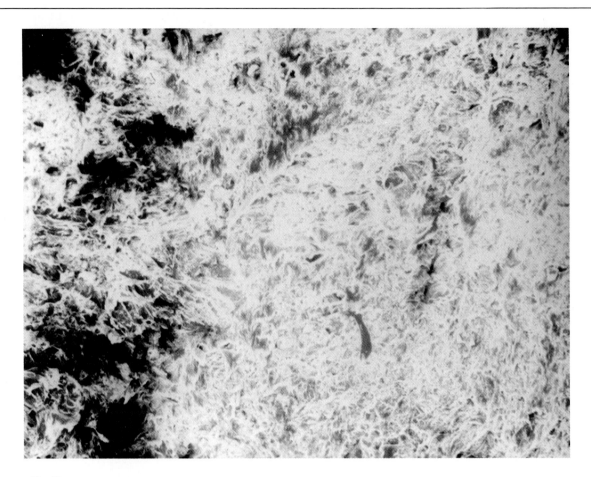

Fig. 10 Scanning electron micrograph of the outer surface of a polyethylene acetabular component showing a finely abraded surface caused by motion against bone and/or bone cement.

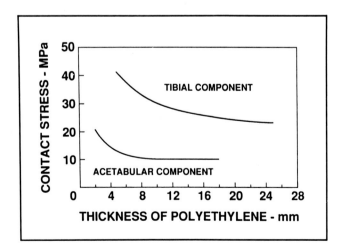

Fig. 11 Contact stress of the polyethylene component of total joint prosthesis as a function of plastic thickness. Note the significant increase in stress as the thickness decreases to less than 8 mm. Higher stresses are observed in the tibial components of the total knee prosthesis because the articulating surfaces conform less closely.

generation of particulate debris after long-term implantation.

Implant Design and Biomaterials

The primary goals in total hip arthroplasty are relief of pain and restoration of function. The long-term realization of these goals depends to a great extent on the longevity of the implants and their fixation, which means that stresses must be minimized. Stress distribution in total hip arthroplasty depends on the magnitude and direction of the loads applied, the design geometry of the prostheses, and the mechanical properties of the material used. Bone quality and surgical technique must also be considered.

Johnston and associates,[53] using finite-element analysis, proposed that an inferior and medial placement of the hip center reduces the resultant forces across the hip joint, in turn minimizing the stresses in the bone-cement interface. High compressive and tensile stresses are generated in the cement mantle when a stem that is narrow in proximal cross section is used.[54] It is, there-

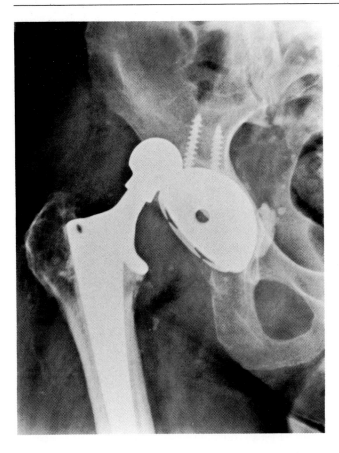 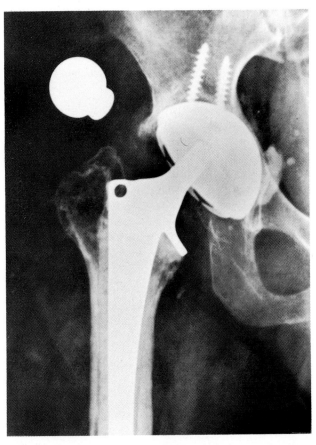

Fig. 12 **Left,** Dislocation of a modular total hip replacement. **Right,** Dissociation of the prosthetic head at the time of reduction under epidural anesthesia. (Reproduced with permission from Pellicci PM, Haas SB: Disassembly of a modular femoral component during closed reduction of the dislocated femoral component: A case report. *J Bone Joint Surg* 1990;72A;619–620.)

fore, recommended that the femoral component should have a broad medial body. Most recently, Huiskes and Boeklagen,[55] using finite-element analysis, concluded that the optimal design for cemented femoral component should include a proximal and distal taper with a belly-shaped middle region.

Oh and Harris,[56] using a well-fixed cemented femoral component, demonstrated in vitro that maximal femoral strain was recorded at the distal stem, and that there was considerable stress reduction proximally. This proximal stress reduction could lead to stress shielding and bone resorption. Larger and stiffer stems did not influence the stress distribution.

Sarmiento pioneered the concept that proximal stress shielding could be reduced by using a more flexible stem composed of titanium-based alloy. However, to do so increases the stress on the cement mantle. Sarmiento and associates[8] described 331 patients who had cemented low-modulus titanium femoral components implanted. The 11-year survival probability was 92.7%. The titanium group had a lower incidence of calcar resorption and distal hypertrophy, but a 56% incidence of bone-cement radiolucencies, compared

with 32% in a similar group of patients who received the stiffer cobalt-chromium alloy Charnley total hip prostheses. The more flexible stem increased the stresses on the cement mantle, leading to a greater incidence of radiolucencies.

Implant materials used in load-bearing components must have suitable mechanical properties to avoid fatigue failure with cyclic loading. The ultimate strength of the prosthesis depends on its material properties as well as its geometry. Fatigue failure of the femoral component is presently uncommon, with reported incidences of 0.23% to 1.15%.[57] Failures are often associated with inferior metallurgy during casting.

To minimize microporosity and crack initiation within the implant material, new manufacturing methods have been adopted. One such process, forging, employs a combination of heat and pressure to produce a superior microstructure with better mechanical properties and fatigue resistance. This process can be applied to both cobalt- and titanium-based alloys.[57,58] The forging process, however, cannot be easily adopted for prosthetic designs of complex geometry. In addition to material improvement, design geometry that minimizes sharp edges, which can act as stress concentration points, also plays an important role in maximizing longevity and minimizing fatigue failure in the implants.

Clinical Results With Newer Techniques

The advances previously discussed have improved the clinical outcome in patients undergoing cemented total hip reconstruction. Harris and McGann[59] reported an incidence of aseptic failure of only 1.7% in 117 stems using distal plug and pressurization that were followed up for at least five years. Harris and Mulroy[60] recently reported a 3% failure rate of the femoral components in the same group of patients after a minimum ten-year clinical follow-up. Yoder and associates[61] found a significantly lower incidence of failure of both components among hips with anatomic reconstruction of the hip center, after a mean follow-up of 9.1 years. Weber[62] reported a 5% incidence of symptomatic failure, seven to 11 years after implantation, in 108 total hip arthroplasties performed using cement pressurization.

Russotti and associates[63] reported an incidence of only 1.7% of definite loosening of the femoral component in 251 primary total hip arthroplasties performed using contemporary cementing techniques. The follow-up period was five years. Only one acetabular component revealed evidence of migration (0.4%). Ninety-eight percent of the patients had excellent results on clinical evaluation. Similarly, Poss and associates,[64] using the T-28 design, compared the early with the modern cementing techniques, after an equivalent mean follow-up of 4 years. Definite femoral loosening was observed in six hips with the early technique as opposed to none with the modern cementing technique. Ranawat and associates[65] demonstrated a significantly lower incidence of acetabular radiolucencies in cups inserted with contemporary cementing techniques, compared with those used in a similar group of patients whose surgery was performed with older techniques.

Conclusion

The long-term results of the earlier series of adequately performed cemented total hip arthroplasties confirm a low incidence of revision surgery and a high long-term prosthetic survival in the older population. In patients whose average age at the time of surgery was 60 years or more, the incidence of revision was less than 10% after ten years. During the past two decades, there have been significant advances in surgical and cementing techniques, prosthetic designs, and biomaterials. The benefits of these improvements are already reflected in better and longer-lasting results.

Cement is not obsolete, and it still has a clear and definitive role in the fixation of prosthetic components, particularly on the femoral side.[66] The accumulated experience of the past 30 years has outlined cement's limitations. Basic and clinical research will continue to overcome these limitations; at the same time, newer avenues of cementless fixation, such as those provided by hydroxyapatite-coated surfaces, must be explored.

Acknowledgments

Foster Betts, PhD, Director of the Trace Metal Laboratory at The Hospital for Special Surgery, provided the metallic and barium levels cited in this chapter.

Maujula Bansal, MD, Pathology Department at The Hospital for Special Surgery, provided Figure 8.

Timothy Wright, PhD, provided Figure 11.

References

1. Charnley J: Arthroplasty of the hip: A new operation. *Lancet* 1961;1:1129–1132.
2. Charnley J, Cupic Z: The nine and ten year results of the low-friction arthroplasty of the hip. *Clin Orthop* 1973;95:9–25.
3. Wroblewski BM: 15–21-year results of the Charnley low-friction arthroplasty. *Clin Orthop* 1986;211:30–35.
4. Older J: Low-friction arthroplasty of the hip: A 10–12-year follow-up study. *Clin Orthop* 1986;211:36–42.
5. McCoy TH, Salvati EA, Ranawat CS, et al: A fifteen-year follow-up study of one hundred Charnley low-friction arthroplasties. *Orthop Clin North Am* 1988;19:467–476.
6. Fowler JL, Gie GA, Lee AJ, et al: Experience with the Exeter total hip replacement since 1970. *Orthop Clin North Am* 1988; 19:477–489.
7. Amstutz HC, Yao J, Dorey FJ, et al: Survival analysis of T-28 hip arthroplasty with clinical implications. *Orthop Clin North Am* 1988;19:491–503.
8. Sarmiento A, Natarajan V, Gruen TA, et al: Radiographic performance of two different total hip cemented arthroplasties: A survivorship analysis. *Orthop Clin North Am* 1988;19:505–515.
9. Collis DK: Long-term results of an individual surgeon. *Orthop Clin North Am* 1988;19:541–550.
10. Kavanagh BF, Dewitz MA, Ilstrup DM, et al: Charnley total hip arthroplasty with cement: Fifteen-year results. *J Bone Joint Surg* 1989;71A:1496–1503.
11. Draenert K: Histomorphology of the bone-to-cement interface: Remodeling of the cortex and revascularization of the medullary canal in animal experiments. *Hip* 1981;9:71–110.
12. Linder L, Hansson HA: Ultrastructural aspects of the interface between bone and cement in man: Report of three cases. *J Bone Joint Surg* 1983;65B:646–649.
13. Ulmansky M, Bab I, Kaznelson D: Primary mineralization in the interface between bone and methyl methacrylate implants in rat mandibles: A correlative light and scanning and transmission electron microscope study. *Arch Orthop Trauma Surg* 1983;101: 171–176.
14. Malcolm A: The pathology of retrieved Charnley total hip replacements. *J Bone Joint Surg* [B], in press.
15. Jasty M, Maloney WJ, Bragdon CR, et al: Histomorphological studies of the long term skeletal responses to well fixed cemented femoral components. *J Bone Joint Surg* 1990;72A:1220.
16. Goldring SR, Schiller AL, Roelke M, et al: The synovial-like mem-

brane at the bone-cement interface in loose total hip replacements and its proposed role in bone lysis. *J Bone Joint Surg* 1983; 65A:575–584.

17. Johanson NA, Bullough PG, Wilson PD Jr, et al: The microscopic anatomy of the bone-cement interface in failed total hip arthroplasties. *Clin Orthop* 1987;218:123–135.

18. Agins HJ, Alcock NW, Bansal M, et al: Metallic wear in failed titanium-alloy total hip replacements: A histological and quantitative analysis. *J Bone Joint Surg* 1988;70A:347–356.

19. Howie DW, Vernon-Roberts B: The synovial response to intra-articular cobalt-chrome wear particles. *Clin Orthop* 1988;232: 244–254.

20. Lombardi AV Jr, Mallory TH, Vaughn BK, et al: Aseptic loosening in total hip arthroplasty secondary to osteolysis induced by wear debris from titanium-alloy modular femoral heads. *J Bone Joint Surg* 1989;71A:1337–1342.

21. Black J: Does corrosion matter? *J Bone Joint Surg* 1988;70B:517–520.

22. Brien WW, Salvati EA, Healey JH, et al: Osteogenic sarcoma in the area of a total hip replacement: A case report. *J Bone Joint Surg* 1990;72A:1097.

23. Bartel DL, Bicknell VL, Wright TM: The effect of conformity, thickness, and material on stresses in ultra-high molecular weight components for total joint replacement. *J Bone Joint Surg* 1986; 68A:1041–1051.

24. Wroblewski BM: Direction and rate of socket wear in Charnley low-friction arthroplasty. *J Bone Joint Surg* 1985;67B:757–761.

25. Livermore J, Ilstrup D, Morrey B: Effect of femoral head size on wear of the polyethylene acetabular component. *J Bone Joint Surg* 1990;72A:518–528.

26. Isaac GH, Atkinson JR, Dowson D, et al: The role of cement in the long term performance and premature failure of Charnley low friction arthroplasties. *Eng Med* 1986;15:19–22.

27. Isaac GH, Wroblewski BM, Atkinson JR, et al: Source of the cement within the Charnley hip. *J Bone Joint Surg* 1990;72B:149–150.

28. Wroblewski BM: Wear and loosening of the socket in the Charnley low-friction arthroplasty. *Orthop Clin North Am* 1988;19:627–630.

29. Howie DW, Vernon-Roberts B, Oakeshott R, et al: A rat model of resorption of bone at the cement-bone interface in the presence of polyethylene wear particles. *J Bone Joint Surg* 1988;70A: 257–263.

30. Michel R, Hofmann J, Löer F, et al: Trace element burdening of human tissues due to the corrosion of hip-joint prostheses made of cobalt-chromium alloys. *Arch Orthop Trauma Surg* 1984; 103:85–95.

31. Pazzaglia UE, Ceciliani L, Wilkinson MJ, et al: Involvement of metal particles in loosening of metal-plastic total hip prostheses. *Arch Orthop Trauma Surg* 1985;104:164–174.

32. Buchert PK, Vaughn BK, Mallory TH, et al: Excessive metal release due to loosening and fretting of sintered particles on porous-coated hip prostheses: Report of two cases. *J Bone Joint Surg* 1986;68A:606–609.

33. Robinson RP, Lovell TP, Green TM, et al: Early femoral component loosening in DF-80 total hip arthroplasty. *J Arthrop* 1989; 4:55–64.

34. Martell JM, Pierson RH, Sheinkop MB, et al: Results of primary total hip reconstruction with a cemented titanium total hip arthroplasty: Minimum four-year results. Presented at the 57th Annual Meeting of the American Academy of Orthopaedic Surgeons, New Orleans, Feb 8–13, 1990.

35. Rae T: The Toxicity of metals used in orthopaedic prostheses: An experimental study using cultured human synovial fibroblasts. *J Bone Joint Surg* 1981;63B:435–440.

36. Blumenthal NC, Cosma V: Inhibition of apatite formation by titanium and vanadium ions. *J Biomed Mater Res* 1989;12 (suppl A1):13–22.

37. Burke DW, Gates EI, Harris WH: Centrifugation as a method of improving tensile and fatigue properties of acrylic cement. *J Bone Joint Surg* 1984;66A:1265–1273.

38. Rimnac CM, Wright TM, McGill DL: The effect of centrifugation on the fracture properties of acrylic bone cements. *J Bone Joint Surg* 1986;68A:281–287.

39. Skinner HB, Murray WR: Variations in the density of bone cement after centrifugation. *Clin Orthop* 1986;207:263–269.

40. Lindén U: Porosity in manually mixed bone cement. *Clin Orthop* 1988;231:110–112.

41. Davies JP, O'Connor DO, Burke DW, et al: The effect of centrifugation on the fatigue life of bone cement in the presence of surface irregularities. *Clin Orthop* 1988;229:156–161.

42. Wixson RL, Lautenschlager EP, Novak MA: Vacuum mixing of acrylic bone cement. *J Arthrop* 1987;2:141–149.

43. Lindén U, Gillquist J: Air inclusion in bone cement: Importance of the mixing technique. *Clin Orthop* 1989;247:148–151.

44. Chin HC, Stauffer RN, Chao EYS: The effect of centrifugation on the mechanical properties of cement: An in vitro total hip arthroplasty model. *J Bone Joint Surg* 1990;72A:363.

45. Oh I, Carlson CE, Tomford WW, et al: Improved fixation of the femoral component after total hip replacement using a methacrylate intramedullary plug. *J Bone Joint Surg* 1978;60A:608–613.

46. Harris WH, White RE Jr: Socket fixation using a metal-backed acetabular component for total hip replacement: A minimum five-year follow-up. *J Bone Joint Surg* 1982;64A:745–748.

47. Harris WH, Penenberg BL: Further follow-up on socket fixation using a metal-backed acetabular component for total hip replacement: A minimum ten-year follow-up study. *J Bone Joint Surg* 1987;69A:1140–1143.

48. Ritter MA, Keating EM, Faris·PM, et al: Metal-backed acetabular components of total hip replacement: Does it reduce loosening? Presented at the 57th Annual Meeting of the American Academy of Orthopaedic Surgeons, New Orleans, Feb 8–13, 1990.

49. Ritter MA, Stringer EA, Littrell DA, et al: Correlation of prosthetic femoral head size and/or design with longevity of total hip arthroplasty. *Clin Orthop* 1983;176:252–257.

50. Morrey BF, Ilstrup D: Size of the femoral head and acetabular revision in total hip-replacement arthroplasty. *J Bone Joint Surg* 1989;71A:50–55.

51. Pellicci PM, Haas SB: Disassembly of a modular femoral component during closed reduction of the dislocated femoral component: A case report. *J Bone Joint Surg* 1990;72A:619–620.

52. Zichner L: In-vivo changes of the dimension of polyethylene acetabuli in total hip replacements. Presented at the Society for Biomaterials Symposium on the Retrieval and Analysis of Surgical Implants and Biomaterials, 1988.

53. Johnston RC, Brand RA, Crowninshield RD: Reconstruction of the hip: A mathematical approach to determine optimum geometric relationships. *J Bone Joint Surg* 1979;61A:639–652.

54. Crowninshield RD, Brand RA, Johnston RC, et al: The effect of femoral stem cross-sectional geometry on cement stresses in total hip reconstruction. *Clin Orthop* 1980;146:71–77.

55. Huiskes R, Boeklagen R: Mathematical shape optimization of hip prosthesis design. *J Biomech* 1989;22:793–804.

56. Oh I, Harris WH: Proximal strain distribution in the loaded femur: An in vitro comparison of the distributions in the intact femur and after insertion of different hip-replacement femoral components. *J Bone Joint Surg* 1978;60A:75–85.

57. Galanté JO: Causes of fractures of the femoral component in total hip replacement. *J Bone Joint Surg* 1980;62A:670–673.

58. Wright TM, Burnstein AH: Musculoskeletal biomechanics, in Evarts CM (ed): *Surgery of the Musculoskeletal System*, ed 2. New York, Churchill Livingstone, 1990, pp 231–274.

59. Harris WH, McGann WA: Loosening of the femoral component after use of the medullary-plug cementing technique: Follow-up note with a minimum five-year follow-up. *J Bone Joint Surg* 1986; 68A:1064–1066.

60. Harris WH, Mulroy RD Jr: Cemented femoral total hip replacement: Eleven-year loosening rate of three percent. Presented at the 57th Annual Meeting of the American Academy of Orthopaedic Surgeons, New Orleans, Feb 8–13, 1990.

61. Yoder SA, Brand RA, Pedersen DR, et al: Total hip acetabular component position affects component loosening rates. *Clin Orthop* 1988;228:79–87.

62. Weber BG: Pressurized cement fixation in total hip arthroplasty. *Clin Orthop* 1988;232:87–95.

63. Russotti GM, Coventry MB, Stauffer RN: Cemented total hip arthroplasty with contemporary techniques: A five-year minimum follow-up study. *Clin Orthop* 1988;235:141–147.

64. Poss R, Brick GW, Wright RJ, et al: The effects of modern cementing techniques on the longevity of total hip arthroplasty. *Orthop Clin North Am* 1988;19:591–598.

65. Ranawat CS, Rawlins BA, Harju VT: Effect of modern cement technique on acetabular fixation total hip arthroplasty: A retrospective study in matched pairs. *Orthop Clin North Am* 1988;19:599–603.

66. Salvati EA: Preface. Is cement obsolete? *Orthop Clin North Am* 1988;19:xv.

Cemented Versus Cementless Hip Fixation

M.A.R. Freeman, MD, FRCS

Robert E. Tennant, MD

Introduction

This chapter considers the use of cemented versus cementless fixation from the mechanical and biologic standpoints. The advantages and possible risks involved in using cement or porous surfaces are outlined on the basis of data gleaned from a number of scientific studies. The properties of hydroxyapatite are mentioned only in passing.

Mechanical Considerations

Mechanically, all prostheses should be designed so as to be intrinsically stable when inserted without cement. In other words, they should be inserted so as to minimize the stresses (in particular in tension and in shear) on the bone at the interface. Once the design of the implant and the surgical procedures have achieved this stability, the following questions arise: Is the resultant fixation adequate in clinical practice, that is to say, is the patient free of symptoms? Does the prosthesis migrate either not at all or at an acceptably slow rate over the years? If the answers to these questions are in the affirmative, it might be thought that no further supplementary fixation is required. The advantages of such a press-fit are ease of insertion and ease of extraction, should that be necessary. If, on the other hand, the optimized press-fit does not provide an appropriately stable implant, the surgeon must attempt to increase the compressive, shear, and tensile strength at the interface by using some form of supplementary fixation. Today three varieties of supplementation are available: The use of polymethylmethacrylate (PMMA) as a cementing agent, the use of porous surfaces in an attempt to gain bone ingrowth into a cementless surface, and the use of hydroxyapatite applied to surfaces having various contours. In this paper, attention is directed particularly toward the use of PMMA and porous surfaces. Although hydroxyapatite is promising, its use is still in the experimental stage, and there are not yet adequate clinical series on which to base an opinion as to its efficacy. Materials other than PMMA have been used as cementing agents, but, once again, there is insufficient experience to make informed comment possible.

Mechanically, cement and the use of a porous surface both rely on the same mechanism to increase tensile and shear strength, namely, the acquisition of microinterlock at the bone-implant interface. Hydroxyapatite may act by encouraging bone to grow into recesses on a prosthesis. This bone ingrowth, which ranges from a fraction of a millimeter up to 2 or 3 mm, also acts to encourage bone-prosthesis interlock. In addition, bone adheres to hydroxyapatite, and this adherence provides shear and tensile strength in the absence of interlock. Insofar as they increase the bone-prosthesis contact area, any of the three might reduce compressive interface stresses.

When cement was first introduced by Charnley, it was not used in a semiliquid condition, and no special effort was made to pressurize it into a bone surface that had been dried and in which the intertrabecular spaces had been opened.[1] The work of Halawa and associates,[2] Lee and associates,[3] and Oh and associates[4] emphasized that, used in this way, cement produces an imperfect interlock, because it is difficult, if not impossible, to drive cement into intertrabecular spaces if the cavity is not closed, if the the cement is viscous, and if the bone surfaces are not cleaned of fat and blood. In contrast, if the bone surface is dried and the marrow tissue between the trabeculae at the cut surface is removed by a water jet or a scrubbing brush, any cement with a low viscosity can easily be pressurized so as to flow into trabecular bone. In the highly convoluted interface so produced, the cement penetrates between the trabeculae and interlocks with the bone.

The reliability with which such interlock can be produced depends to some extent on surgical technique and to some extent on the particular interface under consideration. For example, interlock is much easier to achieve below a tourniquet at the knee than it is at the acetabulum. Despite these difficulties, it is usually possible with modern techniques to produce interlock over the whole of the cement surface, certainly at all three components of the knee and at the proximal femur. A number of studies have now demonstrated that this interlock can be maintained with direct bone-PMMA contact over many years, and this subject is discussed in greater detail below.

In contrast to the relatively reliable interlock that can be achieved at a cement interface, the ingrowth of bone into porous surfaces has proved less easy to achieve. This is hardly surprising when one remembers that cement interlock is directly under the surgeon's control and depends on certain principles of physics. In contrast, the growth of bone into a porous surface is not entirely under the surgeon's control and is a biologic process analogous to fracture healing. Most porous surfaces have a pore size on the order of 0.25 to 0.5 mm in diameter, and micromotion of this magnitude occurring at the interface immediately after implantation can prevent the ingrowth of any tissue into the pores and, in particular, can prevent the ingrowth of bone. Thus it would seem, paradoxically, that a prerequisite for bone ingrowth is almost perfect fixation of the implant in the first place. If that has been achieved, one might ask what the ingrowth is intended to accomplish.

Published estimates of the amount of bone present in porous surfaces of various components vary widely. The retrieval studies of Cook and associates[5] at the proximal femur and the acetabulum show that one third of components, in particular at the acetabulum, exhibit no bone ingrowth at all and that, in general, the maximum ingrowth covers only about 10% of the interface surface. It should be remembered that in any porous surface only about 30% of the surface is actually pore (the remainder being metal), and that in a pore that has bone ingrowth, only about 30% of the ingrown tissue is actually bone, the remainder being soft tissue. Therefore, in an interface in which 10% of the available pore volume has bone ingrowth, only about 1% (that is, 10% × 30% × 30%) of the total surface is actually occupied by bone. The remaining 99% has no bone in it whatsoever. Furthermore, in many components the porous surface does not cover the whole implant, but involves only limited sections, such as, for example, those on the front and back of the femoral neck. This means that the total amount of bone that has entered such an implant when ingrowth has occurred is so small as to raise questions as to whether or not it will function effectively over time.

Notwithstanding the above, it has been demonstrated that bone will grow into a porous-coated femoral component and that, after ingrowth, the component can remain clinically stable over time.[6] However, in Engh and Bobyn's[6] view, only if the implant is fully porous-coated can this be achieved with reliability sufficient to give clinical results comparable to those produced by cement. If the implant is fully porous-coated, however, two dangers present themselves: extraction of the implant may be difficult[7] and, because the load is transferred to the most distal point of bone ingrowth, proximal stress protection may lead to proximal bone loss.[6] Furthermore, stress analysis using the finite-element method at the acetabulum suggests that partial ingrowth can produce high peak stresses where the bone has grown in and low stresses elsewhere, rather than the more even distribution of stress that probably occurs in the normal hip.[8]

In summary, from the mechanical point of view it appears that microinterlock can be obtained more reliably by the use of PMMA cement than it can by bone growth into a porous surface. Cement may someday be supplanted as a preferred material by hydroxyapatite,

which appears to be capable of inducing bone to grow into defects in a prosthetic surface. Interestingly, hydroxyapatite has this effect when used to coat defects as much as several millimeters in depth and width. Thus, a macrotextured surface coated with hydroxyapatite may be capable of providing interlock as reliably as does cement and more reliably than is achieved with a porous-coated surface. If this is true, there may be no need in the future to use a microporous surface, thus avoiding the disadvantages outlined above. Porous-coated surfaces are not easy to coat with hydroxyapatite, because the hydroxyapatite can block the pores. Also, adequate coating cannot be achieved in the deeper layers, because plasma spraying is a "line-of-sight" process.

The Long-Term Loss of Microinterlock

Microinterlock, once achieved, can subsequently be lost for a number of reasons. PMMA as used clinically is relatively weak in fatigue. The fatigue strength can be increased by centrifuging, which eliminates porosities,[9] but even then the weakness of PMMA in tensile fatigue is such as to raise the possibility that in the long term the material may fracture. Unfortunately, it is equally possible for a porous coating to fail in fatigue. This is true both of pure titanium, which is inherently weak in fatigue, and of (at least early) sintered cobalt-chromium porous surfaces, in which the point of sintering was also weak. Hydroxyapatite is weak in fatigue both in tension and in shear and is biodegradable. Thus, none of the available interlocking materials can be relied on with certainty in the long term. Perhaps the most reliable configuration would be bone ingrowth into a macrotextured hydroxyapatite-covered surface in which the hydroxyapatite was not relied on as an adhesive.

Not only can microinterlock be lost because of failure of the interlocking implant material, the bone itself can fail. Two mechanisms can cause this failure. One of these is stress protection, in which, ingrowth having been achieved remotely from the joint with a rigid component, the bone between the point of ingrowth and the articular surface is offloaded and becomes porotic. This porosis may lead to critical weakening of the bone at the interface. The second possible cause of bone failure occurs when polyethylene debris generated from the articular surface moves into the area between the implant and the bone, starting from the juxtasynovial region of the interface. As this happens, granulation tissue, evoked by the debris, induces osteolysis at the interface, loosening the implant from the bone. These mechanisms apply to prostheses fixed both with and without PMMA. In favor of cement, it may be argued that, because part of the implant is made of a relatively low-modulus acrylic, the degree of stress protection at such interfaces is typically less than with all-metal prostheses. Furthermore, the use of PMMA may obstruct the access of high-density polyethylene debris to the interface. On the other hand, once an acrylic interface loosens, acrylic debris may add its osteolysis-inducing properties to those of high-density polyethylene.

In summary, it is not clear that there is a striking mechanical advantage for cementless over cemented supplementary fixation. Cement fixation can achieve a more reliable bone interlock initially, and the mechanisms that lead to the loss of interlock apply no more and perhaps less in cemented fixation.

Biologic Considerations

The argument here hinges on whether PMMA is more or less bioinert than metals, either in the form of a block or as particles or solutes. For the purposes of this discussion, the alloys to be considered are cobalt-chromium (CoCr) and titanium-aluminum-vanadium (TiAlV). Stainless steel is practically never used in direct contact with bone, although in fact there is little evidence that it has any marked disadvantage compared with the other two alloys. In view of the disadvantages associated with CoCr and TiAlV interfaces against bone, some of which will be discussed below, there is increasing interest in using these materials coated with other chemicals, such as hydroxyapatite or titanium nitride. In the future, these coating techniques may minimize some of the disadvantages discussed here, but at present they are experimental.

Materials in the Form of a Block

With regard to the long-term response of human bone to the presence of PMMA, two critical facts are now clear. These are, first, that there are quiescent macrophages at the well-fixed PMMA-bone interface and, second, that living bone is regularly seen in direct contact with PMMA at such interfaces (at least at the proximal femur).[10]

Charnley[1] drew attention to the fact that histiocytes were present at the interface with cement in well-fixed implants, and he commented that "histiocytes (macrophages and foreign body giant cells) represent a tissue reaction which no implant surgeon can lightly dismiss." Freeman and associates[11] reported that at some tibial interfaces composed partly of metal and partly of PMMA, a radiolucent line was seen beneath the cement but not around the metallic portions of the interface. Histologically, the radiolucent line contained fibrous tissue with macrophages and osteoclastic resorption cavities at the bone interface, whereas the metallic portion of the interface demonstrated bone-to-metal contact. These authors suggested that this difference represented a specific, adverse response of bone to PMMA. Subsequent work suggests that this conclusion may not have been justified by the observations. The PMMA

portion of the interface was accessible to the synovial cavity, whereas the metallic portion, although theoretically accessible, was less so. Further histologic study of interfaces similar to those studied by Freeman and associates shows that they contain numerous particles of high-density polyethylene debris, and that it is particularly in relation to these that the macrophage reaction occurs (Freeman and Revell, unpublished data). Thus, the observed difference between the metallic and PMMA interfaces may have been caused as much by their relative accessibility to high-density polyethylene debris as by any specific response to PMMA as against metal. The relatively benign nature of PMMA has been emphasized by Linder and Hansson,[10] who, although they reported the presence of (inactive) macrophages at the interface, demonstrated that cement could be seen to be in direct contact with living bone in the human femur at the ultramicroscopic level. Similar findings have been reported by A. Malcolm (personal communication), who studied long-term (average, ten years) specimens implanted by Charnley. Although Linder and Hansson[10] reported inactive macrophages and bone contact at the femoral interface in humans, they also reported that active macrophages were present in the same hips at the acetabulum and that all acetabular specimens displayed a fibrous interface. These findings raise the question, also suggested by the difference in clinical outcome between cement fixation at the acetabulum and at the femur, as to whether it is possible to generalize about all interfaces fixed with PMMA or whether comments can only be made specifically about a particular interface, such as the femur, and about a particular design of prosthesis.

Histologically, human bone has been observed in direct contact with both CoCr[12] and pure titanium in block form.[13] Contact with TiAlV is said to occur but is not so well documented.[14] Whether there is a preference for either of the alloys from the point of view of their acceptability to bone is unclear. However, it has been suggested that pure titanium, which presents a surface of titanium oxide to bone, can form a chemical link with bone,[15] a process that has been neither sought nor described for CoCr.

It may be concluded that in block form there is relatively little difference between the bone response to PMMA on the one hand and to CoCr or TiAlV on the other. All three of these materials have been seen in direct contact with bone in humans. The ease with which a direct bone-implant material contact is formed may depend on the interface under study. Contact with any of these materials can be lost if high-density polyethylene debris gains access to the interface.

Materials in the Form of Particulate Debris

In general, the tissue response to a particular substance depends not only on its chemistry but also on its surface topography, size, and shape. Thus, a rough surface and a polished surface can evoke different responses, and particulate debris can evoke a response different from that evoked by the same material implanted as a block. PMMA as a block is capable of long-term direct contact with bone. In contrast, particulate PMMA debris evokes a macrophage response. Depending on the size of the particles and their number, macrophages may fuse to form giant cells. The ingested PMMA, which cannot be degraded by lysozymal enzymes, therefore accumulates in the cell. Eventually the saturated cell dies, and the ultimate tissue response becomes one of necrosis and chronic inflammation. Bone in the vicinity undergoes osteolysis. Thus, although PMMA in solid form is not perfectly bioinert, in that quiescent macrophages can be seen on its surface, it is acceptably so. In contrast, particulate PMMA evokes a chronic inflammatory response that eventually leads to osteolysis and implant loosening. This process may be exacerbated by cyclical pressure changes and micromotion and becomes worse the longer it is neglected. It is the end stage of this process that gave rise to the term "cement disease." In our view, this term is misleading because the disease is not specifically a disease of cement, it is a disease of debris. It was observed by Charnley[16] in connection with Teflon, and it can be observed today by any implant surgeon in connection with high-density polyethylene. Thus, the problems attributed specifically to cement, which led in part to the attempt to achieve cementless fixation, are in reality a nonspecific response to particulate debris, a response exacerbated by surgical neglect.

Because CoCr is harder than PMMA, it is less readily abraded when used as an implant. Significant quantities of CoCr debris are produced clinically only when CoCr is articulated with itself, as in the all-metal McKee-Ferrar prosthesis or in certain of the early hinged-knee prostheses. CoCr debris generated in this way evokes the same macrophage response that particulate PMMA does. In addition, skin sensitivity to cobalt has been reported with such implants.[17]

In contrast to CoCr, TiAlV is easily abraded. In this respect, the corrosion resistance of TiAlV needs to be carefully qualified. TiAlV resists corrosion because, in a physiologic environment, a layer of titanium oxide forms on the surface of the alloy. Because this oxide is chemically inert, no further chemical reaction, that is, no further corrosion, takes place once it has formed. Unfortunately, the oxide layer is only weakly adherent to the underlying alloy. Thus, if the implant is subjected to fretting or wear while it is in a corrosive environment, the oxide layer will be rubbed off, will reform, and will once again be rubbed off. As a consequence, the tissues adjacent to a TiAlV component subjected to fretting in an environment of biologic fluids can become blackened by accumulated titanium particles. It is now known that these particles evoke a macrophage and giant cell response and that, as happens with particles of PMMA, this can lead to osteolysis.[18,19] Recent work, as yet unconfirmed, suggests that, in addition, T-helper lymphocytes may be found in titanium-containing tissue, suggesting some form of immune response.[20]

Thus, in debris form, all three implant materials—PMMA, CoCr, and TiAlV—are bioactive. The response to all three takes the form of a macrophage reaction that can lead to osteolysis. There appears to be little difference between PMMA and TiAlV in terms of abradability. Because it is harder, CoCr, unless rubbed against itself, is less likely to produce debris than are PMMA or TiAlV.

Materials in the Form of Solutes

Abrasion and corrosion not only can produce particulate debris, they can also produce biologically active solutes. In the case of PMMA, the only possible solutes are unpolymerized methylmethacrylate and small quantities of certain additives. To date no evidence has been obtained for the release of such solutes. Acute methylmethacrylate toxicity is outside the scope of this paper.

Unfortunately, the biologic effects of CoCr in solution may be of significance, because hexavalent chromium is known to be a carcinogen in humans.[21] Chromium in solution may induce tumors locally or remotely, and studies supporting the possibility that both can occur clinically are now in the literature.[22,23] Nonetheless, it should be recognized that CoCr has been used for many years in such forms as endoprostheses and onlay plates and in cup arthroplasties with no substantial risk of malignancy having been demonstrated. The risk from a smooth block of the material may therefore be very slight. Unfortunately, it is not safe to extrapolate from this relatively benign clinical experience to what might be expected if expanded surfaces of CoCr were to be implanted, especially into younger individuals. Porous CoCr surfaces increase the exposed surface area of the alloy per unit area of prosthetic surface by a factor of about ten. The rate of release of solutes from such surfaces is proportional to the surface area and may be increased further if the surface is stressed mechanically.[24] Thus porous-surfaced implants may be releasing chromium ten times more rapidly than their smooth-surfaced predecessors. This might be likened to a person smoking 100 cigarettes a day rather than ten. Furthermore, porous-surfaced implants are used particularly for younger individuals, in whom the smooth-surfaced implants (such as endoprostheses for femoral neck fractures and cup arthroplasties) are rarely employed. This situation might be compared with the effect of starting to smoke 100 cigarettes at the age of 20 years compared with ten cigarettes at the age of 60 years.

Titanium in solution appears to be biologically inert in the long term.[25] Aluminum, one of the constituents of TiAlV, has been implicated in the pathogenesis of

Alzheimer's disease and in osteoporosis following dialysis.[26,27] In this connection, it should be appreciated that the normal intestinal mucosa, which prevents the absorption of much of the aluminum in food, is bypassed when an implant containing aluminum is used. Vanadium is cytotoxic but no adverse effects attributable to this metal have been demonstrated clinically.

Summary

These considerations do not appear to prove that either CoCr or TiAlV is certain to provide an implant surface preferable to that provided by PMMA from either the mechanical or the biologic point of view. It does not follow from this that we should abandon the goal of clinically successful cementless fixation, but it does follow that to dismiss cement as being in some way dangerous or as having failed is not justified by the facts as they are known today.

References

1. Charnley J: Anchorage of the femoral head prosthesis to the shaft of the femur. *J Bone Joint Surg* 1960;42B:28–30.
2. Halawa M, Lee AJ, Ling RS, et al: The shear strength of trabecular bone from the femur, and some factors affecting the shear strength of the cement-bone interface. *Arch Orthop Trauma Surg* 1978;92:19–30.
3. Lee AJ, Ling RS, Vangala SS: Some clinically relevant variables affecting the mechanical behaviour of bone cement. *Arch Orthop Trauma Surg* 1978;92:1–18.
4. Oh I, Carlson CE, Tomford WW, et al: Improved fixation of the femoral component after total hip replacement using a methacrylate intramedullary plug. *J Bone Joint Surg* 1978;60A:608–613.
5. Cook SD, Thomas KA, Haddad RJ Jr: Histologic analysis of retrieved human porous-coated total joint components. *Clin Orthop* 1988;234:90–101.
6. Engh CA, Bobyn JD: *Biological Fixation in Total Hip Arthroplasty.* Thorofare, Slack, 1985.
7. Lord G, Marotte JH, Blanchard JP, et al: Cementless madreporic and polarized total hip prostheses: A ten year review of 2688 cases. *Fr J Orthop Surg* 1988;2:82–92.
8. Rapperport DJ, Carter DR, Schurman DJ: Contact finite element stress analysis of porous ingrowth acetabular cup implantation, ingrowth, and loosening. *J Orthop Res* 1987;5:548–561.
9. Burke DW, Gates EI, Harris WH: Centrifugation as a method of improving tensile and fatigue properties of acrylic bone cement. *J Bone Joint Surg* 1984;66A:1265–1273.
10. Linder L, Hansson HA: Ultrastructural aspects of the interface between bone and cement in man: Report of three cases. *J Bone Joint Surg* 1983;65B:646–649.
11. Freeman MAR, Bradley GW, Revell PA: Observations upon the interface between bone and polymethylmethacrylate cement. *J Bone Joint Surg* 1982;64B:489–493.
12. Engh CA, Bobyn JD, Glassman AH: Porous-coated hip replacement: The factors governing bone ingrowth, stress shielding, and clinical results. *J Bone Joint Surg* 1987;69B:45–55.
13. Linder L, Carlsson A, Marsal L, et al: Clinical aspects of osseointegration in joint replacement: A histological study of titanium implants. *J Bone Joint Surg* 1988;70B:550–555.
14. Lintner F, Zweymüller K, Brand G: Tissue reactions to titanium endoprostheses: Autopsy studies in four cases. *J Arthroplasty* 1988;1:183–195.
15. Albrektsson T, Brånemark PI, Hansson HA, et al: Osseointegrated titanium implants: Requirements for ensuring a long-lasting, direct bone-to-implant anchorage in man. *Acta Orthop Scand* 1981;52:155–170.
16. Charnley J: *Low Friction Arthroplasty of the Hip: Theory and Practice.* Berlin, Springer-Verlag, 1979, p 34.
17. Evans EM, Freeman MAR, Miller AJ, et al: Metal sensitivity as a cause of bone necrosis and loosening of the prosthesis in total joint replacement. *J Bone Joint Surg* 1974;56B:626–642.
18. Agins HJ, Alcock NW, Bansal M, et al: Metallic wear in failed titanium-alloy total hip replacements: Histological and quantitative analysis. *J Bone Joint Surg* 1988;70A:347–356.
19. Lombardi AV Jr, Mallory TH, Vaughn BK, et al: Aseptic loosening in total hip arthroplasty secondary to osteolysis induced by wear debris from titanium-alloy modular femoral heads. *J Bone Joint Surg* 1989;71A:1337–1342.
20. Lalor PA, Revell PA, Railton GT, et al: Implant failure and contrast hypersensitivity to titanium (Ti): A report of five cases. *J Bone Joint Surg* 1990, in press.
21. Black J: Does corrosion matter? *J Bone Joint Surg* 1988;70B:517-520.
22. Bagó-Granell J, Aguirre-Canyadell M, Nardi J, et al: Malignant fibrous histiocytoma of bone at the site of a total hip arthroplasty: A case report. *J Bone Joint Surg* 1984;66B:38–40.
23. Gillespie WJ, Frampton CM, Henderson RJ, et al: The incidence of cancer following total hip replacement. *J Bone Joint Surg* 1988;70B:539–542.
24. Bundy KJ, Luedemann R, Cooper K: Factors affecting metal ion release from porous implant materials. *Trans Orthop Res Soc* 1986;11:101.
25. Woodman JL, Jacobs JJ, Galante JO, et al: Metal ion release from titanium-based prosthetic segmental replacements of long bones in baboons: A long-term study. *J Orthop Res* 1984;1:421–430.
26. Perl DP, Brody AR: Alzheimer's disease: X-ray spectrometric evidence of aluminum accumulation in neurofibrillary tangle-bearing neurons. *Science* 1980;208:297–299.
27. Ward MK, Ellis HA, Feest TG, et al: Osteomalacic dialysis osteodystrophy: Evidence for a water-borne aetiological agent, probably aluminium. *Lancet* 1978;1:841–845.

Why Cement Is Weak and How It Can Be Strengthened

William H. Harris, MD

Jeffrey P. Davies, MS

Introduction

The critical issue in assessing the mechanical properties of bone cement is its fatigue strength. In total joint arthroplasty bone cement is required to undergo an average of 1 million loading cycles a year. Thus, within the cement itself, the dominant mode of failure is fatigue failure. This is particularly important because until recently most of the testing of cement has been static testing, not fatigue testing. The data from static testing are not helpful. Only fatigue testing is useful in assessing the mechanical strength of bone cement as it is used clinically. Not only is static testing inappropriate, we have now shown that static testing can be misleading.[1]

Fatigue Testing

There are a variety of different conditions used in fatigue testing. The conditions we have adopted involve fully reversed, tension-compression loading at a frequency of 2 Hz with a maximum stress range of ± 15 MPa with the specimen submerged in a saline bath at 37 C.[1-5]

From our extensive testing of Simplex P, Palacos R, LVC, Zimmer Regular, and CMW cements, it is clear that not all cements have the same fatigue strength. They differ in fatigue strength because of intrinsic differences in such variables as polymer bead size, the addition of copolymers, and the presence of radiopacifiers.[2-4]

In our fatigue testing system, the average fatigue lives of bone cements as supplied by the manufacturer are Simplex P, 15,147 cycles to failure; Palacos R, 11,500 cycles; LVC, 2,575 cycles; Zimmer Regular, 879 cycles; and CMW, 7,043 cycles. Thus, as these cements are commonly used, Simplex P is significantly stronger than CMW, LVC, and Zimmer Regular and has the same fatigue strength as Palacos R.

The next major determinant of fatigue strength is porosity. The porosity of the cements vary. For example, the porosity of Zimmer Regular is 12.3%, that of Palacos R is 9.7%, that of Simplex P is 9.4%, and that of LVC is 5.1%.

It is clear that porosity is not the sole determinant of fatigue strength. For example, uncentrifuged LVC has a porosity of 5.1% and a mean fatigue life of only 2,575 cycles. Uncentrifuged Simplex P has a larger porosity, 9.4%, but its mean fatigue life is 15,147 cycles. However, when each cement is compared with itself, reduction of porosity increases the fatigue strength. For example, for both LVC and for Simplex P, reducing the porosity increases the fatigue life. Optimal porosity reduction for Simplex P reduces its porosity to 4.3% and increases its mean fatigue life to 71,479 cycles.[2] Palacos, however, is so viscous that its porosity cannot be reduced effectively.

Porosity Reduction

Examination of retrieved specimens from revision surgery and of specimens studied in the laboratory indicates that the initiation of fatigue failure within cement itself is almost always associated with a pore. Therefore, porosity reduction is essential.

There are two clinically useful methods of doing this, centrifugation and vacuum mixing. It should be pointed out, however, that chilling the monomer substantially reduces the fatigue strength of the cement.[2] It does so because it increases the porosity. Thus, chilling the monomer, a widely used technique, particularly in revision surgery, carries with it the adverse effect of making the cement weaker. Therefore, it becomes even more important to carry out porosity reduction if the cement being used has been made with chilled monomer.

The optimum porosity reduction involves either centrifugation or vacuum mixing, but under specific conditions. We examined the IEC clinical centrifuge, the Zimmer centrifuge, and the J & J centrifuge, which is activated with a power tool. The Zimmer centrifuge was clearly the most effective.[2]

Of all of the combinations of different cements and porosity reduction techniques studied, the optimum method was to use Simplex P, to centrifuge two packs mixed with the chilled monomer, and to centrifuge at full speed for 60 seconds. Centrifugation for shorter periods did not produce the optimum increase in fatigue life. Centrifugation for longer than 60 seconds did not significantly increase the fatigue strength above that achieved by 60 seconds. With this optimum combination, the fatigue life of surgical Simplex P was increased by nearly a factor of five.

Of the vacuum mixing techniques, we examined the Mixevac II, the Enhancement System, and the Mitab.[4] Of special interest is the fact that when any of these three vacuum techniques was used to prepare a single pack of cement, there was no significant increase in the fatigue life of the cement. In other words, vacuum mixing just one pack of cement is not useful. However, with two packs of cement per syringe and chilled monomer, it was possible to increase mean fatigue life significantly with any of the three vacuum systems.

Therefore, our first major recommendation in making cement stronger is to start with the strongest cement, namely Simplex P, and then to carry out porosity reduction either with centrifugation of two packs or with the vacuum mixing of two packs. These techniques provide improved Simplex P bone cement that is five times stronger than untreated Simplex P and is ten or 15 times stronger than some other types of cement commonly used.

Cement-Metal Interface

The next major issue in terms of failure of fixation of cemented implants is the cement-metal interface. Charnley thought that the cement was not a glue and that nothing could be done to enhance the cement-metal interface. Our recent studies of cemented total hips retrieved at autopsy after as much as 17 years after insertion have shown that the major initiation of failure of fixation of a cemented femoral component is debonding at the cement-metal interface,[6] not failure at the cement-bone interface or fracture of the cement itself.

In a series of laboratory studies from a variety of research units, it has been shown that the industrial application of a thin layer of bone cement to the metal surface at the factory (precoating) substantially enhances the strength of this vulnerable cement-metal interface.[7] In in vitro tests that we conducted to study fatigue of this interface at a maximum stress of 1.25 MPa at a frequency of 2 Hz, the standard cement-metal interface without precoating failed at an average of 9,486 cycles, whereas the precoated interface failed at an average of 224,251 cycles.[8] Many other studies have confirmed observations of this nature. The fatigue life of this interface can also be improved by creating a rough surface on the metal. Optimum enhancement of the strength of the interface requires precoating and a rough surface.

Cement-Bone Interface

What about the cement-bone interface? Here, pressurization is a key issue,[9,10] and this process begins by plugging the medullary canal.[11–14] It is our belief that a cement plug is preferable to either a bone plug or a plastic plug. The use of a femoral seal[9] enhances the pressure that can be generated, driving the cement into the trabecular bone. Not only is the pressure in the cement higher when a plug is used, it can be sustained over a longer period.[9,15] With the pressurization, the cement can be driven more successfully deeper into the trabecular bone.[10] Centrifugation makes no difference in terms of the penetration of cement into the cement-bone interface.

Thus, a number of steps are now available that significantly enhance the durability of cemented femoral components for total hip replacement surgery. These steps include the use of a medullary plug and delivery of the cement with a cement gun, pressurization of the cement to increase the penetration into bone, selection of the strongest cement (Simplex P) and further strengthening of the fatigue life of that cement by porosity reduction (centrifugation or vacuum mixing).

When these changes are combined with improved design of the femoral component and the specific enhancement of the cement-metal interface by precoating and a rough surface, the likelihood of prolonged successful fixation of a cemented femoral component is substantially enhanced.

References

1. Gates EI, Carter DR, Harris WH: Comparative fatigue behavior of different bone cements. *Clin Orthop* 1984;189:294–299.
2. Davies JP, O'Connor DO, Burke DW, et al: Comparison and optimization of three centrifugation systems for reducing porosity of Simplex P bone cement. *J Arthroplasty* 1989;4:15–20.
3. Davies JP, Jasty M, O'Connor DO, et al: The effect of centrifuging bone cement. *J Bone Joint Surg* 1989;71B:39–42.
4. Davies JP, Harris WH: Optimization and comparison of three vacuum mixing systems for porosity reduction of Simplex. *Clin Orthop*, in press.
5. Carter DR, Gates EI, Harris WH: Strain-controlled fatigue of acrylic bone cement. *J Biomed Mater Res* 1982;16:647–657.
6. Maloney WJ, Jasty M, Burke DW, et al: Biomechanical and histologic investigation of cemented total hip arthroplasties: A study of autopsy-retrieved femurs after in vivo cycling. *Clin Orthop* 1989;249:129–140.
7. Ahmed AM, Raab S, Miller JE: Metal/cement interface strength in cemented stem fixation. *J Orthop Res* 1984;2:105–118.
8. Davies JP, O'Connor DO, Harris WH: Fatigue strength of cement-metal interfaces: Comparison of porous, precoated and smooth specimens. *Trans Orthop Res Soc* 1988;13:367.
9. Oh I, Bourne RB, Harris WH: The femoral cement compactor: An improvement in cementing technique in total hip replacement. *J Bone Joint Surg* 1983;65A:1335–1338.
10. Rey RM Jr, Paiement GD, McGann WM, et al: A study of intrusion characteristics of low viscosity cement Simplex-P and Palacos cements in a bovine cancellous bone model. *Clin Orthop* 1987;215:272–278.
11. Geim GM, Lavernia CJ, Convery FR: A comparison of intramedullary plugs used in total hip arthroplasty. *Trans Orthop Res Soc* 1989;14:396.
12. Bourne RB, Aitken GK, Finlay JB, et al: Femoral cement pressurization in vitro: The effect of intramedullary plugs. *Trans Orthop Res Soc* 1985;10:244.
13. Oh I, Carlson CE, Tomford WW, et al: Improved fixation of the femoral component after total hip replacement using a meth-

acrylate intramedullary plug. *J Bone Joint Surg* 1978;60A:608–613.

14. Amstutz HC, Markolf KL, McNeice GM, et al: Loosening of total hip components: Cause and prevention. *Hip* 1976;4:102–116.

15. Bourne RB, Oh I, Harris WH: Femoral cement pressurization during total hip arthroplasty: The role of different femoral stems with reference to stem size and shape. *Clin Orthop* 1984;183:12–16.

The Optimum Cement Mantle for Total Hip Replacement: Theory and Practice

Philip C. Noble, MS

Hugh S. Tullos, MD

Glenn C. Landon, MD

Introduction

In recent years, debate has raged over the comparative virtues of cemented and cementless fixation in total hip replacement. Central to this issue is the assumption that a significant incidence of osteolysis, sometimes referred to as cement disease, is an inevitable consequence of the use of cement, particularly in the femur (Fig. 1). In fact, however, the incidence of loosening of cemented femoral components reported at long-term follow-up has varied by a factor of approximately 20-fold, even when relatively similar components have been in use. This suggests that the longevity of cemented hip replacements is determined by the integrity of the bone-cement mantle and its interfaces rather than by the presence or absence of cement.

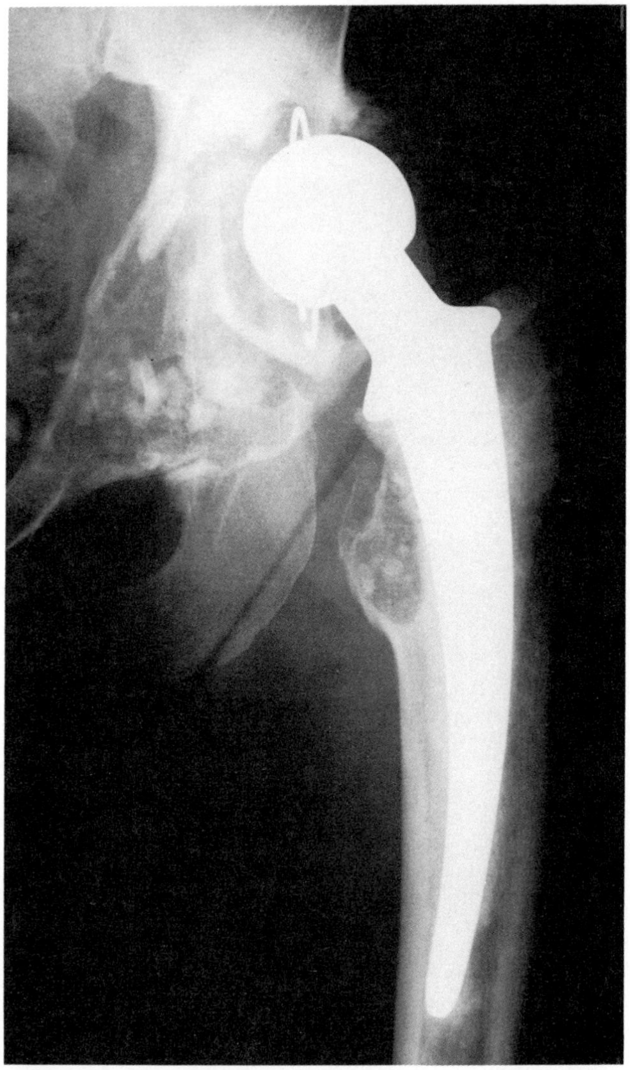

This conclusion has been borne out by the recent studies of Huddleston,[1] who examined 51 cases of focal femoral lysis associated with cemented prostheses. He found that lysis was frequently initiated at points where the metal of the prosthesis was in direct contact with the medullary canal or where the cement mantle was deficient or fractured. In this series, 76% of cement-deficient hips developed an associated resorptive cyst. This correlation was particularly pronounced in the mid and distal thirds of the cement mantle where cortical resorption was most prevalent (Fig. 2). Huddleston cited several sources of mantle deficiency, principally implantation of the femoral component in varus or valgus and failure to center the femoral stem within the cement mantle. Both of these technical errors frequently led to areas of direct impingement of the prosthesis with the femoral cortex. These observations suggest that in the femur, cystic lysis occurs as a biologic response to the particulate debris generated by fragmentation of the cement mantle. Thus, cement disease is actually particulate disease and is observed in cemented and cementless joint replacements when a source of particulate debris is present.

Fig. 1 An extreme example of focal osteolysis of the femur and acetabulum following cemented hip replacement.

Mantle Geometry

A key factor in preserving the integrity of the cement mantle is control of mantle geometry (Fig. 3). The durability of cement fixation is a function of two factors: (1) the inherent strength of the cement itself, and (2) the magnitude of internal stresses developed in response to loading. In joint replacement, the enhancements that can be made to the first of these factors, the strength of acrylic cement, are relatively modest, amounting, at most, to only 20% to 30%. In comparison, by controlling mantle geometry, it is possible to achieve a 50% to 90% reduction in cement stresses.

Several biomechanical studies have shown that the strongest cement mantle is not of uniform thickness.[2] The relationship between stress and geometry of the cement mantle has been studied in detail, using a variety of computer models.[3] These and other studies have shown that during normal weightbearing activities the

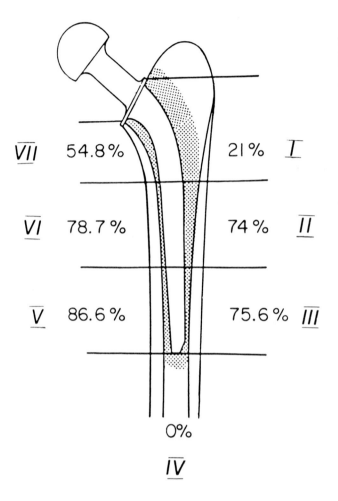

$\overline{VII}$ 54.8%   21% $\underline{I}$

$\overline{VI}$ 78.7%   74% $\underline{II}$

$\overline{V}$ 86.6%   75.6% $\overline{III}$

0%

$\overline{IV}$

Fig. 2   The incidence of osteolytic lesions in cement-deficient zones in cases of femoral osteolysis. (Reproduced with permission from Huddleston HD: Femoral lysis after cemented hip arthroplasty. *J Arthroplasty* 1988;3:285–297.)

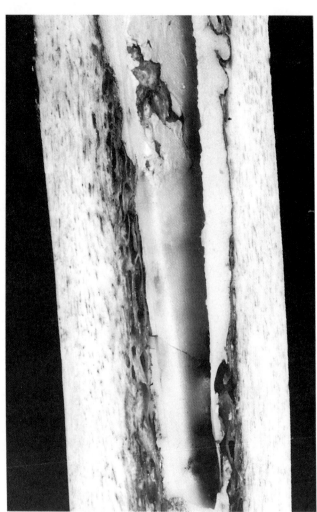

Fig. 3   Laboratory specimen showing areas of fissuring and fragmentation of the cement mantle in regions where the stem passed close to the endosteal surface during implantation.

stresses borne by the cement mantle are very uneven, tending to concentrate over the proximal end of the femur and the distal tip of the prosthesis where the greatest discontinuities in stiffness are present. Thus, the key to designing implants that generate the least cement stress lies in understanding how mantle geometry may be varied to minimize these peak stress concentrations in the proximal and distal mantle.

During loading of the prosthetic joint, the femoral stem tends to bend, thereby dissipating load to the proximal- and mid-stem regions of the femur via the cement mantle. The bending of the femur is concentrated about the distal end of the prosthesis, at the point where the stiffening effect of the implant ceases. The magnitude of the stress concentrated at the distal tip of the prosthesis increases dramatically with the bulk of the distal stem filling the canal (Fig. 4, *left*). Thus, the thinner the cement mantle, the higher the cement

stress and the greater the risk of fracture and fragmentation of the cement column. Conversely, as the thickness of the mantle increases, the stresses on the cement become less.

In practice, because any reduction in the distal diameter of the femoral stem is limited by the strength of the stem itself, a compromise must be reached so that both the cement mantle and the implant are bulky enough to prevent failure of either structural element. The area of optimum compromise corresponds to 70% to 80% filling of the medullary canal by the prosthesis, leaving a distal mantle that is 1 to 2 mm in thickness.

Proximal cement stresses follow different guidelines (Fig. 4, *right*). In the proximal-medial area of the cement mantle, minimum cement stresses occur with stems that are 80% to 90% canal-filling. These stresses increase gradually as the mantle becomes thicker and increase catastrophically as the mantle gets thinner.

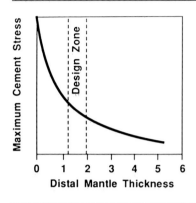

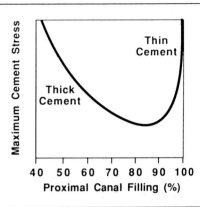

Fig. 4 **Left**, The dependence of cement stress on the thickness of the mantle (in millimeters) adjacent to the distal tip of the prosthesis, according to thickness. **Right**, Proximal cement stresses are minimum in mantles 3 to 6 mm thick, which lie between the extremes of thin and thick cement. (Modified with permission from Huiskes R: Some fundamental aspects of human joint replacement: Analysis of stresses and heat conduction in bone-prosthesis structures. *Acta Orthop Scand* 1980;185:109–200.)

Thus once again, the highest cement stresses are associated with thin cement mantles and conditions that approach direct impingement of stem on bone.

Several clinical studies have related the radiographic performance of cemented femoral components to the thickness of the proximal cement.[2-4] Of particular interest is the work of Sarmiento and Gruen,[4] who showed that once the proximal mantle became thinner than 2 mm, the incidence of subsidence and calcar resorption increased significantly. In a review of older implant designs and cement techniques, Beckenbaugh and Ilstrup[5] found that the thinner the proximal cement mantle, the higher the incidence of loosening as evidenced by medial migration of the femoral component. As severe calcar resorption may be a response to particulate debris, this observation is particularly interesting and is consistent with the studies of Vives and associates,[6] who examined the results of a series of 110 press-fit prostheses, implanted with bone cement to augment distal fixation. In this study, five cases of early radiographic failure occurred in association with focal osteolysis of the proximal-medial femur. In every case, a thin layer of cement was interposed between the implant and the bone. Thus, the conclusion of a variety of clinical and biomechanical studies is that the optimum cement mantle is distinctly asymmetric and that thin cement carries with it a high risk of fragmentation, particle generation, and osteolysis.

Stem Design

The presence of thin and inadequate cement mantles is attributable to (1) the use of femoral stems whose geometry does not fit the canal properly and (2) the lack of an effective means of centering the stem within the cement mantle. In years past, designs of femoral stems were generally based on scant anatomic data. Thus, it was initially assumed that femoral stems should be designed with a fixed medial shape representative of the average femur. In these systems, all femoral stems were designed with the same medial and distal profile, without taking into account the width of the femoral canal. Larger and smaller bones were accommodated by increasing or decreasing the total medial-lateral width of the component, without altering the shape of the external surfaces of the stem.

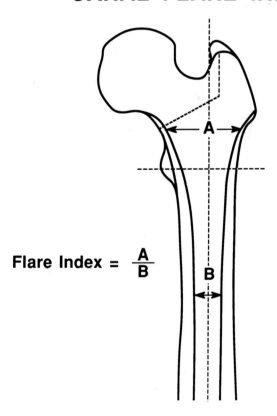

CANAL FLARE INDEX

Flare Index = $\dfrac{A}{B}$

Fig. 5 The Canal Flare Index is a simple measure of the shape of the femoral canal in the anteroposterior view. (Reproduced with permission from Noble PC, Alexander JW, Lindahl LJ, et al: The anatomic basis of femoral component design. *Clin Orthop* 1988;235:148–165.)

Although implants of this fixed design will fit average femurs, the shape of the femoral canal varies dramatically within the human population from a straight, stove-pipe shape to markedly flared, champagne-flute geometries (Figs. 5 and 6).[7] Moreover, there is a loose relationship between the size of the canal and its contours, with smaller bones tending to be more fluted and larger bones tending toward the stove-pipe extreme. Thus, when components of average shape are implanted into the wide range of femurs seen in total joint replacement, shape mismatches are common. These mismatches lead to large gaps between stem and bone and to areas where the stem impinges on bone. The most common form of malfitting arises when the femoral canal has a straighter medial curvature than the implant. Ironically, canals of this shape are more common in older patients, the age group in whom cement is used most frequently. Consequently, inadequate cement mantles resulting from mismatches in bone and implant geometry occur most frequently in older patients.

Proportional Sizing of Implants

In an attempt to improve their match with femoral geometry, several implant systems have been designed with proportionally sized femoral components. These implants also use an average femoral geometry, but one that has been scaled proportionally to predict the geometry of smaller and larger femurs. The concept of proportionality arose from forensic science and physical anthropology, in which the correlation between the external dimensions of bones has been used as a basis for calculating the height of the skeleton. However, this observation is completely unrelated to variations in endosteal bony architecture, which is not proportional and which is subject to the multiple influences of age, sex, race, and activity. Consequently, there are wide variations in the shape of the metaphysis in the coronal, sagittal, and transverse planes.

Because of these multiple factors, proportional implants also present significant misfits of stem to canal, leading to a substantial incidence of inadequate cement mantles. An additional, detrimental feature of proportional stems is excessive length. This occurs because the distance to the anterior bow from the proximal femoral osteotomy is not proportional to canal width. Thus, a frequent occurrence with proportional femoral stems is distal impingement of the tip of the prosthesis on the anterior cortex, leading to a longitudinal fissure in the cement mantle during implantation of the stem. Thus, implants of proportional designs tend to violate the cement column both proximally and distally in the regions of highest stresses.

To overcome these problems, femoral stems may be designed with anatomically devised contours in which each size of component has a unique shape that is based on the geometry of bones within each size range. This method of implant design requires a detailed knowledge of the shapes of a large sample of femurs, because each size of component is designed individually.

Somatyping

One way of implementing this design strategy is termed "somatyping."[8] Each somatype is a unique canal shape. Through mathematical techniques, it is possible to represent the anatomic range of femurs by a finite

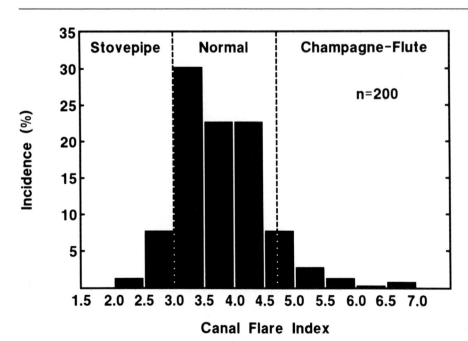

Fig. 6 The anatomic distribution of values of the canal flare index demonstrates that the femur varies continuously in shape from "stove-pipe" to "champagne-fluted." One single shape cannot be proportionally scaled to represent the majority of canals. (Reproduced with permission from Noble PC, Alexander JW, Lindahl LJ, et al: The anatomic basis of femoral component design. *Clin Orthop* 1988;235:148–165.)

set of unique shapes or somatypes, the number depending upon the acceptable error of fit between any one bone and its closest somatype. This analysis predicts that 17 unique prostheses would be required to match virtually all femurs, but that only eight sizes would be needed if errors of the order of $\pm$ 2 mm could be tolerated in matching the proximal medial contour. If this tolerance is relaxed to $\pm$ 3 mm, as in a cemented hip replacement, only five unique geometries are required to provide acceptable canal fit.

Once the somatypes of the femurs in the cemented hip cases are determined, implant shapes may be devised by allowing for the optimal, asymmetric shape of the cement mantle. This results in components that have less medial curvature than is customary in cementless hip replacement, because of the necessary allowance for a mantle that is thicker proximally than distally.

The benefits of "somatype-devised" femoral stems remain theoretical unless the stem can be positioned centrally within the cement mantle. The recent emergence of centralizing devices now makes this possible (Fig. 7). Detailed study of the mantles of femurs harvested from cadavers shows that areas of fissuring and perforation of the cement mantle are extremely common in cemented hip replacement. This is not surprising, given that the position of the stem in the canal is difficult to control by feel alone and that the surgeon often forces the component into anteversion to maximize joint stability and into valgus to avoid a varus stem position. However, both these deviations almost inevitably cause stem impingements in some area of the canal, a situation that often goes unnoticed during implantation.

Centralizing

Centralizing devices prevent stem impingement by fixing the minimum possible thickness of the cement mantle. Although various designs are available, all commonly used devices are fabricated from polymethylmethacrylate, which, by bonding chemically with the wet cement, avoids stress concentrations through mechanical or structural discontinuities. The use of proximal and distal centralizers, like the dual sights of a gun barrel, is strongly recommended, because laboratory experiments have shown that accurate positioning of the femoral stem is not readily achieved with a distal centralizer used alone, although stem impingement is at least avoided distally.

The effect of centralizers on stem position and mantle thickness was examined in a recent study of 288 cemented hip cases in which three patient groups were compared.[8]

Group 1 consisted of 46 cases of fixed stems or stems with proportional geometry implanted by experienced hip surgeons without centralizing devices. Group 2 consisted of 201 cases of a somatype-devised cemented stem implanted by the same experienced surgeons us-

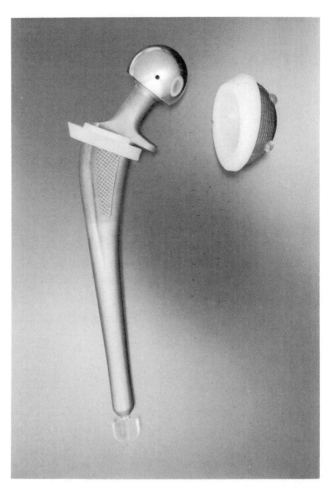

Fig. 7 Centralization and mantle thickness can be controlled through the use of proximal and distal devices fabricated from polymethylmethacrylate.

ing distal centralizers alone. Group 3 consisted of 41 cases of the same somatype-devised stem implanted by orthopaedic residents using both distal and proximal centralizers.

The orientation of the femur and the prosthesis and the distribution of mantle thickness was measured in each case on the first postoperative anteroposterior radiograph. In group 1, the incidence of significant stem misalignment ($>$2 degrees varus or valgus) was 20%. An inadequate cement mantle was present proximally in 35% of cases and distally in 49% of cases. Some 37% of hips had direct impingement of stem on bone. In group 2, average stem alignment improved, but the incidence of significant misalignment was still 17%. Although 19% of proximal mantles were inadequate, only 3% of distal mantles were thinner than 1 mm. Because a distal centralizer was used, there were no cases of distal stem-bone impingement, but benefits in the proximal stem area were minimal.

In group 3, in which both proximal and distal centralizers were used, there were no cases of significant

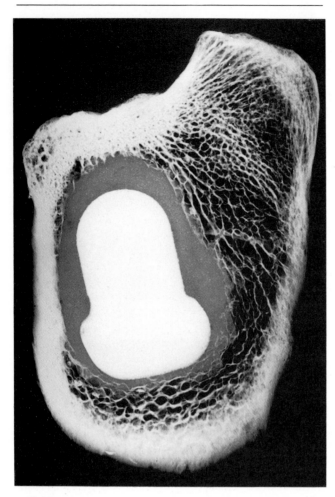

Fig. 8 Cement enables the surgeon to prepare the best possible foundation for component fixation regardless of the shape of each individual femur.

stem misalignment, no cases of stem-bone impingement, and all components had acceptable cement mantles despite the relative inexperience of the operating surgeons. In one case, a distal centralizer fractured during implantation of stem in slight valgus, but this did

not significantly compromise the position of the distal stem.

A comparison of the results of the three patient groups demonstrates that centralization of the femoral stem and prevention of stem-bone impingement may be achieved through the use of proximal and distal centralizing devices in combination with prosthetic components derived from femoral somatypes. Using this approach, excellent technical results become less dependent on the individual skill and personal experience of each surgeon. This dependency has been the fundamental shortcoming of previous implant systems and is a key factor in the variability of the clinical results of cemented hip arthroplasty reported in the past. It is our belief that this approach represents a substantial advance in the design of cemented hip replacements, which enables every surgeon to achieve an ideal radiologic result on a routine, reproducible basis (Fig. 8).

References

1. Huddleston HD: Femoral lysis after cemented hip arthroplasty. *J Arthrop* 1988;3:285–297.
2. Bocco F, Langan P, Charnley J: Changes in the calcar femoris in relation to cement technology in total hip replacement. *Clin Orthop* 1977;128:287–295.
3. Huiskes R: Some fundamental aspects of human joint replacements: Analysis of stresses and heat conduction in bone-prosthesis structures. *Acta Orthop Scand* 1980;185:109–200.
4. Sarmiento A, Gruen TA: Radiographic analysis of a low-modulus titanium-alloy femoral total hip component: Two to six-year follow-up. *J Bone Joint Surg* 1985;67A:48–56.
5. Beckenbaugh RD, Ilstrup DM: Total hip arthroplasty. *J Bone Joint Surg* 1978;60A:306–313.
6. Vives P, de Lestang M, Jarde O, et al: Interet du contact direct entre la tige femorale et l'os diaphysaire dans les prostheses totales cimentees. *Rev Chir Orthop* 1987, suppl 2, pp 218–220.
7. Noble PC, Alexander JW, Lindahl LJ, et al: The anatomic basis of femoral component design. *Clin Orthop* 1988;235:148–165.
8. Scheller A, Levy RN, Noble PC, et al: A comparative analysis of total hip component position and cement technique. Presented at the 56th Annual Meeting of the American Academy of Orthopaedic Surgeons, Las Vegas, Feb 14, 1989.

Why Cemented Femoral Components Become Loose

Murali Jasty, MD

Introduction

Total hip replacement using cement for fixation of the prosthetic components has provided dramatic relief of pain and improvement of function for millions of patients in the world with end-stage arthritis of the hip.[1] Late mechanical loosening of the prosthetic components, however, has been a problem with these procedures.[2,3] Additional surgery to revise the loose components is possible, but the technical difficulties, complications, and failure rates are all greater with revision surgery than with the primary arthroplasty. It is therefore of critical importance to minimize the failure rates of primary arthroplasty.

To improve the success of the cemented total hip arthroplasties, it is important to evaluate the mechanisms that initiate the processes that ultimately lead to failure of fixation. In the case of cemented femoral components, the surgeon creates a composite structure made up of the prostheses, the cement, and the femur, and it is important to know which critically weak member or members of this structure are involved in initiating the failure. The cement-prosthesis interface, the cement, the cement-bone interface, or the bone can fail first and be the initiating event in the failure of the entire composite structure. Many of the observations on the failure of cemented femoral components, however, have been based on clinical follow-up studies of patients with total hip replacements or on studies that used histologic material obtained at revision surgery.[1-7] The information from such studies has limited use in elucidating the events that initiated the failure, because clinical radiographs are inadequate to identify the initiating cause of failure, and by the time a patient has come to revision surgery most of the critical information on the initiation of failure has been obscured.

Early investigators using cement believed that cemented femoral components loosened primarily because of mechanical factors, and that cement was tolerated by the skeleton very well over the long term.[1] Other studies, based on radiographic and clinical observations, have since suggested that a fibrous tissue membrane forms at the cement-bone or cement-metal interface as a result of biologic reactions to the implanted foreign materials, and that these biologic events lead to loosening of cemented prostheses.[4,6,8-10] Thus, a great deal of controversy has been generated about whether the failure of the cemented femoral components is related to mechanical factors or biologic factors. Even proponents of the concept that mechanical factors are important in prosthetic loosening have argued about the specific events that initiate the loosening process. The role of the strength of bone cement, the strength of the cement-prosthesis interface, the strength of the cement-bone interface, the alignment of the prosthetic components in the cement mantle, the thickness of the cement mantle, the design of the prosthetic components, and the moduli of the implant devices have each been implicated as the principal determinant in the loosening of cemented prostheses.[1-3,11-17] Likewise, the proponents of a biologic basis for loosening have also debated on whether the adverse tissue responses around cemented femoral components are caused by bulk polymethylmethacrylate, particulate polymethylmethacrylate, monomer toxicity, or polyethylene wear debris.[4,6,8-10]

The many secondary changes that take place with loosening of cemented prostheses confuse the information gained from the radiographic and clinical evaluation of patients who come to revision surgery. For this reason, morphologic and experimental investigation of femurs obtained from patients who had undergone cemented total hip arthroplasty, but whose prosthetic components had not yet loosened, can provide many valuable insights into the specific events that initiate the loosening of prosthetic components. Therefore, my colleagues and I carried out mechanical, morphologic, and fractographic studies of successful cemented femoral components retrieved at autopsy from patients who had undergone cemented total hip arthroplasty between two weeks and 17 years earlier. It was possible in these specimens to evaluate both the biologic and mechanical changes that occur in vivo. Specifically, we investigated long-term implant stability and the mechanical parameters involved in loosening, including detailed studies of the cement-bone and cement-metal interfaces and fractographic evaluation of the bone cement, in order to understand the sequence of events that leads to the loosening of cemented femoral components.

Studies on Femurs Retrieved at Autopsy

Sixteen femurs were harvested from 12 patients who died between two weeks and 17 years after undergoing cemented total hip arthroplasty. Seven of the patients were women; five were men. Their ages ranged from 43 to 98 years at the time of death. In the majority of the patients, the initial diagnosis necessitating the total hip arthroplasty was osteoarthritis. Seven different types of prostheses had been inserted into these femurs for time periods ranging from 0.5 months to 17.5 years. Four intact contralateral femurs were also available, which allowed the skeletal architecture in the femurs with arthroplasty to be compared with that in the normal femurs. The treating physicians, medical records, and family members provided the clinical information on these patients.

The femurs were subjected to mechanical,[18] morphologic, and fractographic studies to elucidate the mechanisms involved in loosening of femoral components. Detailed radiographic examination carried out on the femurs included evaluation of radiolucencies[5] at the cement-bone and cement-prostheses interfaces on the anteroposterior, lateral, and right- and left-oblique radiographs. Criteria described by Harris and McGann[15] were used to evaluate the radiographic evidence of loosening of the femoral components.

Biomechanical Testing for Implant Stability

In order to assess implant stability more rigorously, we carried out detailed mechanical testing of the femoral components using a torque wrench-micrometer device.[19] As the wrench applied a torsional load to the femoral components, the resultant micromotion was measured by a micrometer attached between the bone and the prosthetic components. Torque, in increments of 25 in-lb up to 150 in-lb, was applied to the prosthetic femoral components, and the rotational micromotion of the prosthesis relative to the anterior femoral cortex was measured by the micrometer at each load increment. Any permanent, irreversible displacement of the femoral component that remained after the torque was released was also recorded. The maximum torque of 150 in-lb was selected on this basis of calculations of the in vivo rotational moment generated in patients implanted with an instrumented total hip replacement.[20]

Morphologic and Fractographic Studies

After the radiographic and biomechanical testing, the femurs were dehydrated in calcium chloride pellets, were embedded in a rectangular block of surgical bone cement, and were cut into serial, transverse sections at 5-mm increments by a high-speed, water-cooled circular saw with an aluminum ceramic blade. Each section was radiographed.

The surfaces of each of the sections were polished and sputter coated with a thin layer of gold. All of the specimens were then examined with a scanning electron microscope equipped with a backscatter detector to assess the bone morphology, with particular attention to the cement-bone interface. The extent and thickness of fibrous tissue at the bone-cement interface and the proximity of the endosteal bone to the cement were evaluated. Representative sections from areas surrounding the proximal, middle, and distal regions of the femoral components were ground further, and the thin sections were stained with hematoxylin and eosin and examined under transmitted light microscopy.

Fractographic studies of the cement were done to assess the presence of fatigue fractures in the cement. The locations and orientation of the fractures in the cement mantle and the integrity of the cement-metal interface were investigated. The prosthetic component was removed from the cement mantle in some sections, and the cement was viewed from the prosthetic surface using scanning electron microscopy. In other specimens, in which fractures through the cement mantle were present, the fractures were completed acutely, and the fracture surfaces were evaluated for the presence of signs of fatigue.

Results

Radiographic Findings

In 15 of the 16 cases, the radiographs showed no evidence of femoral component loosening. On the contact radiographs, only one of the femoral components showed evidence of subsidence and radiolucencies at the cement-metal interface. No cement fractures or radiolucencies at the cement-metal interface were present on any of the radiographs of the other 15 femurs. Radiolucencies at the cement-bone interface, however, were common (Fig. 1). All of the specimens showed radiolucencies at the cement-bone interface in at least some areas. Seven of the femurs showed radiolucencies surrounding the entire cement mantle and were considered possibly or probably loose on the basis of radiolucencies criteria of Harris and McGann.[15] Three additional femurs showed focal areas of osteolysis at the cement-bone interface. In one of these specimens, the focal osteolysis was small and confined to the cortex surrounding the distal tip of the femoral component. In the other two, the areas of osteolysis were more diffuse and involved a major portion of the cement-bone interface.

Mechanical Stability of the Femoral Components

All but one of the femoral components demonstrated exceptional stability with micromotion at the cement-bone interface measuring less than 0.25 mm. Only the femoral component that was diagnosed to be loose on the basis of radiolucencies seen at the cement-metal interface on the radiographs was also loose on mechanical testing. The stability of the remaining femoral components was remarkable even though most of these femurs had been exposed to functional loading in vivo for many years. The higher micromotions (50 to 300 μ) occurred in those four femurs (118 months, 58 months, 40 months, and 13 months) with marked osteoporosis caused by advanced age, disuse, or chronic steroid therapy. The remainder of the specimens showed even lower rotational micromotion (less than 50 μ). Even the two specimens retrieved as late as 209 and 210 months after surgery showed elastic or reversible rotational micromotion of 15 μ and 3 μ, respectively, at a torque of 150 in-lb. In almost all cases, the micromotion was the result of the elastic deformation of the bone and the femoral components returned to the original position when the force was removed.

Morphologic Observations

There was no evidence of loosening at the cement-bone interface in 15 of the 16 cases, even though extensive radiolucencies were present at the cement-bone interface on the radiographs of seven of these specimens. The trabecular bone was intimately associated and interdigitated with the cement mantle, with no evidence of significant fibrous tissue formation at the cement-bone interface in these cases (Figs. 2 to 4). Exhaustive histologic examination of all the cement-bone interfaces showed no significant fibrous tissue formation in 90% of the sections. In the other sections, small areas of fibrous tissue formation at the cement-bone interface could be recognized, but these patchy areas of fibrous tissue occurred in conjunction with excellent interdigitation of the bone and the cement everywhere else. These areas of fibrous tissue did not exceed four to five cell layers thick, did not surround the cement mantle, and did not significantly interfere with cement-bone interdigitation. Evidence for significant fibrous tissue at the cement-bone interface was found in only one case, retrieved at 101 months. In this case the component was shown to be loose radiographically and biomechanically.

In the 15 cases without femoral component loosening, normal-appearing viable marrow elements, without evidence of adverse cellular response, were frequently found directly adjacent to the cement mantle. There was little or no evidence of the foreign body giant cells and macrophage cellular aggregates that have been reported at the cement-bone interface of a loose prosthesis.

Evidence of extensive intramedullary trabecular remodeling was seen in the femurs that were retrieved five to 17 years after surgery (Fig. 3). In the specimens that were retrieved in less than five years, the cement had intruded into trabecular bone. These trabeculae showed viable osteocytes, and their architecture in the metaphysis of these specimens was similar to that normally found at the corresponding locations in the intact femur. However, the trabecular pattern in the proximal metaphysis and the proximal diaphysis of the longer-term specimens (five to 17 years) had changed, and was characterized by thick trabeculae running circumferentially around the cement mantle. Thinner trabeculae surrounded these thick trabeculae, gradually merging with the original outer cortex. The most central of these

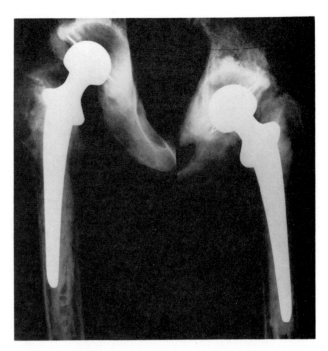

Fig. 1 Femurs retrieved from a patient who had undergone total hip arthroplasty ten years earlier. Note extensive radiolucencies at the cement-bone interface. However, there were no radiolucencies at the cement-metal interface and no cement fractures visible on the radiographs. The femoral components were found to be rigidly fixed on mechanical testing. Histologic sections demonstrated no evidence of fibrous tissue in the areas of radiolucencies at the cement-bone interface.

remodeled trabeculae formed a shell of dense bone that completely encircled the cement mantle.

In specimens in which components had been in place for ten to 17 years, a secondary medullary canal was seen to have formed outside the condensation of dense bone surrounding the cement mantle (Fig. 3). Thick trabeculae running circumferentially around the cement mantle resembled the formation of a secondary "neocortex" in the endosteal canal. It was this remodeling—not the bone resorption and membrane formation—that led to the radiographic appearance of radiolucencies at the cement-bone interface in these specimens. In several areas, the cement mantle was completely encircled with these circumferentially oriented trabeculae. The surrounding original cortex had undergone extensive remodeling and was markedly porotic and thinned. Supporting trabeculae (formed from the resorption and remodeling of the endosteal cortex), which were thinner than the circumferentially oriented lamellae surrounding the cement mantle, connected the inner shell of dense bone to the porotic outer cortex. The "neocortex" was not discernible on either the clinical or contact radiographs because the density of the barium-filled bone cement was similar to that of the bone in the "neocortex."

Backscatter scanning electron microscopy, as well as

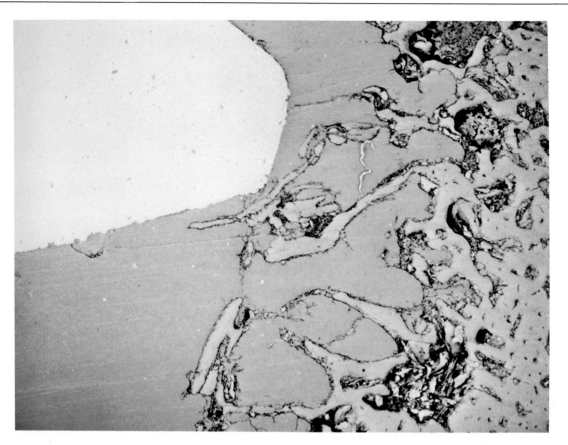

Fig. 2 High-power scanning micrograph of a proximal section through the cement-bone interface showing excellent interdigitation between the cement and the trabecular bone.

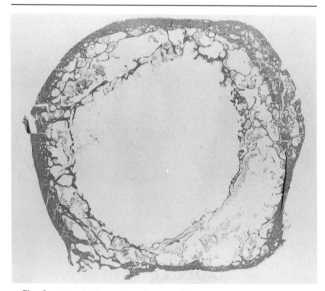

Fig. 3 Histologic section from a femur containing a cemented femoral component inserted 12 years earlier. The cement was dissolved out of the section during the processing. Note however, the development of a dense shell of new bone (a "neocortex") surrounding the cement mantle, and extensive osteoporosis and thinning of the cortex on the outside of the dense shell of new bone.

light microscopy, confirmed the intimate association of the bone with the cement in all of the femurs. Fine bony trabeculae were frequently noted to be growing into the porous surface of the cement without any intervening fibrous tissue. Although it could not be proven that the presence of these trabeculae represented bone ingrowth into the cement mantles of the specimens retrieved early after the surgery, the persistence of the trabeculae in the porous surfaces of cement, along with extensive alterations in the architecture of the surrounding bone after many years of in vivo service, established that bone remodeling and ingrowth into the surface undulations of the cement continue to support the cement mantle.

Fractographic Observations of the Cement Mantles

Although the vast majority of the hips showed no clinical, radiographic, or physical evidence of loosening and showed excellent cement-bone interdigitation, separation of the cement-prosthesis interface (debonding) was identified on the microscopic evaluation of the cross sections in every specimen (Figs. 5 and 6). This separation was complete in two hips, one of which was retrieved at 118 months and the other at 156 months.

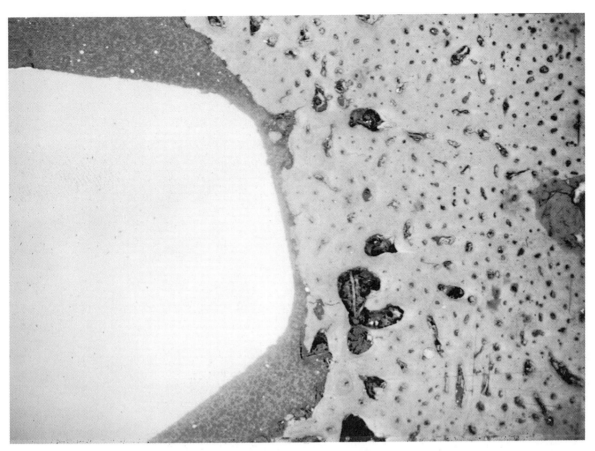

Fig. 4 High-power scanning micrograph of a section through the cement-bone interface at the diaphyseal region. Note the excellent interdigitation of the cement with the bone and lack of fibrous tissue formation at this interface.

The contact radiographs showed loosening at the cement-metal interface in only one of these femurs. The debonding at the cement-metal interface had progressed to the point where it involved the entire circumference of the cement mantle in these two specimens. In the others, it was focal and involved the most proximal and distal ends of the prosthetic components. A thin layer of collagenous and fibrous tissue measuring approximately 50 to 100 μ in thickness was present between the femoral component and the surrounding cement in four specimens, which established that the gaps had existed in vivo and were not artifacts of cutting the femurs into sections.

Despite the absence of radiographic evidence for loosening in 15 of the 16 specimens, fractures in the cement mantle were present around all prostheses that had been in use for over three years (Fig. 5). In some cases, the fractures in the cement mantle were small and incomplete. In others, with more than ten years of in vivo service, the fractures were large and involved the entire thickness of the cement mantles. The fractures were oriented both circumferentially, at the cement-metal interface, and radially, propagating away

from the cement-metal interface. The radial fractures were more numerous and were usually located at the sharp corners of the prosthesis on the medial, anterior, and posterior surfaces. The fractures were wider at the prosthetic side and seemed to originate at the cement-metal interface.

Defects in the cement mantle were also frequently associated with fractures in the cement and debonding at the cement-prosthesis interface. Defects in the cement mantles at the proximal medial regions and distal lateral regions were frequently associated with fractures in the cement mantle in regions adjacent to the defect and with debonding at the cement-metal interface. In one case (the implant that was loose by radiographic criteria), the defect in the proximal medial cement mantle led to the development of several radial fractures and migration of the prosthetic component into retroversion (Fig. 6).

Although most fractures through the cement originated at the prosthesis-cement interface, other smaller fractures associated with voids in the cement mantle and with trabecular bone interdigitation with the cement mantle were also observed. In the 3.3-year spec-

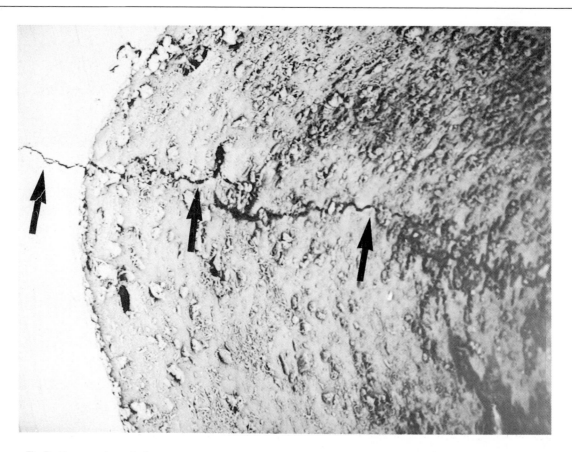

Fig. 5 Fracture through the cement mantle on the medial side near a sharp corner of the prosthesis. The prosthesis had separated from the cement mantle in this section and was easily removed. The arrows show the fracture in the cement mantle.

imen, the prosthesis tip had debonded from the cement mantle. When the tip was removed and the adjacent cement surface was examined, numerous fractures were seen that originated at voids in the cement where the tip had resided.

The specimen that contained the loose femoral component showed many interesting features. The prosthesis in this femur was completely debonded from the cement mantle and was surrounded with a layer of fibrous tissue, even though this specimen showed an excellent cement-bone interface with only minimal and sporadic fibrous tissue formation. There were numerous radial fractures within the cement mantle, and the prosthesis had subsided into retroversion by opening these cement fractures.

Another specimen with an area of focal endosteal osteolysis at the tip of the femoral component also illustrated many features that characterize the adverse biologic response to cemented femoral components. The tip of the femoral component had debonded from the cement mantle in this specimen. The cement mantle in this region was thin, with numerous voids and numerous fractures through the voids. Near the region

of the osteolysis, the cement had fragmented (Fig. 7). There was focal loss of bone in the region where the cement had fragmented, even though the cement-bone interface was pristine, with no evidence of fibrous tissue formation elsewhere. Such bone loss suggests that mechanical factors, such as cement fractures and fragmentation of the cement, lead to the focal osteolysis sometimes seen around prostheses that are otherwise firmly fixed to the bone.

Discussion

The cemented femoral components retrieved from patients who had undergone total hip replacement surgery up to 17 years earlier provide valuable insight into the mechanisms that lead to the failure of cemented femoral components. A realistic picture of the long-term mechanical and biologic behavior of these components can be obtained from these femurs, which had been subjected to physiologic loads in vivo for many years. The sequence of events that initiates the process of failure of fixation in these cemented femoral components can be elucidated from these observations.

The cement in all of these cases was tolerated very well in vivo, in most of them over a very long term. Excellent apposition with the trabecular bone and intimate osseointegration with the surface of the cement without evidence of intervening fibrous tissue at the cement-bone interface is possible with the cemented femoral components over the long term. The fibrous tissue at the cement-bone interface may be secondary to prosthetic loosening rather than the cause of loosening in well-done cemented femoral components.

In every one of the femurs retrieved from three to 17 years after surgery, despite the absence of symptoms or radiographic evidence for loosening, localized areas of separation of the cement-metal interface were detected. In a few cases, fibrous tissue had formed at the cement-metal interface rather than at the cement-bone interface. In the one prosthetic component in which there was radiographic evidence of femoral component loosening, the prosthetic component was found to have loosened completely from the cement mantle even though excellent interdigitation had been maintained everywhere between the cement and bone.

These data suggest that loosening at the cement-bone interface is a late event in the failure of femoral component fixation and follows the mechanical events that originally initiated the loosening process. With time, fragments of polymethylmethacrylate or polymeric debris may be released, and it is these particles that are responsible for the membrane formation at the cement-bone interface and for the bone lysis that often accompanies loosening.

Of special interest are the numerous large and small fractures in the cement found in several cases in the absence of radiographic or clinical evidence of loosening at the cement-bone interface. These fractures occurred in the presence of intimate cement-bone apposition and in the absence of fibrous tissue formation at the cement-bone interface, indicating that the cement can undergo accumulated fatigue damage in vivo for some time before gross loosening manifests itself radiographically or clinically.

The demonstration of local debonding at the cement-metal interface seen in almost all of these cases is important. Debonding at the cement-prosthesis interface may be a primary feature in the initiation of prosthetic loosening. This debonding may lead to secondary changes and a marked increase in the stresses within the cement, causing additional mechanical failures of the cement mantles.[14] Experimental studies by Ahmed and associates[11] have shown cement to be a poor adhesive material, which means that the cement-metal interface is not very strong. Clinical studies by Fornasier and Cameron[4] and Stauffer[2] have shown failure of the cement-metal interface as a cause for loosening. Recent improvements aimed at increasing the strength of the

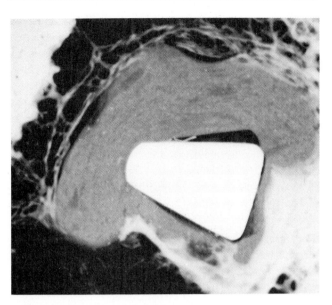

Fig. 6 Specimen radiograph of a section from a femur 13 years after total hip arthroplasty. The prosthesis had separated from the cement mantle and migrated into retroversion but most of the cement-bone interface was intact. There were fractures in the cement mantle at the corners of the prosthesis.

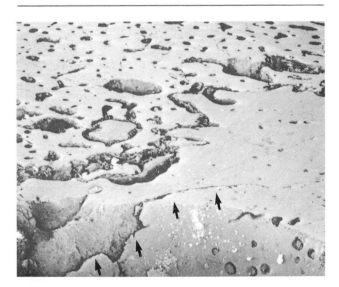

Fig. 7 Section from a femur with focal osteolysis in the cortex. Arrows mark fractures through the thin cement mantle in this region. The fragmentation of the cement and the liberation of the particulate debris may have led to the osteolytic process locally, even though the cement-bone interface was intact elsewhere.

cement-metal interface include precoating the metal prosthesis with polymethylmethacrylate and texturing the implant surfaces. These changes may help to minimize the failures at these interfaces, improving the longevity of the fixation.

Improvements in the design of the femoral component, such as eliminating the sharp corners of the prosthesis,[1] strengthening the cement-metal interface by techniques such as precoating or creating a roughened surface,[11] reducing the porosity of bone cements by techniques such as centrifugation[12] or vacuum mixing, curetting the fine trabecular bone in the proximal metaphysis, and maintaining adequate thickness of the cement mantle,[1,17] are all of paramount importance in improving the long-term success of cemented femoral components. Evidence of the value of these improvements already exists in clinical studies. The success rates of total joint replacements have been markedly improved by the use of newer components without sharp corners and by modern cementing techniques.[15]

Recommended Techniques for Femoral Arthroplasty Using Cement

Femoral components should be made of superalloy metals such as cobalt chromium-based alloys. They must not have sharp borders. Femoral components with rounded corners and broad lateral surfaces are preferred. A broad medial collar on the femoral component is recommended for maximizing load transfer to the calcar and for reducing the stresses in the proximal femoral cement mantle. The largest component that will fit the canal should be used, but the component must leave room for a cement mantle 2 to 3 mm thick all around the prosthesis.

The femoral canal must be prepared meticulously before the femoral component is cemented. The femoral canal is irrigated with radial pulsatile lavage and dried thoroughly before cementing. Plugging the canal, injecting the polymethylmethacrylate with a gun, and then pressurizing the cement in the canal after delivery by using femoral seals are important steps in improving the intrusion of cement into the bone. A cement plug to occlude the canal is recommended. Special calibrated medullary plug syringes make insertion of the cement plug much easier. The cement is mixed to make the plug and is loaded into the plug syringe. Once the cement reaches the dough state, 4 cc of it is inserted 3 cm below the planned level of the tip of the stem using the calibrated syringes. This insures that the femoral implant will pass down the canal unobstructed by the cement plug. After the cement has been injected, the nozzle is rotated back and forth several times to detach the plug from the tip of the syringe. Avoid further manipulation inside the femoral canal until the plug is completely hardened.

Once the methacrylate plug has hardened, the medullary canal is meticulously cleaned to remove blood, marrow fat, and residual bone debris with pulsatile (radially directed) jet saline lavage and suction. After irrigation, the canal is packed with sponges to make it thoroughly dry. Alternatively, special polyethylene intramedullary brushes can be used to mechanically remove medullary debris. To reduce bleeding from the cancellous bone of the endosteal surface, another sponge soaked in dilute adrenaline solution (0.5 ml of 1:1000 adrenaline in 250 ml of saline) is inserted into the femoral canal. A final dry sponge is passed down the canal just before inserting the cement, and the distal end of the canal near the plug is suctioned to remove any pooled blood. The combination of these techniques should leave the interstices of the cancellous bone clean and dry, which promotes maximal cement interdigitation and a superior cement-bone interface.

In mixing the bone cement, techniques are used to reduce its porosity, improve its fatigue strength, and maximize its intrusion into the bone. Chilled monomer is used to mix the cement, which is poured into cartridges and centrifuged to give it a low viscosity and high fatigue strength. Alternatively, the cement can be mixed in a vacuum. The cartridge of cement is inserted into a cement gun and is ready for injection into the canal. The cement should be inserted just before it becomes doughy, at the moment the cement will not stick to the surgeon's glove. Introducing the cement into the femoral canal in a retrograde fashion using a cement gun with a long nozzle inserted to the level of the plug will prevent air entrapment. The cement gun, by pressurizing the cement, improves its mechanical properties and diminishes the likelihood of entrapping blood and air, a problem commonly encountered during finger packing.

The cement must then be pressurized with a femoral canal seal or a compactor. An effective way to pressurize the cement is to occlude the proximal femoral canal opening with a femoral canal seal that attaches to the end of the cement gun nozzle, and continuing to inject the cement slowly into the femoral canal. Occluding the opening of the medullary canal proximally and forcing the cement against the closed outlet distally generates high sustained pressures and promotes interdigitation of the cement with the bone. Because more polymethylmethacrylate is used when the cement is pressurized (as a result of the more complete filling of the trabecular spaces), it is wise to mix one more pack of cement than is customarily used without pressurization. Greater resistance to passing the stem is usually felt when this technique is used, because the space available is more completely filled with polymethylmethacrylate. The additional pressure generated during insertion of the femoral component improves the intrusion of the cement into the endosteal surface of the femoral diaphysis.

The femoral component should be put in neutral orientation relative to the long axis of the medullary canal. Varus or valgus positioning should be avoided to prevent defects in the cement mantle. A preformed centralizer made of polymethylmethacrylate can be attached to the distal end of the prosthesis to help center the femoral component within the medullary canal. It is important to hold the femoral component steady until the cement has hardened completely. Moving the femoral component while the cement is in the dough phase will produce separation at the cement-metal interface.

The combination of techniques discussed above will insure void-free cement of high fatigue strength with excellent interdigitation with the endosteal trabecular bone. Ideally, the cement mantle is uniform and void-free and is 2 to 3 mm thick around the entire circumference of the femoral component. No radiolucencies should be seen at the cement-bone interface on the radiographs.

Summary

These studies of femurs retrieved at autopsy from patients who had undergone cemented total hip arthroplasty up to 17 years earlier show that cemented femoral components can be tolerated exceptionally well by the skeleton over a long period of time. In all of these specimens, the cement-bone interface was found to be intact, with rare fibrous tissue formation. Failures of cemented femoral components are related primarily to mechanical changes that occur with time, specifically separation of the cement from the metal prosthesis and fractures in the cement. The cement mantles are surrounded and supported by a dense shell of new bone in the medullary cavity (a "neocortex"), which develops as a consequence of the long-term skeletal remodeling in response to the prosthesis. The most common early feature of failure was debonding of the cement from the metal prosthesis, specifically at the most proximal and distal ends of the prosthesis. Subsequent developments are circumferential fractures in the cement near the cement-metal interface and radial fractures extending from the cement-metal interface into the cement and the cement-bone interface. The most extensive cement cracks arise from the corners of those prostheses with sharp corners and in areas where the cement mantels are thin and incomplete. Cracks can also arise from the voids in the cement and, occasionally, at the cement-bone interface.

These studies also showed that, in these successful cemented femoral components, failure of fixation is not initiated primarily by biologic processes. The initiating mechanisms of failures were mechanical, and involved debonding at the cement-metal interface and fractures of the cement. Improvement in prosthetic designs and cementing techniques are therefore of paramount importance in attempting to improve the longevity of cemented femoral components.

References

1. Charnley J: *Low Friction Arthroplasty of the Hip: Theory and Practice.* Berlin, Springer-Verlag, 1979.
2. Stauffer RN: Ten-year follow-up study of total hip replacement. *J Bone Joint Surg* 1982;64A:983–990.
3. Sutherland CJ, Wilde AH, Borden LS, et al: A ten-year follow-up of one hundred consecutive Muller curved-stem total hip-replacement arthroplasties. *J Bone Joint Surg* 1982;64A:970–982.
4. Fornasier VL, Cameron HU: The femoral stern/cement interface in total hip replacement. *Clin Orthop* 1976;116:248–252.
5. Gruen TA, McNeice GM, Amstutz HC: "Modes of failure" of cemented stem-type femoral components: A radiographic analysis of loosening. *Clin Orthop* 1979;141:17–27.
6. Jasty MJ, Floyd WE III, Schiller AL, et al: Localized osteolysis in stable, non-septic total hip replacement. *J Bone Joint Surg* 1986;68A:912–919.
7. Jasty M, Goldring SR, Harris WH: Comparison of bone cement membrane around rigidly fixed versus loose total hip implants. *Trans Orthop Res Soc* 1984;9:125.
8. Goldring SR, Jasty M, Roelke MS, et al: Formation of a synovial-like membrane at the bone-cement interface: Its role in bone resorption and implant loosening after total hip replacement. *Arthritis Rheum* 1986;29:836–842.
9. Willert H-G, Ludwig J, Semlitsch M: Reaction of bone to methacrylate after hip arthroplasty: A long-term gross, light microscopic, and scanning electron microscopic study. *J Bone Joint Surg* 1974;56A:1368–1382.
10. Willert H-G, Semlitsch M: Tissue reactions to plastic and metallic wear products of joint endoprostheses, in Geshwend M, Debrunner HU (eds): *Total Hip Prosthesis.* Baltimore, Williams & Wilkins, 1976, pp 205–239.
11. Ahmed AM, Raab S, Miller JE: Metal/cement interface strength in cemented stem fixation. *J Orthop Res* 1984;2:105–118.
12. Burke DW, Gates EI, Harris WH: Centrifugation as a method of improving tensile and fatigue properties of acrylic bone cement. *J Bone Joint Surg* 1984;66A:1265–1273.
13. Crowninshield RD, Brand RA, Johnston RC, et al: An analysis of femoral component stem design in total hip arthroplasty. *J Bone Joint Surg* 1980;62A:68–78.
14. Crowninshield RD, Tolbert JR: Cement strain measurement surrounding loose and well-fixed femoral component stems. *J Biomed Mater Res* 1983;17:819–828.
15. Harris WH, McGann WA: Loosening of the femoral component after use of the medullary-plug cementing technique: Follow-up note with a minimum five-year follow-up. *J Bone Joint Surg* 1986;68A:1064–1066.
16. Lewis JL, Nicola T, Keer LM, et al: Failure processes at the cancellous bone-PMMA interface. *Trans Orthop Res Soc* 1985;10:144.
17. Tarr RB, Clarke IC, Gruen TA, et al: Predictions of cement-bone failure criteria: Three-dimensional finite element models versus clinical reality of total hip replacement, in Callahan RF, Simon BR, Johnson PC, et al (eds): *Finite Elements in Biomechanics.* New York, John Wiley, 1982, p 345.
18. Maloney WJ, Jasty M, Burke DW, et al: Biomechanical and histologic investigation of cemented total hip arthroplasties: A study of autopsy-retrieved femurs after in vivo cycling. *Clin Orthop* 1989;249:129–140.
19. Harris WH, Mulroy RD Jr, Maloney WJ, et al: Intraoperative measurement of rotational stability of femoral components of total hip replacement. *Clin Orthop*, in press.
20. Davy DT, Kotzar GM, Brown RH, et al: Telemetric force measurements across the hip after total arthroplasty. *J Bone Joint Surg* 1988;70A:45–50.

Introduction

Dennis K. Collis, MD

At the 57th Annual Meeting of the American Academy of Orthopaedic Surgeons, in 1990, the five authors of this published Instructional Course were charged with the impossible task of covering the subject of revision total hip arthroplasty in two hours. An equally impossible task is that of covering such a voluminous subject in writing in the few short pages that follow. Each of the authors is an expert in the field of revision total hip arthroplasty, but, in the scope of this volume, they will only be able to touch on the highlights of their segment of this broad subject. These chapters will, however, encourage readers to seek further information by reading the articles and books listed in the excellent bibliographies that follow each section.

In the first of the five chapters, Moreland concisely covers the subject of how to remove aseptically loose cemented prostheses, both acetabular and femoral components. This is an extremely technique-related topic and, unfortunately, it is not possible to include all of the visual aids that were available in a live presentation. In the next chapter, Rubash and associates cover the techniques for removal of uncemented acetabular and femoral components. Because this type of revision is a new challenge in orthopaedic surgery, the special tips included in this chapter are very helpful. Goldberg includes a detailed discussion of the basic science of bone grafting, both allografting and autografting, and then covers the surgical techniques used to treat various bone deficits with different types of

bone graft. This, again, is a relatively new area in hip revision surgery, and Goldberg reports his personal short-term results with the use of bone graft.

Callaghan discusses the results of revision total hip arthroplasty using cement. As he clearly points out, these results were obtained using the older cement techniques and prostheses available in the 1970s. Newer prosthetic components and cement techniques will improve on these results, and Callaghan describes other surgical techniques that are expected to achieve additional improvements.

Engh and Glassman give an excellent presentation of the methods and results of the use of an extensively coated, uncemented stem in revision total hip replacement. Although they do not include any results with femoral components coated only in the proximal area, the reader is referred to pages 161 through 163 of *Instructional Course Lectures, XXXV*, published in 1986, in which Raymon B. Gustilo reported the early results using such prostheses.

Throughout these five chapters, each of the authors points out the high degree of difficulty involved in performing this type of surgery. The extreme importance of extensive preoperative planning is emphasized as is the value of having available in the operating room the appropriate pieces of equipment to allow the surgery to be accomplished most expediently. Each author also points out the need for extensive exposure in order to accomplish these demanding operations.

Techniques for Removal of the Prosthesis and Cement in Hip Revisional Arthroplasty

John R. Moreland, MD

Removal of the prosthesis and cement of the failed total hip replacement should be accomplished without additional damage to the remaining bone stock and in a reasonable time frame. Several techniques for prosthesis and cement removal have been described and are in current use.[1-20] In this chapter, these techniques will be described and the advantages and disadvantages of each given. In addition, I will outline the techniques I prefer.

Exposure

Because adequate exposure is essential for safe and efficient prosthesis and cement removal, the preferred approach must give adequate exposure. Leaving the greater trochanter in place obstructs orientation somewhat and limits vision, but most authorities on hip revisional surgery currently recommend avoiding trochanteric osteotomy during most revisions. When the trochanter is not osteotomized, additional soft tissue is usually released, which may contribute to a high rate of dislocation. Disadvantages of trochanteric osteotomy include difficulty in obtaining union, bursitis caused by wires and other devices used for trochanteric fixation, and compromise to the integrity of the proximal femur, which may be needed for the press-fit of the prosthesis, as well as to contain bone graft. I routinely use trochanteric osteotomy in revisional hip surgery, because I believe that the added exposure gained outweighs the disadvantages of osteotomy and that the dislocation rate is lower with trochanteric osteotomy.

Femoral Component Removal

After the hip is dislocated, removal of the femoral component should be performed next. Most prostheses have a curved area proximally, and the presence of cement and bone proximal to this curved portion of the prosthesis can block direct exit of the femoral component. If this bone and cement are not removed, forceful extraction of the femoral component can fracture the metaphyseal region of the femur. This proximal cement and bone can be removed with osteotomes, a rongeur, and/or high-speed burrs. I prefer to use hand tools for the task. After these impeding structures have been removed, the femoral component can usually be extracted from the cement by applying a mild ex-

traction force. Extraction force can be applied with a punch inserted underneath the collar or the inferior aspect of the head. This can be done more elegantly with a device that loops over the prosthetic femoral head. This device is then attached to a sliding hammer mechanism used to apply the extraction force. Some prostheses have a proximal hole through which a hook can be placed and then attached to this same sliding hammer mechanism. Access to this hole can be difficult because of metaphyseal bone anterior and posterior to the hole. Thus, insertion of the hook can be problematic without some bone removal. Most of the latest generation of femoral prostheses have modular heads, and these complicate application of extraction force because the modular head usually comes off when forces are exerted underneath it. If a prosthesis of this type does not have a collar, an extraction hole, or some other ledge under which to exert an impacter, it will be necessary to use a special extraction device. Such devices are usually available from the manufacturer of the prosthesis. A relatively universal extraction device has been devised that directs extracting force against the ledge usually located just underneath the Morse taper on the femoral prosthetic neck. If the femoral component lacks such a ledge, one can be made with a high-speed burr on the prosthetic neck in order to gain adequate purchase with this universal femoral extraction device (Fig. 1). Once locked into place, this device minimizes the damping of the extraction force through vibration, because, after firm tightening, the extraction device and the prosthesis to be extracted have no potential for movement between them.

Most of the older generation of femoral components will release easily from the cement bed. Some prosthetic designs, however, trap cement in various irregularities in the stem itself and, thus, the stem cannot easily exit the cement bed. Any cemented porous-coated or rough-surfaced implant will not release easily from the cement bed unless the cement-prosthesis interface is disrupted first. Prostheses precoated with methylmethacrylate are also difficult to release from the cement bed, and the prosthesis-cement interface must be directly interrupted. Both hand tools and small high-speed burrs can be used for this maneuver. Removal of the trochanter will facilitate exposure. In areas of cancellous bone, thin osteotomes can be used to disrupt the prosthesis-cement interface. In areas where the prosthesis is directly apposed to the cortical bone, usually proximally and anteriorly, insertion of even a thin

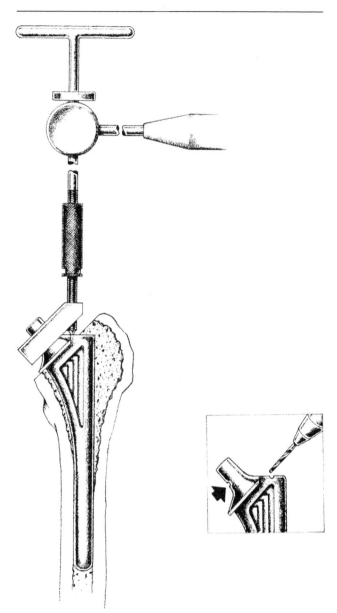

Fig. 1 Universal femoral extraction device. Metal-cutting burr may be needed to create notch for purchase.

osteotome runs a high risk of fracture. All osteotomes have a wedging effect and if the bone's capacity to absorb this wedging effect is limited, fracture will occur. Thin high-speed burrs, unlike osteotomes, have the advantage of creating space as cement is removed, and these burrs are usually preferred over osteotomes for disrupting the femoral prosthesis-cement interface and for disrupting the prosthesis-bone interface in prostheses with bone or fibrous ingrowth, particularly with canal-filling prostheses.

Broken Stems

Several different techniques are used to remove broken stems.[3,4,6–8,20] I prefer to create a small controlled

femoral window and use a carbide punch to remove a broken stem (Fig. 2). This window should be positioned on the anterior cortex just below the level at which the prosthesis was broken, not at the tip of the stem. Windows made at the tip of the stem, because they are more distal, will require a much longer replacement stem to bypass the stress riser created by the window. Also, with a distal window, extraction can be difficult because, as the stem is pushed proximally, access through the hole becomes more difficult and the stem still may not be extractable. The anterior window requires little muscle stripping in order to gain adequate access for making a longitudinal oval window approximately 5 by 15 mm. A high-speed burr will pass easily through the cortex and the cement, until the gray metal is seen. A carbide punch made of hard steel with a sharpened tip is then impacted into the femoral stem until a small divot is made. The punch is then angled proximally, and usually enough purchase is gained to push the stem fragment proximally. A series of divots is then made in the stem as it moves past the femoral window.

If the broken stem has indentations or irregularities, is a porous-coated ingrown stem, or has osseointegration, the carbide punch technique will not work if the forces holding the stem in the femur are greater than the force that can be applied with the carbide punch. In this situation, I prefer to use hollow drills (trephines) to core out the broken fragment, as described by Collis

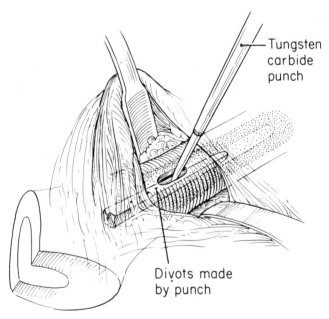

Fig. 2 Method of broken stem extraction gaining purchase via tungsten carbide punch through femoral window. (Reproduced with permission from Moreland JR, Marder R, Anspach WE Jr: The window technique for the removal of broken femoral stems in total hip replacement. *Clin Orthop* 1986;212:245–249.)

and Dubrul.[7] This technique can also be applied to other broken stems.

A third technique for broken stem removal was first described by Wroblewski[3] and later improved by Harris and associates.[4] This technique, which does not require a window, involves machining a hole in the broken end of the distal prosthetic fragment from above. This task is made difficult by exposure problems, problems in holding the carbide drills still during drilling, the problem of finding an adequate area for hole creation in stems with small cross sections, and, at times, the lack of adequate purchase for extraction.

Acetabular Revision

After the femoral component has been extracted, thus facilitating acetabular exposure, acetabular revision should be performed next, before the femoral cement is removed. This avoids the risk of stirring up bleeding in the femoral canal during acetabular extraction and reconstruction. Acetabular component removal can be fairly simple because, in many cases, the prosthesis is grossly loose. If fixation is secure, or if there has been significant protrusion of the acetabular component into the pelvis, removal may involve special procedures. The acetabular component can be transected into pieces to facilitate removal. High-speed burrs are best for this task, but it may take some time to cut through the thicker components, and large amounts of polyethylene particulate matter are created as the cup is transected. I rarely find this maneuver to be necessary. In some cases, however, in which preservation of the cement-bone interface is desirable, transecting the component usually allows removal of the component without disturbing the cement-bone interface.

The best tool for loosening a well-fixed acetabular component is a thin, spoon-like acetabular osteotome. This is used at the prosthesis-cement interface in an attempt to release the polyethylene from the cement bed, leaving the cement to be extracted later. In many instances, some cement is accessible around the periphery of the acetabulum. This cement should be removed first with the V-shaped osteotome to expose the interface between the component and the cement where the curved spoon-like osteotome is to be inserted. While using this osteotome, the surgeon must take care not to fracture the weakened acetabular rim. After the osteotome has been inserted several times, a moderately forceful twisting motion of the handle will often pop the component from the cement bed.

Often the component has protruded centrally and, although grossly loose, cannot be extracted easily without some means of attachment for application of an extraction force. The corkscrew, usually used for femoral head extraction in femoral neck fractures, has been used for this purpose, and devices that wedge on the inside of the polyethylene have also been used. A specific acetabular extractor has been designed that obtains purchase by threading into a hole previously drilled in the polyethylene. An important feature of the extractor is a mechanism for protecting the thread purchase on the polyethylene by transferring the force to the rim of the prosthetic acetabulum as it is rocked back and forth to loosen the remaining fixation points before final extraction. Because the acetabular extractor has a large mechanical advantage, care must be taken to avoid fracturing the acetabular rim (Fig. 3).

This acetabular extractor, when applied to metal-backed components, can be used to separate the polyethylene from the metal backing. A hole is drilled through the polyethylene down to the metal backing and the threads of the extractor are placed into the polyethylene. As the tip of the extractor passes through the other side of the polyethylene, it presses against the metal wall and forces the polyethylene out of the metal shell. Removal of the polyethylene from the metal shell exposes the prosthetic rim, which facilitates removal of the shell itself.

All-plastic components are usually relatively easy to extract from the cement bed. The new generation of metal-backed components can be more difficult to extract, because the cement often is fixed very firmly to

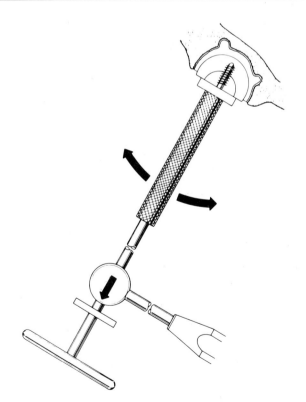

Fig. 3 Device for gaining purchase on a plastic acetabular component for extraction.

the metal backing. If cement has leaked through holes in the floor of the bony acetabulum and is firmly attached to the metal shell, forceful extraction of the metal shell, without first disrupting the cement-prosthesis interface, can contribute to acetabular bone stock damage. The curved spoon-like acetabular osteotome is the best instrument for gradually working around the metal shell, disrupting the cement-prosthesis interface.

After the metal-backed component has been loosened, special tools that fit in the screw holes and other irregularities in the interior of the prosthesis are used to apply force to further loosen it and pull it from the bony bed (Fig. 4). A controlled rocking motion of the prosthesis with these tools will complete the disruption of the prosthesis-bone interface and facilitate extraction.

Often the cement comes out with the acetabular component or can be easily removed. In other instances, the cement remains somewhat fixed to the bone and must be fragmented before removal. The V-shaped osteotome and the pointed osteotome are better than a regular osteotome for fragmenting this cement. Cement that is interdigitated with metal reinforcing mesh can be quite difficult to remove because the mesh prevents the cement from fragmenting. High-speed burrs can be used to thin cement when it cannot be easily fragmented. Mesh that has interdigitated with bone or soft tissue also can be difficult to remove. It is not necessary to remove cement that has leaked through the floor of the acetabulum unless sepsis has occurred. There is danger of injuring internal structures when manipulating such cement fragments. In some instances, the cement fragment is larger than the hole in the floor, because the cement polymerized after it exited through a relatively small hole in the bony floor. Cement in fixation holes is best removed by fragmenting it with the V-osteotomes.

After the acetabular cement has been removed, fibrous tissue must also be removed before reconstruction. Long-handled curettes are useful for scraping fibrous tissue from the bone. Angled curettes used in a scraping motion beginning in the central area and continuing toward the rim will facilitate fibrous tissue removal. At times, if the membrane is thick, it can be removed in one piece like a carpet. I usually complete the acetabular reconstruction before returning to the femur for cement removal and reconstruction.

Femoral Cement Removal

Cement must be removed from three parts of the femur, the proximal (metaphyseal) zone, the middle

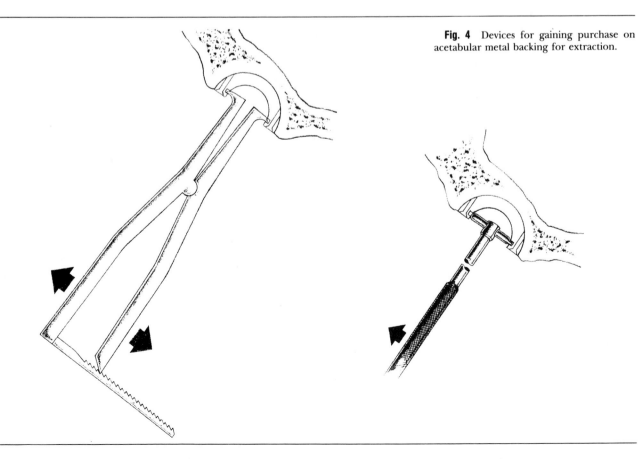

Fig. 4 Devices for gaining purchase on acetabular metal backing for extraction.

hollow zone, and the distal solid-plug zone. Proximal cement is relatively accessible and is easily removed. In the metaphyseal region of the femur, however, the cortex is thin and proximal cement removal may fracture this weak metaphyseal bone. I usually use osteotomes for cement removal, but the force used must be carefully calibrated and directed to preserve the metaphyseal bone integrity. If the cement is thinned first with a high-speed burr, less force will be needed for fragmentation.

If the trochanter has been removed, a trough should be created into the trochanteric bed, through the bone and cement fragments, to allow a direct view down the femoral canal. If the trochanter has not been removed, the surgeon must ensure that enough bone is removed laterally in the trochanteric area to permit direct sighting down the canal. Inadequate lateralization of the entrance hole to the femur will increase the risk of perforating the femoral canal in the lateral cortex as more distal cement is approached.

As the proximal cement is removed, the accompanying fibrous tissue and overhanging bony ledges that obstruct the view should be removed also. Careful cleaning of the metaphyseal region will make it easier to see into the more distal canal.

The second zone of cement is that part distal to the metaphyseal region down to the distal solid-plug zone. The cement in the middle zone is a hollow shell created by the femoral component. In some instances, this cement mantle is relatively intact and is loose in the bone. One can predict cement mantle loosening if the radiographs show a complete cement-bone radiolucency surrounding the cement. In some instances, with this preoperative radiograph finding, the cement will come up with the femoral component. In other cases, the femoral component will exit the cement cocoon, leaving an intact mantle of cement. If this mantle of cement can be grasped, the cement may exit as one large piece. One can at times obtain a purchase on this cement mantle by inserting a metal tap into the cement bed (Fig. 5). These taps are available in various sizes depending on the size of the space left by the original femoral prosthesis. Several turns of the sharp tap threads will cut into the polymethylmethacrylate, and a mallet can then be used to exert an extraction force on the instrument. At times the cement mantle will come up intact. At other times, only the most proximal cement is retrieved, in which case the tap can be used again to extract more cement from the distal cement bed. Cement that is interdigitated with the bone and, thus, is not grossly loose, can come out in small fragments with the tap technique. If the cement is not loose or if there are bony ledges that obstruct passage of the cement, excessive force may result in femoral fracture. A variation of the tap technique for cement removal has recently been introduced in which new cement is

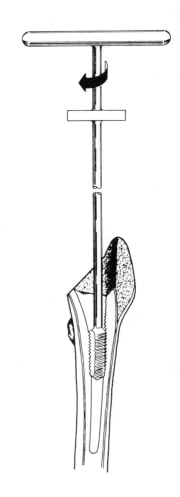

Fig. 5 Metal tap used to gain purchase on intact but loose mantle of cement for extraction.

injected into the prosthesis cement bed to gain purchase on the old cement for extraction.

If the tap technique is unsuccessful, I prefer to fragment the cement in the mid-region gradually, using hand tools. Special T-shaped and V-shaped osteotomes of various lengths will fragment the cement more effectively than will plain osteotomes. Placing the patient in the lateral position with the trochanteric osteotomy and with the hip rotated in external rotation will enable the surgeon to see down the canal more easily, and the operating room table can be raised, with the surgeon standing or sitting. A headlight can be used, but I prefer to aim the operating room light over my right shoulder. Further lighting of the canal can be done with fiberoptic attachments to osteotomes. I prefer to use a special irrigating lighted sucker (Fig. 6). With the push of a button, this versatile instrument irrigates the canal and cleans the blood from the cement, aiding cement identification. Simultaneously, the suction removes the fluid as the light illuminates the area. After the canal

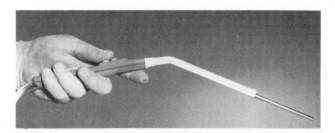

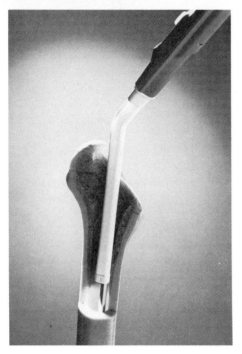

Fig. 6 Lighted irrigating sucker and its use in femoral canal.

has been cleaned of cement fragments and fibrous membrane, the next fragmentation step is planned and is carried out with the hand tools. Cement-grasping forceps are necessary for removing cement fragments as they are created. The cement forceps, which must not be too bulky to open in small bones, are used to pick up small pieces of cement that fall into the bed where the femoral component previously lay. Both short and long heavy-duty cement-grasping forceps should be used for larger cement fragments, in larger femurs, and when some mild force needs to be applied. All cement-grasping forceps will break if used too forcefully. The fibrous tissue in the canal must also be removed. This can be accomplished with curettes and hook-like reverse scrapers. If the cement-grasping forceps have a rongeur tip, it also is effective for removing soft tissue.

Although high-speed burr removal of cement has been advocated by many authorities,[10] the perforation rate has been high even in the hands of the most experienced surgeons.[13] Cement is harder than bone, and when a power burr, either high- or low-speed, is placed

between cement and bone, it will always preferentially cut the softer bone. Control of the high-speed burr far down the canal can be improved by using image intensification, as advocated by Turner and Emerson.[13] Uncontrolled perforation is decreased with this technique, but is not eliminated. Drawbacks of this image intensification technique are the necessity to wear lead aprons, the radiation exposure to the patient and the operating room personnel, the time needed to set up the equipment, and the possible contamination of the operating field by the equipment. Unless biplanar image intensification is available, the extremity must be constantly rotated in order to see the two different planes as the burr is advanced. Much practice is needed with this technique in order to minimize the perforation rate.

Sydney and Mallory[1] described a controlled perforation technique in which one or more anterior windows are made in the femur to help with orientation of the high-speed burr and to allow light into the femoral canal. The more proximal these windows, the less they will damage the bone integrity.[15] Any window created must have the tip of the new prosthesis at least two cortical diameters past it to prevent fracture from the stress riser created from the combination of the stem tip and the window. I do not routinely use controlled windows as described by Sydney and Mallory, but I agree that this procedure will speed cement removal and that controlled windows are much better than uncontrolled windows. With the high-speed burr, holes can be made inadvertently in regions difficult to expose and bypass with the stem tip, and such holes can at times even go unnoticed.

At present, a number of new techniques for cement removal are being evaluated. In a few centers, the laser is being used to remove the cement.[17-19] Problems with laser use include the inability to see clearly, creation of toxic gases, flaming, and bone damage. Also the instrument is expensive, as is the ultrasound-powered osteotome, another device being investigated for cement fragmentation. Various sheaths have also been used to guide saws and burrs during cement fragmentation, in the attempt to keep the working end of the instrument away from the bone.

Each case can present different problems for cement removal. Preoperative radiographic evaluation of the thickness and position of the cement relative to the canal and the stem will help in planning the attack on the cement mantle. When the bone is osteoporotic, much less force can be used to fragment the cement without bone fracture. Thick cement requires more force to crack than thin cement. If sharp osteotomes are used, less force will be necessary for cement fragmentation, making bone fracture less likely. It is more difficult to remove cement from small intramedullary canals and narrower osteotomes are needed.

As cement removal proceeds down the canal, the surgeon finds it more difficult to see clearly. Offset-handled osteotomes will facilitate cement removal at this point, because they keep the handle and the surgeon's hands out of the line of vision.[16] Having the working end of the osteotome at an angle is also useful when working far down the canal, because it allows a more aggressive presentation of the osteotome end into the cement-bone interface (Fig. 7, *left*).[16] This is necessary because the walls of the canal may limit the angle at which the instrument can be held in distal regions.

After all the hollow cement has been removed down to the tip of the prosthesis, there may remain a solid cement plug. These plugs vary in length and difficulty of removal. The high-speed burr and image intensification can be used to grind through this solid cement plug. Drill guides, made up of graduated hollow cones, can be used while drilling through the distal cement plug. The image intensifier or radiographs can assist with orientation of these. If a hole can be drilled through the distal cement plug, a hook can be placed through the hole to pull up the plug, or a tap can be

placed into the hole to gain purchase for extraction. Because a power tool inserted in the canal at this level is very difficult to control, perforation may occur.

I prefer trying to fragment the cement gradually using a combination of T-, V-, and X-ended osteotomes of a long length. This technique, which is laborious, requires practice and the use of the lighted irrigating sucker. Perforation and fracture can also occur with this technique.

In some instances, a hook can be placed between the cement plug and the femoral canal wall and pushed past the cement plug (Fig. 7, *center*). The preoperative radiographs will show where there is the most room between the cortex and the cement plug. A curved osteotome is then placed in this portion of the bone-cement interface, tapped gently, and wedged between the cement plug and the cortex, pushing the cement plug farther away from the cortex. If this is done forcefully, an explosion fracture of the cortex can occur. A thin curved hook is tapped into the channel created, pushed past the cement plug, turned 90 degrees, and

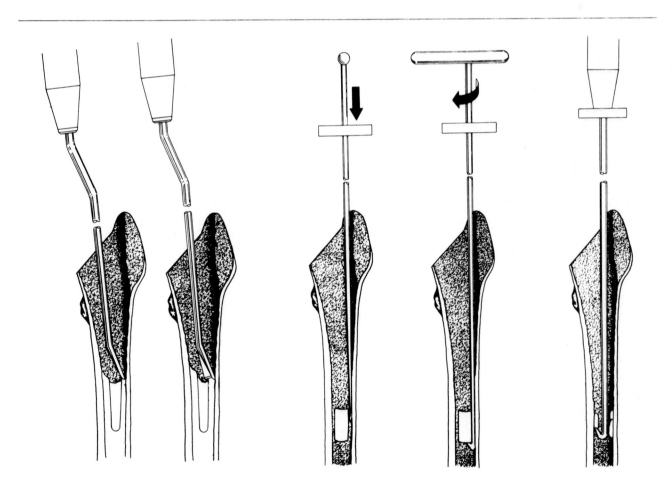

Fig. 7 Left, Long offset-handled osteotomes with angled ends for deep extraction of femoral cement. **Center,** Thin curved hook being used to extract distal cement plug. **Right,** Special curette being used to remove remaining plaques of cement and fibrous debris.

impacted up. At times, only portions of the cement will come up, but a thicker hook can be inserted into the larger passageway that has been created to pull up additional cement.

Canal Preparation

As the surgeon looks down the canal, various ledges will be seen, which may be defects in the endosteal cortex or ledges created by residual plaques of cement on the canal wall. An osteotome placed in the ledge will perforate if the ledge is a defect in the cortex. A hook-like curette inserted far down the canal and pulled proximally to scrape the canal walls, in contrast, is unlikely to cause perforation (Fig. 7, *right*). These instruments should first be used carefully, however, to probe the femoral canal walls for perforations. If the hook goes out a perforation in the cortex and the instrument then is pulled proximally with force, the bone can be damaged. Any obstruction felt by the hook is probably either a cement plaque or bone formed in response to loosening. The curette, used with controlled force, can remove this cement plug or bone with relative safety compared with approaching it from above with an osteotome. Thus, the final step of femoral canal preparation is to use these hook-like curettes repeatedly until the canal walls are completely clean of cement plaques, fibrous tissue, and bony ledges.[16]

In some cases, a bone ledge (pedestal) forms below the tip of the prosthesis. A high-speed burr under image intensification or drills under radiographic control can be used to remove this obstructing bone. I prefer to break through this bony distal plug by rotating a carefully oriented V-shaped osteotome back and forth to grind gradually through this bony obstruction. Orientation of this instrument is ascertained by the preoperative radiographs. After the distal canal has been entered, hooks can be pushed past the obstructed area. The hooks are brought proximally until they catch on the edges of remaining material and are then forcefully pulled up to remove the material. Inserting reamers into the canal before this bone obstruction has been removed may result in off-center reaming of the canal.

References

1. Sydney SV, Mallory TH: Controlled perforation: A safe method of cement removal from the femoral canal. *Clin Orthop* 1990; 253:168–172.
2. Wroblewski BM: Revision surgery in total hip arthroplasty: Surgical technique and results. *Clin Orthop* 1982;170:56–61.
3. Wroblewski BM: A method of management of the fractured stem in total hip replacement. *Clin Orthop* 1979;141:71–73.
4. Harris WH, White RE Jr, Mitchel S, et al: A new technique for removal of broken femoral stems in total hip replacement: A technical note. *J Bone Joint Surg* 1981;63A:843–845.
5. Miller ME, Davis ML, MacClean CR, et al: Radiation exposure and associated risks to operating-room personnel during use of fluoroscopic guidance for selected orthopaedic surgical procedures. *J Bone Joint Surg* 1983;65A:1–4.
6. Moreland JR, Marder R, Anspach WE Jr: The window technique for the removal of broken femoral stems in total hip replacement. *Clin Orthop* 1986;212:245–249.
7. Collis D, Dubrul W: The removal of fractured prosthetic components from medullary cavities: A new technique. *Contemp Orthop* 1984;8:61–65.
8. Mollan RAB, Watters PH, Luney W, et al: New technique for removal of broken femoral stems in THR. *Orthop Rev* 1983;12(2): 77–80.
9. Eftekhar NS: Rechannelization of cemented femur using a guide and drill system. *Clin Orthop* 1977;123:29–31.
10. Harris WH, Oh I: A new power tool for removal of methylmethacrylate from the femur. *Clin Orthop* 1978;132:53–54.
11. Razzano CD: Removal of methylmethacrylate in failed total hip arthroplasties: An improved technique. *Clin Orthop* 1977;126: 181–182.
12. Bierbaum BE: Acetabular revision arthroplasty, in Turner RH, Scheller AD Jr (eds): *Revision Total Hip Arthroplasty.* New York, Grune & Stratton, 1982, pp 119–120.
13. Turner RH, Emerson RH Jr: Femoral revision total hip arthroplasty, in Turner RH, Scheller AD Jr (eds): *Revision Total Hip Arthroplasty.* New York, Grune & Stratton, 1982, pp 75–106.
14. Müller ME: Total hip prostheses. *Clin Orthop* 1970;72:46–68.
15. Dennis DA, Dingman CA, Meglan DA, et al: Femoral cement removal in revision total hip arthroplasty: A biomechanical analysis. *Clin Orthop* 1987;220:142–147.
16. Stühmer G, Weber BG, Mathys R: Special instruments and prosthetic cups for the removal and replacement of a total hip prosthesis. *Arch Orthop Trauma Surg* 1979;93:191–199.
17. Sherk HH, Kollmer C: Revision arthroplasty using a CO_2 laser, in Sherk HH (ed): *Lasers in Orthopaedics.* Philadelphia, JB Lippincott, 1990, pp 75–103.
18. Booth RE, Gordon SL, Carney MD: Use of the CO_2 laser in revision hip surgery. *Contemp Orthop* 1987;15:17–22.
19. Choy DS, Kaminow IP, Kaplan M, et al: Experimental Nd:YAG laser disintegration of methylmethacrylate: Analysis of gaseous products. *Clin Orthop* 1987;215:287–288.
20. Eftekhar NS: *Principles of Total Hip Arthroplasty.* St. Louis, CV Mosby, 1978, pp 475–531.

Removal of Cementless Hip Implants

Harry E. Rubash, MD

Thomas Huddleston, MD

Anthony M. DiGioia III, MD

A major goal in revision total hip arthroplasty is to preserve sufficient bone stock to provide a suitable osseous bed for reimplantation of components. The technical problems associated with removing well-ingrown or press-fit prostheses are unique to revision surgery and provide a challenging task for the revision surgeon. Additional surgical strategies must be developed and refined to facilitate the removal of these cementless unstable and stable implants.

Situations that can require removal of a cementless implant include infection, component malposition and instability, and chronic thigh pain. Even in the presence of both acute and chronic joint sepsis, porous implants may become rigidly stabilized by bone or fibrous tissue and will prove difficult to remove. When dealing with stable malpositioned implants, the surgeon must analyze carefully the positions of the femoral and acetabular components, because at the time of surgery it may be necessary to remove one or both components. Conversely, a component with evidence of migration or subsidence is usually not bonded extensively by osseous integration but rather by a reactive fibrous membrane and may be easily removed. However, a femoral implant without radiographic evidence of migration or subsidence but that causes thigh pain is usually rigidly fixed to bone and difficult to remove.

In general, the information needed to develop an adequate plan for implant removal includes the type and geometry of the implant, the mode of fixation (press-fit or porous surface), the stability of the components, and the reaction of the bone to the implant (fibrous tissue or bone ingrowth). In addition, a careful analysis of serial radiographic findings is frequently helpful in predicting the level of difficulty that will be encountered during implant removal. For instance, a press-fit femoral component with expanding radiolucencies is often easily extracted by means of techniques developed for the removal of cemented components. Removal of a malpositioned porous component with evidence of bone ingrowth and no bone-implant radiolucencies represents a distinct challenge. However, because clinical and radiographic findings can be unreliable predictors of how difficult an implant will be to remove, it is often necessary to prepare for many different surgical contingencies.

Surgical Approach

The bone-implant interface must be completely visible during revision of uncemented components. The authors prefer to use a modified Hardinge[1] lateral approach to the hip[2] with a complete or near complete removal of the pseudocapsule. This approach gives adequate exposure and mobilization of the femur as well as the dome and both columns of the acetabulum. Osteotomy of the greater trochanter is usually not necessary. However, when the femur must be mobilized for a wider exposure of the acetabulum or when improved access to the femoral component is needed, a trochanteric osteotomy should be performed.

After adequate exposure of the hip and dislocation of the components, attention is directed first to the femoral component. If the femoral component is modular, the head is removed (Fig. 1). Various instruments are available to break the lock of the Morris taper. Frequently, repeated tapping on the implant neck or shoulder will cause the femoral head to vibrate free. If removal of the modular head provides adequate exposure to the acetabulum, the femoral stem is left in place until the acetabular reconstruction is completed. If the stem is grossly unstable, it can be removed and the femoral canal packed with a sponge to prevent bleeding. However, if the exposure is inadequate, then the femoral component must be removed first.

Acetabular Component

Before attempting to remove the acetabular component, the surgeon must expose the perimeter of the implant to bring the peripheral portion of the bone-implant interface into view. If the implant is not of modular design, the bone-implant interface is carefully disrupted to free the component from the underlying bone. This process is begun with straight and curved narrow osteotomes and is greatly facilitated by curved acetabular gouges (Fig. 2, *left*). The surgeon must take care to direct the cutting edge of the instrument toward the implant to avoid removing excessive bone from the soft cancellous part of the acetabulum. Countertraction, applied by grasping the component with pliers, a

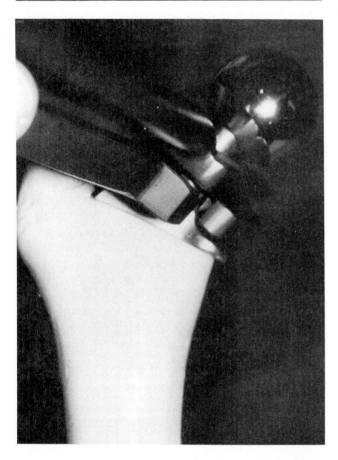

Fig. 1   Removal of a modular femoral head with an inclined plane.

vice grip, or a levering bar, may help expose the bone-implant interface after the periphery has been freed. Next, progressively wider and longer swan-neck gouges are inserted into the interface to break the fibrous or osseous bond (Fig. 2, *right*). The narrow 180-degree gouge can be used to free the medial and inferior bone before complete socket extraction. Great care must be taken to avoid forceful maneuvers, such as excessive levering against the acetabular columns or strong blows with the mallet, because these can have catastrophic consequences, with loss of bone stock or acetabular fracture. If the socket is well ingrown, its removal is a slow and painstaking process.

If the acetabular component is modular, the polyethylene insert is removed by prying at the implant-polyethylene interface with a narrow periosteal elevator. If screws are present beneath the polyethylene, the screw heads should be thoroughly cleaned to remove any fibrous tissue from the screw slot. A new screwdriver is carefully inserted into the head and great care is taken to avoid stripping the screw head. If the head is stripped, the screw head can be removed with the high-speed burr so that the socket can slide over the screw shank. After the socket has been extracted, the broken portion of the screw can be grasped with heavy needleholders or pliers and removed. If the shaft is broken at the surface of the bone, it can be removed using the ASIF technique—core around the screw threads and remove the shaft with a reverse-threaded instrument.[3] Before the socket is removed, the empty

Fig. 2   **Left,** A curved acetabular gouge is used to disrupt the interfaces between bone and the acetabulum. **Right,** Progressively wider and longer swan-neck gouges may be used to further disrupt the bony interface around the acetabulum.

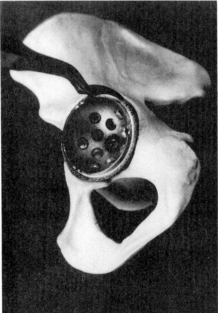 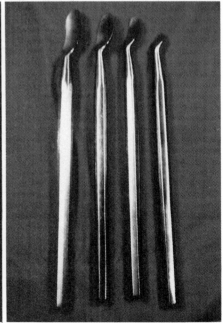

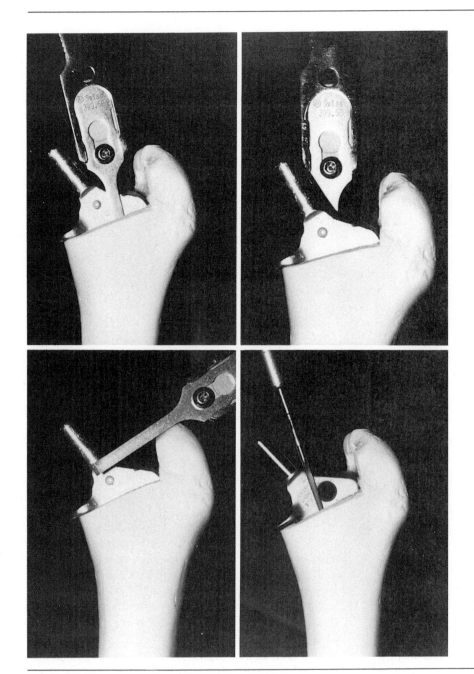

Fig. 3 Narrow, flexible osteotomes (**top left, top right,** and **bottom left**) and high-speed tools (**bottom right**) may be passed along all proximal surfaces of the femoral component. Care must be taken to clear the lateral shoulder of the implant.

screw holes in the socket must be freed of bone and fibrous tissue.

Acetabular components that do not have provisions for screws usually have some modifications in socket geometry, such as blunt plugs, peripheral spikes, or circumferential rims, that provide supplemental fixation and rotational control. With these socket modifications, the surgeon may encounter areas of ingrowth that are difficult to disrupt. Small osteotomes or cutting instruments specific for each socket may be available,

and the surgeon must be familiar with the techniques specific for each component.

The Femoral Component

It is essential that the proximal portion of the femoral component be exposed before starting implant revision. All fibrous or osseous tissue that has grown over the edges of the femoral stem or collar must be resected

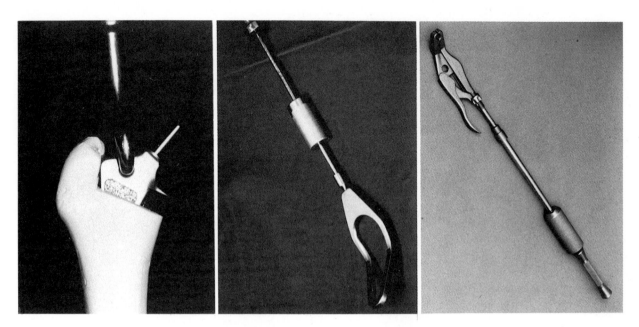

Fig. 4 **Left,** A hook is used to extract a femoral component with an extraction hole. **Center,** A loop may be used to extract nonmodular femoral components. **Right,** Specialized grip pliers with an attached slap hammer may be used to remove modular femoral components.

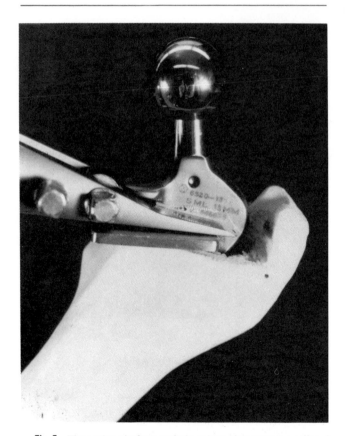

Fig. 5 The wedge-platform technique is used to extract a collared femoral component without an extraction hole.

to provide access to the anterior, posterior, medial, and lateral sides of the component. In particular, the medial aspect of the greater trochanter, near the shoulder of the implant, must be prepared to allow access to the most lateral aspect of the femoral stem and also to avoid fracturing the greater trochanter during stem extraction.

Removal of the cementless femoral component is facilitated by specialized instruments, such as narrow osteotomes, flexible osteotomes, high-speed cutting instruments, extraction hooks and loops, and specialized implant-specific stem removal sets. The bone-implant interface must be disrupted on all sides of the femoral stem. Narrow straight and flexible osteotomes are passed along the proximal aspects of the implant, taking great care to keep the cutting edge of the osteotome directed toward the implant to avoid loss of bone stock from the femoral canal or unplanned perforation or femoral fracture (Fig. 3). Usually the part of the bone-implant interface where the metal is porous is particularly tenacious and a high-speed tool with a small burr or long narrow cutting attachment is used to remove the cancellous bone adjacent to the metal (Fig. 3). When extracting collared stems with medial porous surfaces under the collar, the collar can be removed with a high-speed cutting wheel to gain access to the medial bone-implant interface.

When the femoral bone-implant interface has been disrupted, a disimpaction device is used to remove the stem from the femoral canal. A hook is used for those

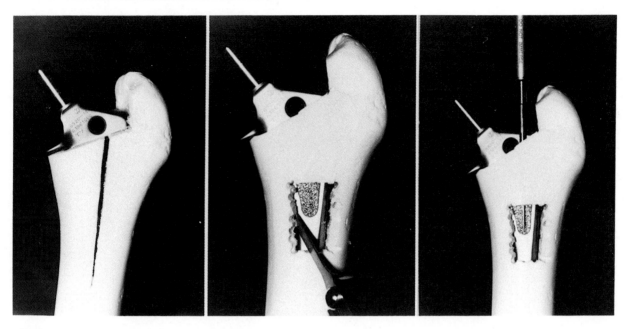

Fig. 6   **Left,** A longitudinal epiphysiotomy is performed on the anterior portion of the proximal femur. **Center** and **right,** A controlled proximal femoral window can be used to facilitate exposure to porous surfaces and to avoid inadvertent femoral fractures.

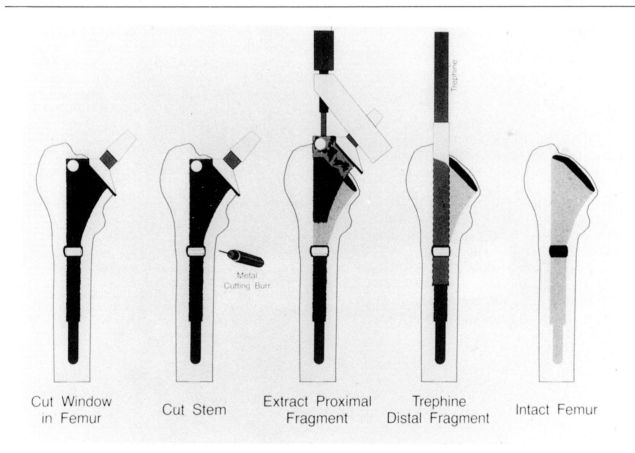

Cut Window in Femur

Cut Stem

Extract Proximal Fragment

Trephine Distal Fragment

Intact Femur

Fig. 7   A cementless removal technique described by Glassman and associates[4] is used to remove implants with extensive porous surfaces.

components with an extraction hole (Fig. 4, *left*). For those nonmodular components without an extraction hole, a loop may be placed around the neck of the component (Fig. 4, *center*). Alternatively, a carbide-tipped punch or blunt impactor can be used to apply a longitudinal extraction force to the implant. For modular components without a proximal hole, different strategies must be used. Specialized implant-specific pliers are available that grasp the femoral neck and proximal part of the implant and attach to a slap-hammer (Fig. 4, *right*). If the collar has been preserved, a mallet and impactor can be used to apply extraction forces via the collar. Alternatively, the wedge-platform technique can be used (D. Burke, D. O'Connor, and W. H. Harris, personal communication). In this system, a metal plate is placed under the collar and rests on the proximal femoral cortex. A wedge is then driven between the plate and the collar to apply extraction forces to the femoral stem (Fig. 5).

When disimpacting the femoral stem, it is essential that the force applied be colinear with the long axis of the stem. Any excessive varus or valgus force applied to the stem can fracture the femur. If the component does not move during attempted disimpaction, the surgeon should direct efforts toward a more complete disruption of the bone-implant interface. In addition, the medial aspect of the greater trochanter above the shoulder portion of a straight component should be rechecked to verify that enough bone has been resected to provide a clear path for the component to exit the femur.

If the implant cannot be removed because of inaccessible areas of porous surfaces, then an osteotomy of the femur can be done to gain access to these regions of the femur. This can be done by splitting the proximal femur over the implant (epiphysiotomy) (Fig. 6, *left*), which may also reduce the circumferential contact of the implant and bone.

Alternatively, a window can be cut in the femur over the area of interest (Fig. 6, *center* and *right*). These later techniques are infrequently used but are preferable to inadvertent femoral fractures. If an osteotomy is performed, the proximal femur must be further stabilized with circumferential cerclage wires before the new implant is inserted.

Some femoral components are particularly difficult to remove either because of peculiar surface geometries (long-stem implants) or distal porous coatings. If a long curved implant is to be removed, the surgeon must be aware of the rotational requirements of the implant. After disruption of implant interface, the surgeon may need to rotate the implant during removal. If an implant has distal porous surfaces that are ingrown with bone, this portion of the implant-bone interface is virtually inaccessible to the surgeon unless the femur is osteotomized. Glassman and associates[4] described a novel and useful technique for removing these implants (Fig. 7). First, the femoral component is transected at its midportion through a small femoral window. The techniques described above are used to remove the proximal half of the component. The distal portion of the implant is then removed with a series of hollow core reamers and broken-stem extraction instruments.

Conclusion

Removal of cementless implants is often very challenging and requires that the surgeon have the proper equipment, surgical exposure with clear access to the areas of prosthetic fixation to the femur and acetabulum, and patience. The surgeon must be prepared to deal with difficult reconstructive problems, such as acetabular or femoral fractures or previously unrecognized or created bony deficiencies. A thorough review of the preoperative radiographs, the implant type, the extraction tools available, and specialized instruments for implant removal will lead to a successful result.

References

1. Hardinge K: The direct lateral approach to the hip. *J Bone Joint Surg* 1982;64B:17–19.
2. Mallory TH: Preparation of the proximal femur in cementless total hip revision. *Clin Orthop* 1988;235:47–60.
3. Müller ME, Allgöwer M, Schneider R, et al: *Manual of Internal Fixation: Techniques Recommended by the AO Group.* Berlin, Springer-Verlag, 1979, p 158.
4. Glassman AH, Engh CA, Griffin WL: Removal of porous-coated femoral hip stems. Presented at the 57th Annual Meeting of the American Academy of Orthopaedic Surgeons, New Orleans, Feb 8–13, 1990.

Bone Grafting in Revision Total Hip Arthroplasty

Victor M. Goldberg, MD

Introduction

The demand for bone grafting procedures in revision total hip arthroplasty is expanding. Although various components are available that provide effective solutions for the problems encountered in revision total hip arthroplasty, there are many circumstances in which bone grafts must be used to correct bone deficiencies. The goal of any procedure must be to prevent further bone loss after the revision total hip replacement. This chapter reviews the basic biology of bone grafting and addresses some of the important issues of bone banking. A practical classification of bone loss of the pelvis and femur is included, along with coverage of the technical aspects of bone grafting in revision arthroplasty. Preliminary results of the outcome of these procedures are discussed.

Basic Biology

Bone grafts serve one or both of two main functions. They provide a source of osteogenesis and act as a mechanical support.[1-6] Osteogenesis refers to bone formation usually either from graft-derived cells or from the host cells that eventually populate the implant. Osteoinduction is another way in which bone grafts can function as a source of osteogenesis.[7,8] In osteoinduction, mesenchymal stem cells are induced to migrate into the bone graft and to differentiate into osteoblasts. This process, which is mediated by glycoproteins, such as bone morphogenetic protein, does not require that viable cells be present.[7] Bone morphogenetic protein activity has been demonstrated in frozen, freeze-dried, and decalcified allografts. Osteoconduction is a function of bone grafts whereby the grafts provide a trellis or scaffold for the ingrowth of new cells and blood vessels. This process ultimately leads to replacement of the bone graft by host-derived tissue. The process of remodeling to a weightbearing structure is prolonged and is enhanced by the strain environment of the graft.

The incorporation of bone grafts takes place in five stages, which are a continuum and are in dynamic equilibrium.[5-7] An inflammatory process is observed very early and is similar to that seen in any wounding process. Revascularization occurs rapidly and soon the osteoinductive process begins to provide precursor cells, which will become osteoblasts. The osteoconductive phase provides the graft with blood vessels and cells.

The last stage, which occurs over many years, results in a mechanically efficient structure. The condition of the host bed significantly affects the healing of bone grafts. The bone-graft environment is optimal when there is little fibrosis and adequate circulation, and when the graft is well fixed and is in close apposition to the host bone.

Cancellous autografts are an effective source for osteogenesis. They are rapidly revascularized and populated by host-derived osteoblast precursors (Fig. 1). Revascularization proceeds in conjunction with resorption by osteoclasts of the non-viable elements of the graft. Graft-derived factors such as bone morphogenetic protein are active during the first few weeks after implantation of the bone graft. These early events occur rapidly and are in dynamic equilibrium. Cancellous autografts are rapidly populated by osteoblasts that line the edges of dead trabeculae upon which osteoid and bone are deposited. This type of graft is usually completely replaced by new viable bone.

Because autografts are in short supply and are associated with other problems, such as donor-site morbidity, cancellous allografts are used in many cases. Fresh allografts have been shown to invoke an immune response, and humoral and cellular immune responses to donor histocompatibility antigens have been noted both experimentally and clinically following implantation of allogeneic bone.[9-14] In order to diminish the immune response and provide a more effective bone graft, processed allografts, which have been frozen or freeze-dried, have been shown to be an effective graft material.[10,11,14] Freeze-drying and freezing diminish the immune response while preserving osteoinduction and osteoconduction. Although the process of bone-graft incorporation observed with these grafts resembles that seen with cancellous autografts, these grafts do not provide active osteogenesis and are primarily useful as fillers for defects. These grafts may remain an admixture of viable and necrotic bone for a long period of time and may never be completely replaced by host bone (Fig. 2).

Cortical autografts provide structural support early in the incorporation sequence.[15-18] Although the pattern of incorporation is similar to that seen in cancellous autografts, the rate of revascularization is markedly slowed. Before vascular invasion can take place, osteoclastic resorption must occur. This bone resorption results in increased porosity, which is first seen at six weeks after cortical autograft implantation and

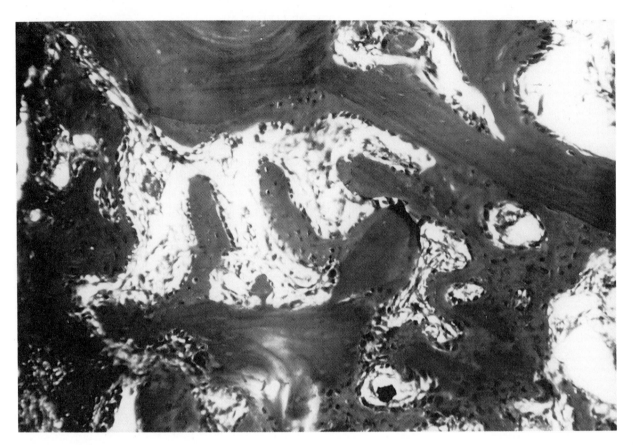

Fig. 1 Photomicrograph of a cancellous autograft three weeks after transplantation demonstrates active new bone formation (hematoxylin-eosin, × 25).

peaks six months after surgery. This has been shown experimentally to provide a weaker construct.[15] If formation and resorption become uncoupled, the graft may remain weaker and fail. Cortical grafts are never completely resorbed and usually remain an admixture of old and new bone for the lifetime of the graft (Fig. 3).

Because cortical autografts are in short supply, freeze-dried and frozen cortical allografts have been used as an effective graft material.[15,19] Although the immune response is markedly inhibited with these allografts, revascularization and resorption are often markedly impaired. New bone formation is usually delayed, compared with fresh autografts, and the graft may be significantly weaker for a prolonged period after transplantation. The slow process of incorporation predisposes the graft to such complications as fatigue fractures, graft-host nonunion or delayed union, and, occasionally, complete resorption. Other methods of preservation, including irradiation and the use of chemical agents, are still controversial and require additional investigation.[20-23]

Combination grafts are often advantageous, depending on the clinical circumstance. One may derive the

advantage of active early osteogenesis by the use of fresh autogenous cancellous bone and mechanical support by the use of cortical autografts or allografts. The clinical outcome of bone grafting depends a great deal on the choice of the graft. Factors that must be considered in choosing a graft are the general nutritional and metabolic status of the host, the specific characteristics of the host bed, the mechanical strains to which the graft will be subjected, and the availability of graft material.

Tissue Banking

Bone banks are required to provide an adequate supply of osteochondral grafts that are safe and have a predictable biologic outcome. Details of the principles and practical applications of bone banking are beyond the scope of this manuscript, but the reader is directed toward more complete sources.[21,24-26] However, some general principles of donor selection and tissue acquisition, preservation, storage, and record keeping will be discussed. The selection of appropriate donors is central to the development of a safe and efficient bank.

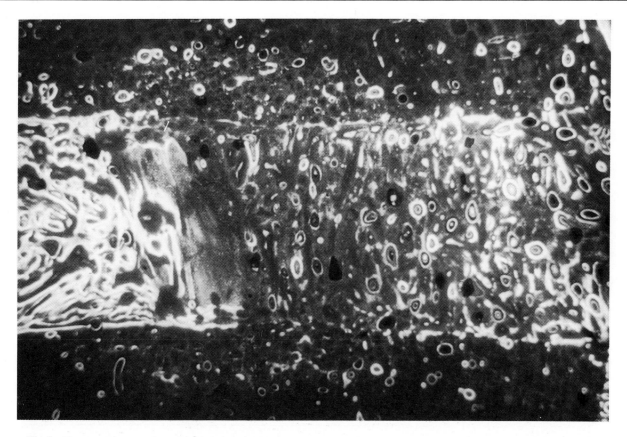

Fig. 2 Photomicrograph of a tetracycline-labeled frozen cancellous allograft nine months after transplantation shows a mixture of viable labeled bone and unlabeled necrotic bone.

The major concern is the elimination of transmissible diseases. Patients with high fevers, positive blood cultures, or viral diseases are not acceptable as donors. Other disorders, such as neurologic diseases, malignancies with metastasis, acquired immune deficiency syndrome (AIDS), history of or active hepatitis, connective tissue diseases, or any metabolic bone disease, are contraindications for donation of tissue. Members of any group that might be at high risk for AIDS should also be screened.

A sterile environment is usually used for procurement of most osteochondral tissue. If a nonsterile retrieval method is used, the sterilization technique must effectively eliminate microorganisms, while providing tissue with biologic and biomechanical functions that have not been compromised. The retrieved bones are cultured, washed in an antibiotic solution, and wrapped in sterile plastic bags. The two most widely used techniques for preserving and storing tissue are deep freezing to −80 C or freeze-drying. There is still controversy concerning the best preservation techniques for articular cartilage. Presently, cryopreservatives such as 10% glycerol and dimethyl sulfoxide are widely used. Other techniques that have been used for either sterilization or preservation include high doses of irradiation and

the use of such chemical agents as thimerosal. Chemosterilization of bone provides tissue that retains osteoinductive functions and may be stored for a prolonged period of time. Documentation of the selected donor, the results of laboratory tests, identification of the recipient, description of the surgical procedure, and appropriate follow-up information is important. The development of networking will improve the availability of tissue for clinical use.

Classification of Bone Loss

Acetabulum

There are many acetabular bone-loss classifications, including that provided by the Hip Committee of the American Academy of Orthopaedic Surgeons.[27] Acetabular defects may be described by anatomic sites. These defects include rim deficiencies, intra-acetabular cavitary defects, protrusion and perforation of the medial wall of the acetabulum, and combined segmental rim defects and cavitary intra-acetabular loss.

A functional classification that can be useful for determining the outcome of bone grafting describes bone loss of the pelvis by specific types. In type I, the medial

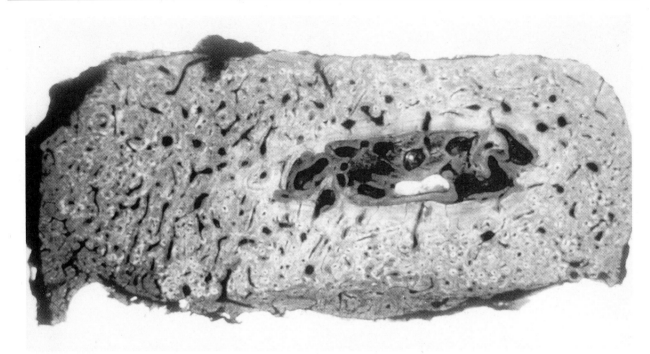

Fig. 3 Photomicrograph of a cortical autograft 11 months after transplantation shows marked resorption and a mixture of viable and nonviable bone (hematoxylin-eosin, × 25).

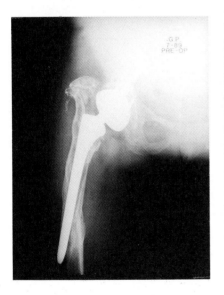 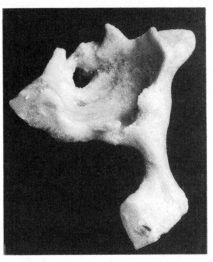 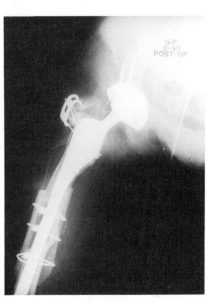

Fig. 4 **Left,** Preoperative radiograph demonstrating severe bone loss. **Center,** Three-dimensional computer-assisted tomogram of acetabulum demonstrating the severe bone loss. **Right,** Postoperative radiograph showing reconstructed socket.

wall and rim of the acetabular structure are intact, and only minimal bone thinning is seen. In type II, thinning of the acetabulum exceeds 50% and there is acetabular enlargement. Type III refers to bone loss of the superior, anterior, and/or posterior rims with central loss or a combination of these. In type IV, there is a massive acetabular collapse with complete inner wall loss and segmental rim defects with extensive bone loss.

Femur

Femoral defects can be classified using descriptive anatomy. This classification includes calcar and tro-

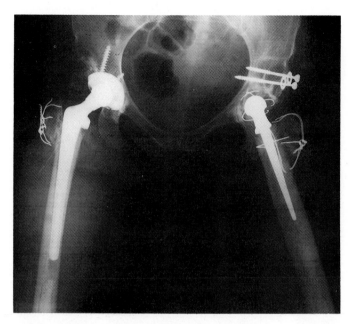
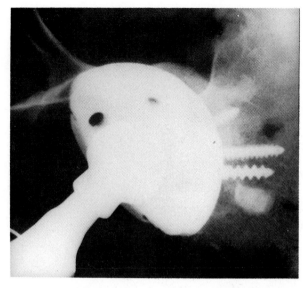

Fig. 5 Left, Preoperative radiograph of a failed acetabular component. **Right,** Reconstructed with morselized cancellous autograft and an uncemented cup.

chanteric deficiency, cortical thinning and/or perforation, segmental femoral loss, circumferential deficiency of the metaphyseal and proximal diaphysis, and, finally, total loss of the proximal femur. As described for the acetabulum, femoral bone loss can be defined by types. This classification also has importance in outcome studies of bone grafting in revision surgery. Type I describes the femur with less than 50% thinning of the proximal femoral cortex and an intact circumferential femoral canal. In type II, there is interface failure, thinning of the proximal femoral cortex of more than 50%, and canal enlargement, but the circumferential wall remains intact. In type III, there is posteromedial bone loss with an unstable proximal femoral canal. In type IV, there is complete proximal circumferential bone loss and/or large segmental diaphyseal defects.

Preoperative Planning

Preoperative bone stock assessment is critical for determining the surgical approach and for selecting proper components.[28] Preoperative planning should include complete medical and orthopaedic examination and, most important, appropriate radiographic assessment. The radiographic options include plain radiographs of the pelvis with the hips in neutral rotation and neutral abduction. Additional radiographic views include obliques of the pelvis, Judet views of the acetabulum, and true lateral radiographs of the involved

hip. Anteroposterior and rotational radiographs of the femur are important to determine femoral bone loss. Tomograms of the involved hip, as well as aspiration arthrograms, can be of help in defining bone loss. Computer-assisted tomography and computer-assisted modeling of the acetabulum and pelvis can be helpful in planning the surgical procedure and selecting the appropriate bone graft and components (Fig. 4).[29] Three-dimensional reconstruction of the proximal femur can aid the surgeon in planning the procedure and can be used for practice before the actual performance of the surgery. Adequate provisions for appropriate bone graft material must be made before the surgical procedure. The use of autografts requires preparation of both iliac crests at the time of surgery. Allografts should be available. Preoperative planning is critical in order to assess the structure of the acetabulum and the size of the bone graft required. In the femur, the quality of bone is determined, as well as the size and shape of the canal and the presence or absence of cortical defects. The outcome of bone grafting in revision total hip arthroplasty is significantly influenced by adequate preoperative planning.

Technical Aspects of Bone Grafting

Specific requirements for bone grafting in revision arthroplasty should be assessed preoperatively. Adequate sources of bone, both autogenous and allogeneic, should be available. Autogenous bone-graft material

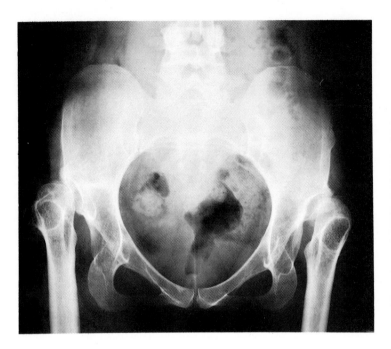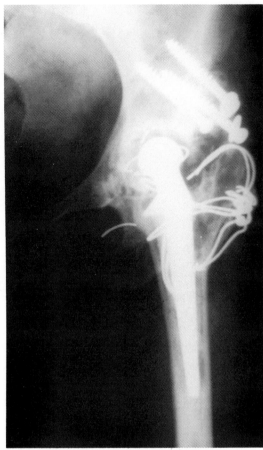

Fig. 6 **Left,** Preoperative radiograph of a deficient acetabulum. **Right,** Reconstruction with a bulk femoral head frozen allograft.

Table 1
Femoral and acetabular bone loss typing vs Harris hip score.*

Type	No. of Hips	Preoperative Average	Postoperative Average
Femoral			
I	7	39	93
II	23	51	83
III	23	46	80
IV	3	36	78
Acetabular			
I	14	44	84
II	18	49	83
III	7	39	76
IV	3	27	64

*Follow-up was 18 months to six years with an average follow-up of 42 months.

may be obtained locally from the greater trochanteric and lesser trochanteric beds; from the anterior and posterior iliac crests or from the fibula and/or tibia when cortical bone is required. Bone-graft material may be used either as a particulate or in bulk. The type and extent of bone grafting depends on the requirements of the reconstruction. Although there are some general technical principles, each individual case is different.

However, the application of basic principles can provide solutions to individual problems.

Cavitary bone defects of the pelvis can usually be managed by the use of autogenous, cancellous bone that has been morselized (Fig. 5).[30-35] These grafts can be used alone or mixed with cancellous allograft to fill intra-acetabular defects. Usually the defect is self-contained and the area affected does not provide signifi-

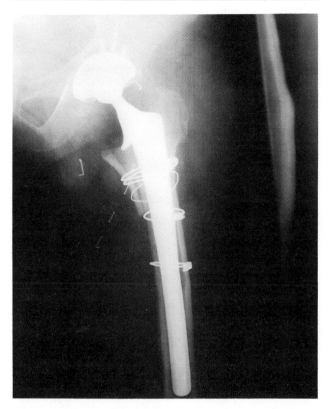

Fig. 7 Radiograph of a frozen cortical allograft used to reconstruct a proximal femoral cortical defect. A long-stem, uncemented femoral component has been used.

cant structural support. Enhancement of osteogenesis may be provided by the use of bone marrow from the reamings or pelvis.

Central wall defects of the acetabulum can be managed by full-thickness autogenous iliac crest grafts.[35] These grafts can be fixed if necessary with such internal fixation devices as pelvic reconstruction plates. Central wall defects of the acetabulum can also be reconstructed using cancellous strips. Major central or superior intra-acetabular defects where structural support is important can be reconstituted with the patient's own femoral head or, if that is not available, allogeneic bone. In most circumstances, when significant segmental loss of either the anterior or posterior pillars is present, and autogenous bone is not available in adequate volume, allogeneic bone must be used. Femoral heads provide excellent material for reconstruction of these rim or major intra-articular defects. They usually are used in bulk and are fixed to the pelvis with appropriate instrumentation (Fig. 6). Significant structural loss of the acetabulum can be corrected by the use of allografts of the distal femoral condyles or proximal tibia. Secure fixation of these grafts is important to ensure the best environment for incorporation.

If noncemented components are used to reconstruct the acetabulum, a viable, bleeding surface must be provided to ensure effective bone ingrowth. Although there are no quantitative studies to indicate the extent of viable bone necessary to support bone ingrowth, clinical experience suggests that if the viable bleeding bone surface area is less than 50%, the outcome will be compromised.

Femoral defects can pose significant technical challenges.[36-40] Cavitary loss can be managed by cancellous morselized autografts or, if these are not available, processed cancellous allografts can be used. In the latter instance, this material acts only as a filler and does not provide active osteogenesis. In a manner similar to that described for acetabular defects, autologous bone marrow can be mixed with the graft in order to provide active induction factors and to serve as a source for osteoblast precursors. Femoral head autografts, when available, or allografts can be used for reconstitution of the calcar or for trochanteric enhancement. Cortical defects of the femur can be reconstructed with cortical onlay grafts. Usually allografts are necessary and, because they must provide some structural support, frozen material is a superior implant. These struts should cover at least one half of the surface of the recipient bone and be securely fixed. When there is circumferential proximal loss of the femur, proximal femoral allografts must be used. These are usually integrated with long-stem implants and must be fixed securely to the host distal femur (Fig. 7).

Femoral components can be either cemented or cementless. However, if one expects bone ingrowth to provide long-term fixation, a bleeding, viable bone surface is necessary. Also, the fate of large, bulk, nonvascularized autogenous or allogeneic cortical grafts is controversial. As previously discussed, these grafts undergo a phase of revascularization that increases their porosity and weakens them structurally. Experimental data suggest that resorption is a major component of the biology of these grafts and predisposes them to long-term failure.[41]

Results of Grafting Techniques

Because each patient has unique problems, it is difficult to predict long-term results. However, some general statements can be made in regard to functional outcomes relative to the bone-loss classifications of the femur and acetabulum outlined previously. Table 1 provides data from 98 hips in which either femoral or acetabular bone grafting was necessary during a revision procedure. The average follow-up of these hips was 42 months with a range from 18 months to six years. The more severe the bone loss, the more compromised the functional outcome as determined by the Harris Hip Score. Bulk grafts that are not subjected to weightbearing tend to resorb as revascularization proceeds. Long-term follow-up is necessary in order to define the role of massive autogenous or allogeneic bone grafts in reconstructing skeletal defects in revision total hip arthroplasty.

A clear understanding of the basic science of bone grafting, extensive preoperative planning, and effective technique in the use of each specific bone graft are critical to maximize successful correction of skeletal loss in revision total hip arthroplasty. Future directions in this field will use alternative biomaterials to reconstruct skeletal defects. These materials include bone substitutes, such as hydroxyapatite, and osteoinductive agents, such as bone morphogenetic protein. Other molecular, cellular, and soluble factor technologies will also help ensure a long-term successful outcome.

References

1. Abbott LC: The use of iliac bone in the treatment of ununited fractures, in Thomson JEM (ed): American Academy of Orthopaedic Surgeons *Instructional Course Lectures, II.* Ann Arbor, JW Edwards, 1944, pp 13–22.

2. Abbott LC, Schottstaedt ER, Saunders JB, et al: The evaluation of cortical and cancellous bone as grafting material: A clinical and experimental study. *J Bone Joint Surg* 1947;29:381–414.

3. Bonfiglio M: Repair of bone-transplant fractures. *J Bone Joint Surg* 1958;40A:446–456.

4. Burwell RG, Gowland G: Studies in the transplantation of bone: I. Assessment of antigenicity. Serological studies. *J Bone Joint Surg* 1961;43B:814–819.

5. Burwell RG: Osteogenesis in cancellous bone grafts: Considered in terms of cellular changes, basic mechanisms and the perspective of growth-control and its possible aberrations. *Clin Orthop* 1965;40:35–47.

6. Goldberg VM, Stevenson S: Natural history of autografts and allografts. *Clin Orthop* 1987;225:7–16.

7. Urist MR: Practical applications of basic research on bone graft physiology, in American Academy of Orthopaedic Surgeons *Instructional Course Lectures, XXV.* St. Louis, CV Mosby, 1976, pp 1–26.

8. Urist MR: Bone transplants and implants, in Urist MR (ed): *Fundamental and Clinical Bone Physiology.* Philadelphia, JB Lippincott, 1980, pp 331–368.

9. Bonfiglio M, Jeter WS: Immunological responses to bone. *Clin Orthop* 1972;87:19–27.

10. Bos GD, Goldberg VM, Zika JM, et al: Immune responses of rats to frozen bone allografts. *J Bone Joint Surg* 1983;65A:239–246.

11. Burwell RG: Studies in the transplantation of bone: V. The capacity of fresh and treated homografts of bone to evoke transplantation immunity. *J Bone Joint Surg* 1963;45B:386–401.

12. Friedlaender GE: The antigenicity of preserved allografts. *Transplant Proc* 1976;8(suppl 1):195–200.

13. Elves MW: Newer knowledge of the immunology of bone and cartilage. *Clin Orthop* 1976;120:232–259.

14. Friedlaender GE, Strong DM, Sell KW: Studies on the antigenicity of bone: I. Freeze-dried and deep-frozen bone allografts in rabbits. *J Bone Joint Surg* 1976;58A:854–858.

15. Burchardt H, Jones H, Glowczewskie F, et al: Freeze-dried allogeneic segmental cortical-bone grafts in dogs. *J Bone Joint Surg* 1978;60A:1082–1090.

16. Lance EM: Some observations on bone graft technology. *Clin Orthop* 1985;200:114–124.

17. Ottolenghi CE: Massive osteo and osteo-articular bone grafts: Technic and results of 62 cases. *Clin Orthop* 1972;87:156–164.

18. Springfield DS: Massive autogenous bone grafts. *Orthop Clin North Am* 1987;18:249–256.

19. Makley JT: The use of allografts to reconstruct intercalary defects of long bones. *Clin Orthop* 1985;197:58–75.

20. Bright RW, Smarsh JD, Gambill VM: Sterilization of human bone by irradiation, in Friedlaender GE, Mankin HJ, Sell KW (eds): *Osteochondral Allografts: Biology, Banking, and Clinical Applications.* Boston, Little Brown, 1983, pp 223–232.

21. Tomford WW, Mankin HJ, Friedlaender GE, et al: Methods of banking bone and cartilage for allograft transplantation. *Orthop Clin North Am* 1987;18:241–247.

22. Urist MR, Hernandez A: Excitation transfer in bone: Deleterious effects of cobalt 60 radiation-sterilization of bank bone. *Arch Surg* 1974;109:486–493.

23. Urist MR, Mikulski A, Boyd SD: A chemosterilized antigen-extracted autodigested alloimplant for bone banks. *Arch Surg* 1975;110:416–428.

24. Friedlaender GE: Guidelines for banking osteochandral allografts, in Friedlaender GE, Mankin HJ, Sell KW (eds): *Osteochandral Allografts: Biology, Banking, and Clinical Applications.* Boston, Little Brown, 1983, pp 177–180.

25. Tomford WW, Doppelt SH, Mankin HJ, et al: 1983 bone bank procedures. *Clin Orthop* 1983;174:15–21.

26. Tomford WW, Ploetz JE, Mankin HJ: Bone allografts of femoral heads: Procurement and storage. *J Bone Joint Surg* 1986;68A:534–537.

27. D'Antonio JA, Capello WN, Borden LS, et al: Classification and management of acetabular abnormalities in total hip arthroplasty. *Clin Orthop* 1989;243:126–137.

28. O'Neill DA, Harris WH: Failed total hip replacement: Assessment by plain radiographs, arthrograms, and aspiration of the hip joint. *J Bone Joint Surg* 1984;66A:540–546.

29. Murphy SB, Kijewski PK, Simon SR, et al: Computer-aided simulation, analysis, and design in orthopedic surgery. *Orthop Clin North Am* 1986;17:637–649.

30. Trancik TM, Stulberg BN, Wilde AH, et al: Allograft reconstruction of the acetabulum during revision total hip arthroplasty: Clinical, radiographic, and scintigraphic assessment of the results. *J Bone Joint Surg* 1986;68A:527–533.

31. Jasty M, Harris WH: Total hip reconstruction using frozen femoral head allografts in patients with acetabular bone loss. *Orthop Clin North Am* 1987;18:291–299.

32. McCollum DE, Nunley JA, Harrelson JM: Bone-grafting in total hip replacement for acetabular protrusion. *J Bone Joint Surg* 1980;62A:1065–1073.

33. Heywood AW: Arthroplasty with a solid bone graft for protrusio acetabuli. *J Bone Joint Surg* 1980;62B:332–336.

34. Mendes DG, Roffman M, Silbermann M: Reconstruction of the acetabular wall with bone graft in arthroplasty of the hip. *Clin Orthop* 1984;186:29–37.

35. Cameron HU: Four methods for reconstruction of acetabular floor deficiencies. *Orthop Rev* 1985;14:71–75.

36. Bargar WL, Paul HA, Merritt K, et al: The calcar bone graft. *Clin Orthop* 1986;202:269–277.

37. Sim FH, Chao EY: Hip salvage by proximal femoral replacement. *J Bone Joint Surg* 1981;63A:1228–1239.

38. McGann W, Mankin HJ, Harris WH: Massive allografting for severe failed total hip replacement. *J Bone Joint Surg* 1986;68A:4–12.

39. Gross AE, Lavoie MV, McDermott P, et al: The use of allograft bone in revision of total hip arthroplasty. *Clin Orthop* 1985;197:115–122.

40. Head WC, Malinin TI, Berklacich F: Freeze-dried proximal femur allografts in revision total hip arthroplasty: A preliminary report. *Clin Orthop* 1987;215:109–121.

41. Goldberg VM, Shaffer JW, Field G, et al: Biology of vascularized bone grafts. *Orthop Clin North Am* 1987;18:197–205.

Results and Experiences With Cemented Revision Total Hip Arthroplasty

John J. Callaghan, MD

Introduction

The number of revision total hip arthroplasties performed in this country has markedly increased over the last 15 years. At The Hospital for Special Surgery fewer than 70 revisions had been performed before 1979; by 1987, 130 were being performed annually, and the number continues to rise.

When discussing revision hip arthroplasty it is important to use the correct terminology. The definition of a revision total hip replacement should be the replacement of a hip in which a previous total hip replacement has undergone mechanical failure (that is, aseptic loosening, disabling dislocation, or component failure). This definition should be distinguished from reimplantation total hip arthroplasty—the replacement of an infected hip prosthesis with another total hip prosthesis—and conversion arthroplasty—the replacement of an endoprosthesis, surface replacement, or cup prosthesis with a total hip replacement. The future will see more terminologic confusion, because revision arthroplasty will include exchange of a cemented prosthesis for another cemented prosthesis, a cemented prosthesis for an uncemented prosthesis, an uncemented prosthesis for another uncemented prosthesis, or an uncemented prosthesis for a cemented prosthesis.

At present, the literature concerning cemented revision total hip arthroplasty is limited to cemented failures replaced by other cemented prostheses. This is the case in all of the studies examined in this chapter.

Results of Cemented Revision Total Hip Arthroplasty

The early results of cemented total hip revisions have been well documented. Four large series included the initial experience at The Hospital for Special Surgery and Robert B. Brigham reported by Pellicci and associates,[1] the UCLA experience reported by Amstutz and associates,[2] the Mayo Clinic experience reported by Kavanagh and associates,[3] and the later experience at The Hospital for Special Surgery reported by Callaghan and associates.[4] Results of these series are summarized in Table 1.

The average follow-up times in the reported series ranged from 2.1 to 4.5 years. According to the criteria used in each study, good or excellent results were reported in 52% to 66% of the cases. Loosening was demonstrated radiographically in 12% to 44% of cases, with

4% to 9% rerevision rates. Femoral fractures occurred in 2.1% to 7.8% of cases, and dislocations occurred in 8.2% to 10.6% of cases. Infection rates (1.2% to 3.4%) were at least double those of primary replacement at the respective institutions. Sciatic nerve palsies occurred in as many as 7%. One should remember, however, that these are all multiple-surgeon studies, and the cases were performed early in the learning curve of this challenging procedure.

The long-term results of revision total hip arthroplasty, documented by Pellicci and associates,[5] and more recently by Marti and associates,[6] are summarized in Table 2. The two series differed in the age of the patients at the time of revision (60 years in Pellicci and associates' series and 71 years in Marti and associates' series). This may account for the differences in revision rates of 19% and 6.7%, respectively. The total loosening rate, however, was more comparable—29% versus 20%, respectively. These results led Pellicci and associates to conclude that, although the early results of revision cemented total hip arthroplasty can be comparable to those of primary arthroplasty, the long-term durability of the result seems to be substantially less. More importantly, the long-term results of revision make all orthopaedic surgeons realize that the best opportunity to obtain a good result is at the initial surgery.

In addition to the early and long-term results of cemented revision hip arthroplasty, the results of multiple cemented revisions have been studied. Kavanagh and Fitzgerald[7] reported that, after an average follow-up of three years, only half of the patients have satisfactory results, with acetabular loosening in 24% and femoral loosening in 31%.

How To Improve the Results of Cemented Revision

Having had the opportunity to review two of the four series of revisions referred to in this chapter, I was able to appreciate the difficult learning curve associated with revision arthroplasty. The remainder of this chapter will address ways of improving the results of revision in general and cemented revision specifically. The results reported in the literature have highlighted the areas of concern in revision surgery—loosening, femoral fractures, infection, dislocation, nerve palsy, and trochanteric problems.

Table 1
Early results of revision cemented total hip arthroplasty

Results	Studies			
	Pellicci et al[1]	Amstutz et al[2]	Kavanagh et al[3]	Callaghan et al[4]
Number	110	66	166	139
Average follow-up (yr)	3.4	2.1	4.5	3.6
Excellent or good results (%)	60	—	52	66
Loosening (%)	13.6	29	20; 44*	12
Rerevision (%)	5.4	9.0	6.0	4.3
Femoral fracture (%)	—	6.0	7.8	2.1
Femoral perforation (%)	—	—	4	13
Dislocation (%)	—	10.6	9.0	8.2
Infection (%)	1.8	1.5	1.2	3.4
Nerve palsy (%)	—	7.0	0.5	0.7
Trochanteric problems (%)	12.7	7.6	6.6	6.2

*Percentages are given for both acetabular (20%) and femoral (44%) loosening.

Table 2
Long-term results of revision cemented total hip arthroplasty

Data	Pellicci et al[5]	Marti et al[6]
Hips	99	60
Average follow-up (yr)	8.1	8.9
Average age at revision (yr)	60	71
Rerevision (%)	19	6.7
Loosening (%)	29	20

Improving Loosening Rates

If cement is to be used in revision surgery, loosening rates must be reduced. As proposed by Marti and associates,[6] patient selection can be an important determinant. Older patients and patients with good quality of bone at the time of revision are the optimal candidates. My colleagues and I have demonstrated that the results of revision surgery are significantly better in patients with better bone quality at the time of revision.[4] In performing the surgical procedure, careful preparation of the sclerotic bone bed, including removal of the "neocortex" (the sclerotic rim of the bone at the margin of the membrane produced by the debris from loosening), is imperative. Reamers and high-speed burrs are useful in obtaining an adequate bone bed after the cement is removed. Stiff (cobalt-chromium) stems with large cross-sectional diameters proximally, smooth medial surfaces, and slightly longer lengths offer better protection for the cement.[8] Metal-backed acetabular components[9,10] positioned inferiorly, medially, and anteriorly (at the anatomic position) also help, by decreasing the joint reaction forces.[11] My colleagues and I documented significantly better clinical results when the hip center was brought to the anatomic location and when slightly longer stems were used.[4] Bone grafting medial wall defects can also produce long-term durability,[12,13] but it remains controversial whether structurally superior weightbearing bone grafts are durable.[14] Pressurization of cement (which may require

the use of three or four packs of cement) by applying a distal plug and using a pressurizing gun has demonstrated markedly improved femoral-side cemented revision results, with only 2% femoral revisions after a follow-up of at least five years.[15] Decreasing porosity of the cement by centrifugation[16] or vacuum mixing[17] may also help lower loosening rates.

Prevention and Treatment of Femoral Fractures

As discussed in other chapters in this section, removal of cement without violating the femoral cortex is imperative in preventing femoral fractures. The surgeon should be aware that most perforations occur anteriorly or laterally because of the natural femoral bow.[4] When perforations do occur, they should be bypassed, with the femoral stem extending at least 1.5 to three outer shaft diameters of the femur distal to the defect.[4,18] If fractures occur, they need anatomic reduction to avoid cement interdigitation between fractured fragments. Bone grafting is also essential, because the endosteal and periosteal blood supply has been compromised.

Prevention of Infection

Infection will always be relatively high during or after revision arthroplasty because of the poor condition of the previously violated tissues and the prolonged surgical times. However, potential ways of decreasing infection rates include identifying indolent infections at the time of surgery and using antibiotic-impregnated cement. Aspiration should be performed preoperatively, antibiotics should be withheld until intraoperative cultures are obtained, and multiple frozen and permanent tissue specimens and cultures should be obtained.[4,7] These steps will help identify any indolent infection as the cause of loosening. Lynch and associates[19] have been able to reduce their infection rate from 3.5% to 0.81% by using gentamicin-impregnated cement in revisions performed for aseptic loosening.

Avoidance of Dislocation

Dislocation rates of 8% to 10% are reported after revision hip replacement. Soft-tissue tensioning problems may account for a number of these dislocations. It is important to have available calcar-type replacements and to use them when needed to restore limb length. More importantly, lateral and distal advancement of the greater trochanter can prevent tissue-tensioning problems. Even when this approach is not used during revision, osteotomy of the trochanter and advancement should be considered if a tissue tensioning problem exists after reduction of the components. If concern over tissue tensioning exists or if the patient is noncompliant with dislocation precautions, bracing or reverse traction can be used.[20]

Avoidance of Sciatic Nerve Palsy

The length of revision surgery alone can lead to sciatic nerve palsy with prolonged retraction. If the leg is brought over the table during the revision surgery, the foot should be placed on a stool or some other measure taken to prevent the leg from hanging in a dependent fashion. The limb should be positioned so that the hip is in extension and the knee is in flexion when possible. Adequate exposure with thorough capsular excision prevents extensive retraction of the posterior soft tissues.

Reduction of Trochanteric Problems

Although the transtrochanteric approach has been abandoned by some surgeons who perform revision total hip arthroplasty, the procedure is still used by many because of the excellent exposure and the ability to improve soft-tissue tensioning by advancing the trochanter. Between the first and second series[4] of revisions that my colleagues and I reported, we reduced our trochanteric problems by 50% by using a three-wire rather than two-wire reattachment technique. Schutzer and Harris[21] studied the use of a four-wire technique with supplemental wire mesh and reported a marked improvement in results. This technique, along with six weeks of brace immobilization in cases with poor trochanteric beds, has markedly reduced trochanteric problems.

In conclusion, elderly patients with reasonably good bone quality at the time of revision can perform well functionally with cemented total hip revisions if the principles of revision surgery outlined above are followed meticulously.

References

1. Pellicci PM, Wilson PD Jr, Sledge CB, et al: Revision of total hip arthroplasty. *Clin Orthop* 1982;170:34–41.

2. Amstutz HC, Ma SM, Jinnah RH, et al: Revision aseptic loose total hip arthroplasties. *Clin Orthop* 1982;170:21–33.

3. Kavanagh BF, Ilstrup DM, Fitzgerald RH Jr: Revision total hip arthroplasty. *J Bone Joint Surg* 1985;67A:517–526.

4. Callaghan JJ, Salvati EA, Pellicci PM, et al: Results of revision for mechanical failure after cemented total hip replacement, 1979 to 1982: A two to five-year follow-up. *J Bone Joint Surg* 1985;67A:1074–1085.

5. Pellicci PM, Wilson PD Jr, Sledge CB, et al: Long-term results of revision total hip replacement: A follow-up report. *J Bone Joint Surg* 1985;67A:513–516.

6. Marti RK, Schuller HM, Besselaar PP, et al: Results of revision of hip arthroplasty with cement: A five to fourteen-year follow-up study. *J Bone Joint Surg* 1990;72A:346–354.

7. Kavanagh BF, Fitzgerald RH Jr: Multiple revisions for failed total hip arthroplasty not associated with infection. *J Bone Joint Surg* 1987;69A:1144–1149.

8. Crowninshield RD, Brand RA, Johnston RC, et al: An analysis of femoral component stem design in total hip arthroplasty. *J Bone Joint Surg* 1980;62A:68–78.

9. Pedersen DR, Crowninshield RD, Brand RA, et al: An axisymmetric model of acetabular components in total hip arthroplasty. *J Biomech* 1982;15:305–315.

10. Carter DR, Vasu R, Harris WH: Stress distributions in the acetabular region: II. Effects of cement thickness and metal backing of the total hip acetabular component. *J Biomech* 1982;15:165–170.

11. Johnston RC, Brand RA, Crowninshield RD: Reconstruction of the hip: A mathematical approach to determine optimum geometric relationships. *J Bone Joint Surg* 1979;61A:639–652.

12. McCollum DE, Nunley JA, Harrelson JM: Bone-grafting in total hip replacement for acetabular protrusion. *J Bone Joint Surg* 1980;62A:1065–1073.

13. Gates HS III, McCollum DE, Poletti SC, et al: Bone-grafting in total hip arthroplasty for protrusion acetabuli: A follow-up note. *J Bone Joint Surg* 1990;72A:248–251.

14. Gerber SD, Harris WH: Femoral head autografting to augment acetabular deficiency in patients requiring total hip replacement: A minimum five-year and an average seven-year follow-up study. *J Bone Joint Surg* 1986;68A:1241–1248.

15. Rubash HE, Harris WH: Revision of nonseptic, loose, cemented femoral components using modern cementing techniques. *J Arthroplasty* 1988;3:241–248.

16. Burke DW, Gates EI, Harris WH: Centrifugation as a method of improving tensile and fatigue properties of acrylic bone cement. *J Bone Joint Surg* 1984;66A:1265–1273.

17. Wixson RL, Lautenschlager EP, Novak MA: Vacuum mixing of acrylic bone cement. *J Arthroplasty* 1987;2:141–149.

18. Panjabi MM, Trumble T, Hult JE, et al: Effect of femoral stem length on stress raisers associated with revision hip arthroplasty. *J Orthop Res* 1985;3:447–455.

19. Lynch M, Esser MP, Shelley P, et al: Deep infection in Charnley low-friction arthroplasty: Comparison of plain and gentamicin-loaded cement. *J Bone Joint Surg* 1987;69B:355–360.

20. Davey JR, Harris WH: Reverse skeletal traction for instability following revision total hip arthroplasty: A report of two cases. *Clin Orthop* 1988;234:110–114.

21. Schutzer SF, Harris WH: Trochanteric osteotomy for revision total hip arthroplasty: 97% union rate using a comprehensive approach. *Clin Orthop* 1988;227:172–183.

Cementless Revision of Failed Total Hip Replacement: An Update

Charles A. Engh, MD

Andrew H. Glassman, MD

Introduction

Although modifications in cementing technique have dramatically decreased the incidence of femoral component aseptic loosening in primary total hip replacement,[1-5] there is to date no evidence demonstrating similar benefits in revision surgery. Published results of revision arthroplasty using cement uniformly dem-

onstrate failure from aseptic loosening at a rate exceeding that reported for primary arthroplasty.[6,7] Moreover, when longer follow-up has been available, continued deterioration has been the rule.[8]

For the past ten years, all revisions of failed cemented total hip stems performed at our institute have used porous-coated femoral components implanted without cement. Cementless techniques have been used in ace-

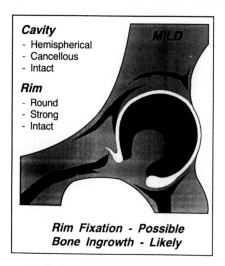
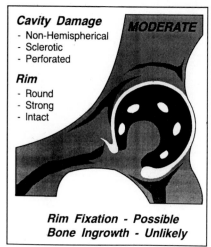
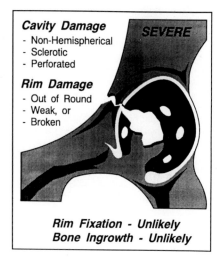

Fig. 1 The three categories of acetabular bone-stock damage.

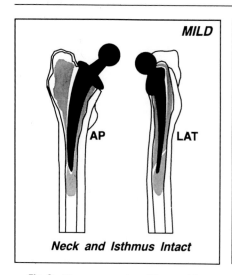
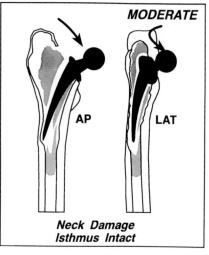
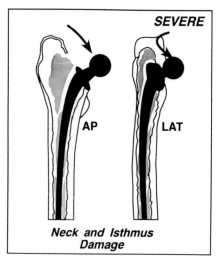

Fig. 2 Three categories of femoral bone-stock damage.

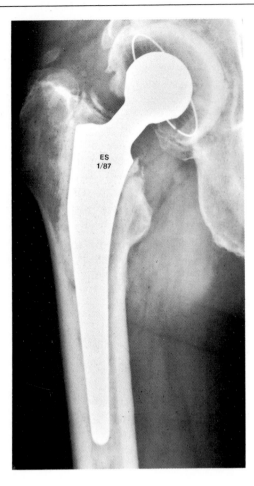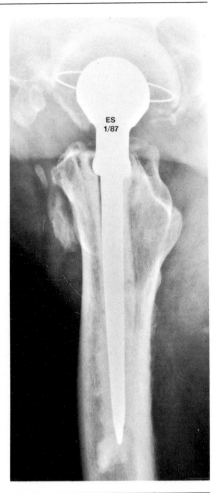

Fig. 3 Aseptic loosening of both components of a cemented total hip replacement. Femoral bone-stock damage is mild because the femoral metaphysis and diaphysis remain intact. Acetabular bone-stock damage is also mild because the bone behind the cemented cup could be reamed to a hemispheric shape and the rim is intact.

tabular revision for the past eight years. During this time, the implant inventory, instrumentation, and surgical techniques have been continuously improved. The results of our initial 127 cases at two-year follow-up were reported previously.[9] Minimum three-year follow-up results for 202 cases are now available and are presented herein. Improved results in the larger current series reflect the technical advancements that have been made. Optimism regarding cementless revision is based on Engh and associates'[10] experience with extensively porous-coated femoral implants in primary arthroplasty over the past 13 years. In primary cases in which bone ingrowth fixation has been achieved, the survivorship probability at ten years exceeds 99%.[10] Therefore, it is reasoned that if biologic stabilization can also be achieved in the revision setting, fixation should be more durable than that reported for cement.

In formulating the methodology for data presentation and analysis, considerable effort has been directed toward facilitating comparison of our results with those of other series, past, present, or in the future, whether they involve cemented or cementless techniques. To that end, four basic principles have been followed. It is hoped that similar reporting methods will be adopted by other orthopaedic surgeons. First, inclusion in the present study was limited to cases in which a cemented, intramedullary femoral component was revised because of aseptic loosening. Cases of concomitant femoral and acetabular revision were included, but isolated revisions of acetabular components were not. Second, the results for revision acetabular and femoral procedures are presented separately. Failure on one side of the prosthesis did not therefore affect the radiographic analysis of the other component, although clinical scores were excluded if follow-up after rerevision was inadequate. Third, an attempt has been made to assess accurately the extent of preoperative bone-stock damage in a fashion that is conceptually simple and reproducible among observers. When series of revision cases are reported, a limited number of categories generally suffice to depict defects, facilitate communication, and avoid creation of multiple subgroups with too few subjects to allow for statistical analysis. Finally, roentgenographic and clinical evaluation was done in a manner that should allow comparison between this and other series of cementless or cemented revisions.

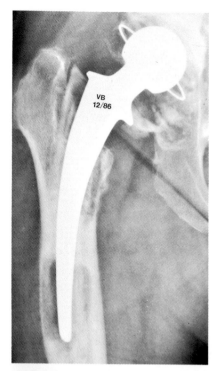
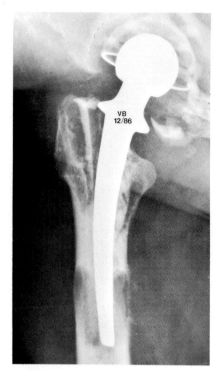
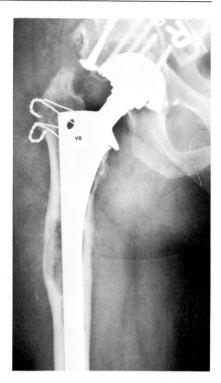
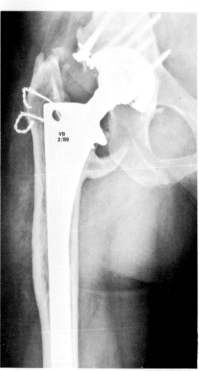

Fig. 4 Anteroposterior **(top left)** and lateral **(top center)** roentgenograms demonstrate loosening of both cemented components. Femoral bone-stock damage is moderate because the femoral stem has migrated into varus and retroversion with resultant damage to the medial and posterior femoral neck. Although there is endosteal resorption below the level of the lesser trochanter, there is an isthmus for distal fixation with a long-stem prosthesis. Acetabular damage is graded as severe because the acetabular cavity has been damaged and the rim is no longer circular. Immediately after surgery, a roentgenogram **(top right)** shows that a structural allograft was necessary for acetabular reconstruction. A fully porous-coated stem, 200 mm in length, has been used to obtain stability distal to the areas of proximal bone damage. These areas were not bone grafted. At two years, a roentgenogram **(bottom)** demonstrates that the acetabular component beneath the supporting allograft remains stable. There appears to be some reconstitution of the proximal femoral diaphysis.

Materials and Methods

Between 1977 and 1987, 202 consecutive revisions of aseptically loosened cemented femoral components were performed in 189 patients. Isolated femoral revisions were performed in 50 cases (49 patients), and combined femoral and acetabular revision was carried out in 152 hips (140 patients). Thus, 202 femoral and 152 acetabular revisions are included. Mean follow-up for the entire group was 4.5 years (range: three to ten years). Thirteen patients underwent bilateral revision. The patients included 102 women (111 hips) and 87 men (91 hips). Mean age at the time of revision was

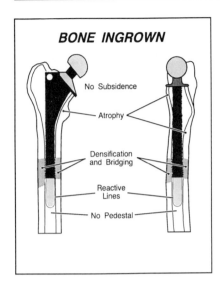
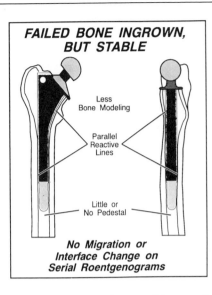
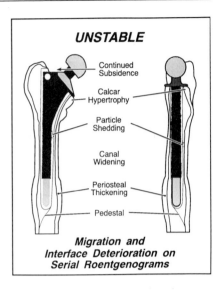

Fig. 5 Schema illustrating the roentgenographic appearance of the three possible types of biologic stabilization of a porous-coated femoral stem.

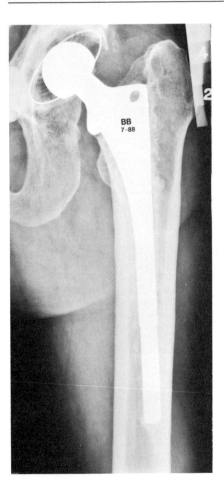
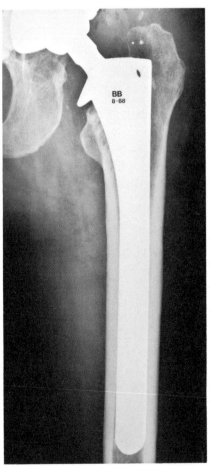
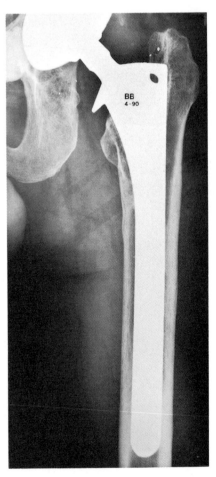

Fig. 6 Remodeling changes after bone ingrowth. Roentgenograms were taken preoperatively **(left)**, immediately after surgery **(center)**, and at two years **(right).** A comparison of the two postoperative radiograms demonstrates densification of the cortex around the distal portion of the stem and proximal cortical atrophy. There is no intramedullary pedestal beneath the stem. The endosteal cortex continues to remain in direct contact with the distal portion of the fully porous-coated stem.

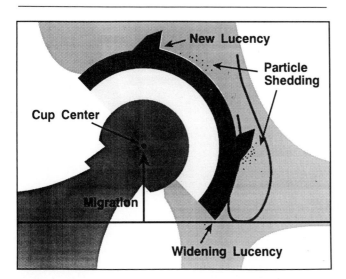

Fig. 7 Schema summarizing the roentgenographic signs of an unstable porous-coated acetabular component. Migration is most frequently confirmed by a change in the vertical distance between the cup center and a horizontal line drawn through the bottom of the teardrops on comparable anteroposterior pelvic radiograms.

57.7 years (range, 21 to 89 years). The average weight for male patients was 81.7 kg (range, 40.4 to 136.4 kg) and that for female patients was 64.9 kg (range, 45 to 124.2 kg). For 153 cases in 146 patients in the study, this revision was their first. The mean number of previous arthroplasties for the remaining 49 hips (43 patients) was 3.2 procedures (range, two to five).

Revision femoral components included 18 proximally porous-coated AMLs and 147 extensively porous-coated AMLs (defined as porous coating extending through the femoral isthmus). Additionally, 37 custom extensively porous-coated long-stem prostheses were used. Seventeen revised acetabular components were recemented early in the study before cementless cups became available. Thereafter, several cementless designs were employed, including 60 porous hemispheric cups and 74 threaded cups. One bipolar prosthesis was used. One cemented, seven porous hemispheric, and 13 threaded components were implanted in combination with major structural allografts.

The surgical technique has been detailed elsewhere.[9,11] In the years 1985 and 1986, proximally porous-coated stems were used in a limited number of cases with mild femoral bone-stock damage. It has otherwise been routine practice to use extensively coated stems that extend several centimeters beyond the endosteal surface previously in contact with polymethylmethacrylate.

The method used to grade preoperative bone-stock damage represents a simplified version of the classification recently devised by the American Academy of Orthopaedic Surgeons Committee on the Hip.[12] For both the femur and the acetabulum, three categories

exist: mild, moderate, and severe bone-stock damage. These are illustrated schematically in Figures 1 and 2. Radiographic examples are shown in Figures 3 and 4.

On the basis of a correlative study of roentgenograms and histologic findings of bone-implant interfaces at multiple sites, we have developed criteria that are now generally accepted for determining the fixation mode of porous-coated femoral components.[10,11] By these criteria, implants are classified as showing bone ingrowth, showing no bone ingrowth but having stable bone-fibrous tissue encapsulation, or being unstable. The features of each in terms of implant migration (or lack thereof), interface appearance, and adaptive remodeling of the surrounding bone are summarized and illustrated in Figure 5. Recognition of adaptive remodeling patterns about porous-coated femoral components is valuable in determining the mode of implant fixation. The typical changes that follow successful diaphyseal bone ingrowth can be appreciated by comparing the immediately postoperative and the two-year follow-up roentgenograms shown in Figure 6.

Because of more uniform implant loading, roentgenographic evidence of adaptive remodeling about acetabular components is minimal compared with that observed about femoral stems. In addition, the geometry of the acetabulum obscures visualization of the bone-implant interface. Together, these factors render the roentgenographic distinction between bone ingrowth and bone-fibrous tissue encapsulation impossible for some acetabular components.[13] As such, acetabular components in the present study are classified as stable, not otherwise specified, or unstable on the basis of the absence or presence of detectable implant migration or interface deterioration. The features of an unstable cementless acetabular component are illustrated schematically in Figure 7 and roentgenographically in Figure 8. Figure 8 also illustrates the features of an unstable cementless stem.

In conformity with published results of cemented arthroplasty, roentgenographic results are presented in the form of both revision rates and mechanical failure rates at specified time intervals. Mechanical failure is defined as implant instability (that is, failure to achieve and maintain biologic fixation, whether or not revised) and stem breakage. Femoral results are also given in the form of survivorship studies[14-16] using rerevision and mechanical failure as the endpoints. Components demonstrating stabilization by bone-fibrous tissue encapsulation are not included with the mechanical failures.

Clinical results are presented in the form of the D'Aubigné and Postel[17] six-point system as modified by Charnley.[18] In addition, the incidence of pain, however slight, when combined with a limp (both pain and walking scores less than 6) is recorded.

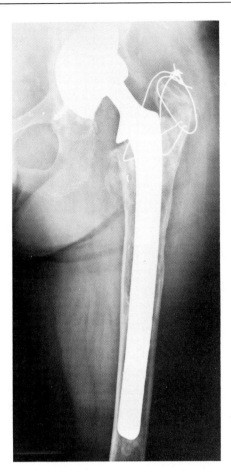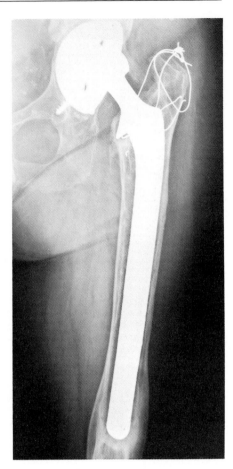

Fig. 8 Roentgenograms of a fully porous-coated prosthesis taken immediately after surgery **(left)** and at four years **(right)**. The four-year roentgenogram demonstrates features of unstable porous-coated femoral and acetabular components.

Table 1
Femoral preoperative bone stock damage/final stem fixation

Fixation	Bone Stock Damage		
	Minimal	Moderate	Severe
Bone ingrowth	52	89	22
Stable fibrous	8	12	5
Unstable	0	4	3
Revised*	2	3	2
Total number of cases	62	108	32

*Six revisions were for failure to achieve bone ingrowth and one was for breakage of a distal bone ingrowth stem.

Roentgenographic Results

Maintenance of Femoral Implant Stability

Preoperative bone-stock assessment (occasionally modified at the time of surgery) resulted in classification of 62 femurs as having minimal, 108 as having moderate, and 32 as having severe bone-stock damage (Table 1).

At last follow-up, 163 hips (80.7%) were classified as having bone ingrowth, 25 (12.3%) as having stable fibrous encapsulation, seven (3.5%) as being unstable, and seven (3.5%) as rerevised. The rerevised hips included one fractured stem—a custom fully porous-coated long-stem device now known to have been weakened by post-manufacturing modification. Six were rerevised because of symptomatic instability. Two of these were proximally coated implants, which we no longer advocate for revision surgery, and the remaining four were early cases grossly undersized at implantation. Among the seven unstable stems not rerevised were six significantly undersized relative to the femoral canal. Combining rerevisions and unstable stems still in situ, the overall femoral component mechanical failure rate was 7% at a mean follow-up of 4.5 years. The effect of preoperative bone stock on the final stability of the implant is also shown in Table 1. Mechanical failure was somewhat higher (P<.10) in those cases with severe bone-stock damage as opposed to cases with lesser damage, but the likelihood of maintaining stability (roentgenographic signs of bone ingrowth or stable bone-fibrous tissue encapsulation) did not differ between cases with moderate and those with severe damage. Two unstable implants subsequently demonstrated localized endosteal resorption.[19] The roentgenographic appearance of the more severe example is age. The incidence of mechanical failure was highest for smooth, threaded (37 of 74 or 50%) and recemented cups (seven of 17 or 41.2%) and lowest for porous hemispheric cups (five of 60 or 8.3%). Table 4 also shows that maintenance of acetabular cup stability is decidedly dependent on the extent of preoperative bone-stock damage, a situation different from that observed on the femoral side. Cup stability was also least apt to be maintained when a threaded cup was placed beneath a structural allograft. This was performed in 13 cases. At the final follow-up evaluation, six were graded as unstable and four have already been revised for instability. Although threaded cups were used in a disproportionate number of cases requiring structural allografting (13 of 21), their rate of failure in cases with even mild acetabular damage was 33.3% compared with 3.9% for porous hemispheric cups. In addition, Table 4 illustrates that the stability of porous hemispheric cups could be equally well maintained in cases with mild and moderate bone-stock damage. High failure rates occurred only when acetabular bone-stock damage was severe.

Clinical Results

Clinical Scores

Clinical scores at most recent follow-up evaluation are presented in Table 5. The mean pain and walking scores were 5.55 and 5.28, respectively. Twenty percent of the patients had mild intermittent thigh pain and limp. Even these patients were satisfied with their results, because their condition was better than their preoperative status and their expectations from revision surgery were not as great as they had been before their first operation.

Complications

The complications included five dislocations, five hips with symptoms related to trochanteric osteotomy, nine femoral fractures, one wound hematoma that required evacuation, and two deep-wound infections.

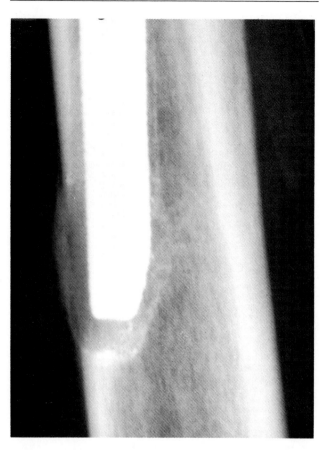

Fig. 9 A roentgenographic example of localized endosteal resorption associated with an unstable, fully porous-coated stem.

shown in Figure 9. Survivorship analysis was possible to eight years (Tables 2 and 3). The probabilities of survival, using revision and mechanical failure as endpoints, were 95.4% and 88.5% respectively.

Maintenance of Acetabular Implant Stability

As shown in Table 4, the maintenance of acetabular stability varied in accordance with both the type of component and the degree of preoperative bone-stock dam-

Table 2
Revision as end point

Time Since Implant (months)	No. at Start of Interval	Failures	Drop-outs	At Risk	Predicted Survival	Cumulative Survivorship	Predicted Failure Rate	Variance	Standard Error
0 to 12	241	0	37	204.0	1	1	0	0	0
12 to 24	202	0	0	202.0	1	1	0	0	0
24 to 36	202	0	1	201.0	1	1	0	0	0
36 to 48	201	5	64	169.0	0.97041	0.9704142	0.02959	0.0002	0.0256794
48 to 60	130	0	43	108.5	1	0.9704142	0	0.0003	0.032049
60 to 72	86	1	47	62.5	0.984	0.9548876	0.016	0.0007	0.0513086
72 to 84	39	0	8	35.0	1	0.9548876	0	0.0012	0.068564
84 to 96	28	0	17	19.5	1	0.9548876	0	0.0021	0.0918572

Table 3
Revision and mechanical loosenings

Time Since Implant (months)	No. at Start of Interval	Failures	Drop-outs	At Risk	Predicted Survival	Cumulative Survivorship	Predicted Failure Rate	Variance	Standard Error
0 to 12	241	0	37	204.0	1	1	0	0	0
12 to 24	202	0	0	202.0	1	1	0	0	0
24 to 36	202	0	1	201.0	1	1	0	0	0
36 to 48	201	9	64	169.0	0.094675	0.9467456	0.05325	0.0003	0.0336123
48 to 60	130	1	43	108.5	0.99078	0.9380198	0.00922	0.0005	0.0448388
60 to 72	86	0	47	62.5	1	0.9380198	0	0.0009	0.0590784
72 to 84	39	2	8	35.0	0.094286	0.8844187	0.05714	0.0026	0.1016477
84 to 96	28	0	17	19.5	1	0.8844187	0	0.0046	0.1361803

Table 4
Acetabular preoperative bone stock damage/final acetabular fixation

Type	Bone Stock Damage		
	Minimal	Moderate	Severe
Cemented cups			
Stable	3	6	1
Unstable	3	1	0
Revised	0	1	2
Mechanical failure rate	50% (3 of 6)	25% (2 of 8)	66.3% (2 of 3)
Smooth-threaded			
Stable	20	11	6
Unstable	7	8	5
Revised	3	9	5
Mechanical failure rate	33.3% (10 of 30)	60.7% (17 of 28)	62.5% (10 of 16)
Porous hemispherical			
Stable	29	19	7
Unstable	0	1	2
Revised	1	0	1
Mechanical failure rate	3.3% (1 of 30)	5% (1 of 20)	30% (3 of 10)
Overall			
Stable	52	36	14
Unstable	11	10	7
Revised	4	10	8
Mechanical failure rate	22.4% (14 of 66)*	35.7% (20 of 56)	51.7% (15 of 29)

*One bipolar cap was used in a case with minimal bone-stock damage and remains in situ.

These did not differ significantly from complications after cemented revision as reported in the literature.

Discussion

The need to revise failed cemented total hip replacements will no doubt continue for some time. Improved cementing techniques that depend on the intrusion of polymethylmethacrylate into the interstices of cancellous bone are unlikely to be of benefit to bone previously damaged by loosened cement. There is growing evidence that when such bone is freshened and placed in direct contact with the porous surface of an implant with immediate and rigid mechanical stability, bone ingrowth and enduring fixation are possible. Experience

Table 5
Clinical evaluation*

Score	Pain	Walking	Pain and Limp (%)
Preoperative	2.81	2.92	100
Final follow-up	5.55	5.28	20.5 (33 of 161)

*Eliminated from the clinical evaluation were those cases already revised, and pain and limp associated with an unstable acetabular component.

using extensively porous-coated femoral components in revision surgery parallels that for primary cases; when postoperative roentgenograms at one year demonstrate clear signs of bone ingrowth fixation, as illustrated in Figure 6, neither interface deterioration nor implant subsidence have occurred. It is our belief that the favorable results reported herein are attributable to the use of extensively coated cylindrical stems and intimate apposition of the porous coating to intact cortical bone over a large area.[20] Moreover, in 12.3% of cases that failed to achieve bone ingrowth, secondary stabilization by bone-fibrous tissue encapsulation and a successful clinical result ensued, again attributable to the large surface area available for tissue ingrowth. Although bone ingrowth is the preferred result, the use of extensively coated stems in which stable bone-fibrous encapsulation occurred was usually associated with a high degree of clinical success. Similar clinical results were not observed when partially porous-coated implants failed to achieve signs of osseointegration. Furthermore, no evidence exists to suggest that bone graft, whether slurried, morselized, or solid, is capable of bridging gaps between the endosteum and implant to provide bone ingrowth into a porous surface. Thus, the same results cannot be expected when proximally porous-coated implants are used in conjunction with bone graft packed into the voids between an expanded metaphysis and the porous surface.[21] With such implants, the potential for subsequent bone ingrowth is markedly limited unless the bone stock is nearly normal. For more severe cases of bone damage, this potential is virtually nonexistent. Moreover, following failure of bone ingrowth or osseointegration, there is little chance of secondary stabilization of proximally porous-coated stems by fibrous tissue ingrowth, and no chance whatever with smooth, press-fit designs.

Femoral results in the present study can be summarized as follows: When an extensively porous-coated implant is used and the distal canal is filled, good results are consistently achieved and fixation is largely independent of preoperative bone-stock damage. Failures early in the series were related to poor canal filling before an adequate inventory of stem sizes had become available. With current implants and surgical techniques, a press-fit into the femoral isthmus is achieved in more than 95% of cases.

The severely damaged acetabulum continues to be a problem. Failures on the acetabular side in this series were associated with poor implant choice (recemented and threaded) and also with extensive acetabular bone-stock damage. In contrast to the femur, in which good distal bone stock is generally available, there is little surplus acetabular bone stock to which the surgeon can resort for fixation when damage is extensive. Bone grafting in its present state is still somewhat unreliable. Custom implants have the potential to allow direct contact between bone and porous surfaces and represent an area where further research would be of benefit.

References

1. Harris WH: Current status of non-cemented hip implants. *Hip* 1986;14:251–256.
2. Harris WH, Davies JP: Modern use of modern cement for total hip replacement. *Orthop Clin North Am* 1988;19:581–589.
3. Harris WH, McGann WA: Loosening of the femoral component after use of the medullary-plug cementing technique: Follow-up note with a minimum five-year follow-up. *J Bone Joint Surg* 1986;68A:1064–1066.
4. Harris WH, McCarthy JC Jr, O'Neill DA: Femoral component loosening using contemporary techniques of femoral cement fixation. *J Bone Joint Surg* 1982;64A:1063–1067.
5. Russotti GM, Coventry MB, Stauffer RN: Cemented total hip arthroplasty with contemporary techniques: A five-year minimum follow-up study. *Clin Orthop* 1988;235:141–147.
6. Callaghan JJ, Salvati EA, Pellicci PM, et al: Results of revision for mechanical failure after cemented total hip replacement, 1979 to 1982: A two to five-year follow-up. *J Bone Joint Surg* 1985;67A:1074–1085.
7. Kavanagh BF, Ilstrup DM, Fitzgerald RH Jr: Revision total hip arthroplasty. *J Bone Joint Surg* 1985;67A:517–526.
8. Pellicci PM, Wilson PD Jr, Sledge CB, et al: Long-term results of revision total hip replacement: A follow-up report. *J Bone Joint Surg* 1985;67A:513–516.
9. Engh CA, Glassman AH, Griffin WL, et al: Results of cementless revision for failed cemented total hip arthroplasty. *Clin Orthop* 1988;235:91–110.
10. Engh CA, Glassman AH, Suthers KE: The case for porous coated hip implants—The femoral side. *Hip*, in press.
11. Engh CA, Bobyn JD: *Biological Fixation in Total Hip Arthroplasty.* Thorofare, Slack, 1985.
12 D'Antonio JA, Capello WN, Borden LS, et al: Classification and management of acetabular abnormalities in total hip arthroplasty. *Clin Orthop* 1989;243:126–137.
13. Bobyn JD, Engh CA, Glassman AH: Radiography and histology of a threaded acetabular implant: One case studied at two years. *J Bone Joint Surg* 1988;70B:302–304.
14. Armitage P: *Statistical Methods in Medical Research.* Oxford, Blackwell, 1971, pp 404–408.
15. Dobbs HS: Survivorship of total hip replacements. *J Bone Joint Surg* 1980;62B:168–173.
16. Engh CA, Massin P: Cementless total hip arthroplasty using the anatomic medullary locking stem: Results using a survivorship analysis. *Clin Orthop* 1989;249:141–158.
17. D'Aubigné RM, Postel M: Functional results of hip arthroplasty with acrylic prosthesis. *J Bone Joint Surg* 1954;36A:451–475.
18. Charnley J: *Low Friction Arthroplasty of the Hip: Theory and Practice.* Berlin, Springer-Verlag, 1979.
19. Lombardi AV Jr, Mallory TH, Vaughn BK, et al: Aseptic loosening in total hip arthroplasty secondary to osteolysis induced by wear debris from titanium-alloy modular femoral heads. *J Bone Joint Surg* 1989;71A:1337–1342.
20. Cook SD, Barrack RL, Thomas KA, et al: Quantitative analysis of tissue ingrowth into human porous total hip components. *J Arthrop* 1988;3:249–262.
21. Hungerford DS, Jones LC: The rationale of cementless revision of cemented arthroplasty failures. *Clin Orthop* 1988;235:12–24.

Instability of the Anterior and Posterior Cruciate Ligaments

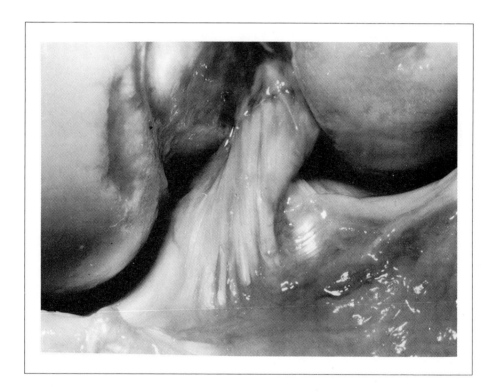

Basic Science of Anterior Cruciate Ligament Repair and Reconstruction

Steven P. Arnoczky, DVM

The anterior cruciate ligament has long been recognized as an important static stabilizer of the knee.[1-5] The functional significance of this structure has provided the rationale for the repair or reconstruction of the anterior cruciate ligament after injury. Techniques of repair and reconstruction vary, but all are predicated on a fundamental understanding of basic science principles. This chapter examines some of the basic science aspects of anterior cruciate ligament repair and reconstruction, including anatomic, physiologic, and biomechanical considerations.

Anatomy

The function of the anterior cruciate ligament as a stabilizer of the knee is directly related to its anatomic structure and orientation within the joint.[3-6] Knowledge of this anatomy, therefore, is a prerequisite to any attempt to repair or reconstruct the anterior cruciate ligament.

The anterior cruciate ligament is attached to a fossa on the posterior aspect of the medial surface of the lateral femoral condyle. The femoral attachment is in the form of a segment of a circle, with its anterior border straight and its posterior border convex (Fig. 1). Its long axis is tilted slightly forward from the vertical, and its posterior convexity parallels the posterior articular margin of the lateral femoral condyle.[1,4,6] The tibial attachment of the anterior cruciate ligament is a fossa in front of and lateral to the anterior tibial spine. At this attachment, the anterior cruciate ligament passes beneath the transverse meniscal ligament, and a few fascicles of the anterior cruciate ligament may blend with the anterior attachment of the lateral meniscus. In some instances, fascicles from the posterior aspect of the tibial attachment of the anterior cruciate ligament may extend to and blend with the posterior attachment of the lateral meniscus. The tibial attachment of the anterior cruciate ligament is somewhat

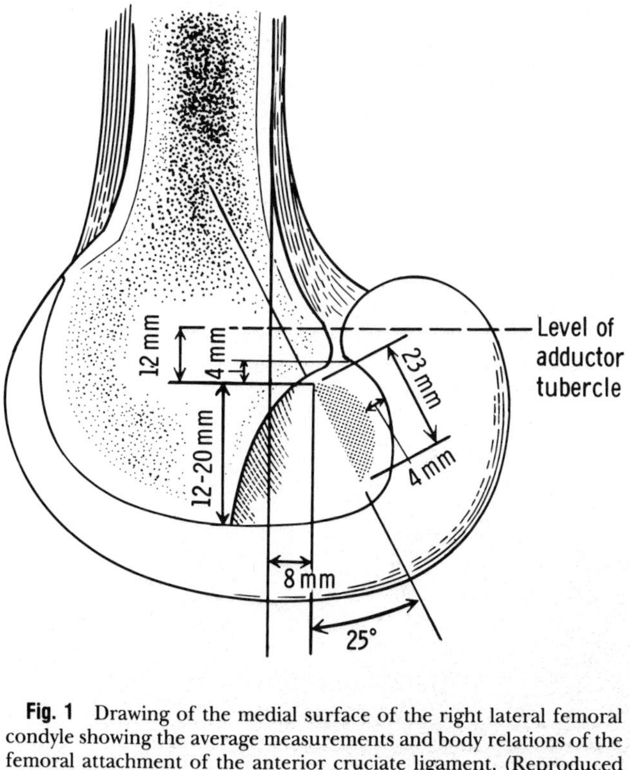

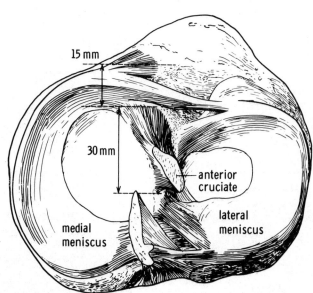

Fig. 1 Drawing of the medial surface of the right lateral femoral condyle showing the average measurements and body relations of the femoral attachment of the anterior cruciate ligament. (Reproduced with permission from Girgis FG, Marshall JL, Al Monajem ARS: The cruciate ligaments of the knee joint: Anatomical, functional, and experimental analysis. *Clin Orthop* 1975;106:216–231.)

Fig. 2 Drawing of the tibial plateau showing the average measurements and relation of the tibial attachment of the anterior cruciate ligament. (Reproduced with permission from Girgis FG, Marshall JL, Al Monajem ARS: The cruciate ligaments of the knee joint: Anatomical, functional, and experimental analysis. *Clin Orthop* 1975;106:216–231.)

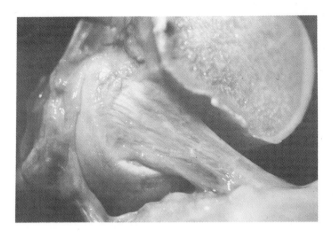

Fig. 3 The femoral attachment of the anterior cruciate ligament, demonstrating its broad attachment area and multifascicular structure. (Reproduced with permission from Arnoczky SP: Anatomy of the anterior cruciate ligament. *Clin Orthop* 1983;172:19–25.)

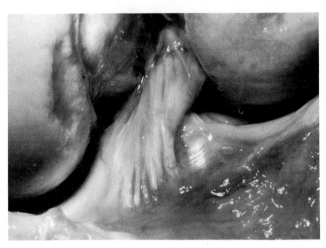

Fig. 4 Photograph of the tibial attachment of the anterior cruciate ligament demonstrating its broad attachment area and the multifascicular nature of the ligament's structure. (Reproduced with permission from Arnoczky SP: Anatomy of the anterior cruciate ligament. *Clin Orthop* 1983;172:19–25.)

wider and stronger than the femoral attachment (Fig. 2).[4,6]

The anterior cruciate ligament courses anteriorly, medially, and distally across the joint as it passes from the femur to the tibia. As it does, it twists on itself in a slight outward (lateral) spiral because of orientation of its bony attachment. The orientation of the femoral attachments of the anterior cruciate ligament, with regard to joint position (flexion-extension), is also responsible for the relative tension of the ligament throughout the range of motion. The anterior cruciate ligament is attached to the femur and tibia not as a single cord but rather as a collection of individual fascicles that fan out over a broad, flattened area (Figs. 3 and 4). These fascicles have been divided into two groups: the anteromedial band, those fascicles that originate at the proximal aspect of the femoral attachment and insert at the anteromedial aspect of the tibial attachment; and the posterolateral band, the remaining bulk of fascicles, which are inserted at the posterolateral aspect of the tibial attachment. When the knee is extended, the posterolateral band is taut, while the anteromedial band is moderately lax. However, as the knee is flexed, the femoral attachment of the anterior cruciate ligament assumes a more horizontal orientation, causing the anteromedial band to tighten and the posterolateral band to loosen (Fig. 5).[4,6] Although this designation provides a general idea as to the dynamics of the anterior cruciate ligament through the range of motion, it is an oversimplification. Although a functional anteromedial band is defined in flexion and a posterolateral band is present in extension, the anterior cruciate ligament is actually a continuum of fascicles, a different portion of which is taut throughout the range of motion.[6] This is of great clinical importance, because in any position of the knee a portion of the

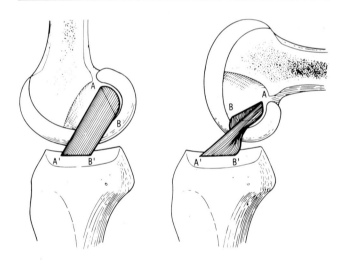

Fig. 5 Schema representing changes in the shape and tension of the anterior cruciate components in flexion and extension. In flexion, the anteromedial band (A-A') is lengthened and the posterolateral aspect of the ligament (C-C') is shortened. (Reproduced with permission from Girgis FG, Marshall JL, Al Monajem ARS: The cruciate ligaments of the knee joint: Anatomical, functional, and experimental analysis. *Clin Orthop* 1975;106:216–231.)

anterior cruciate ligament remains under tension and functional. This aspect of anterior cruciate ligament function is very difficult to duplicate with a single, cord-like graft, as will be discussed later, in the section on graft orientation.

Blood Supply to the Anterior Cruciate Ligament

Although the anterior cruciate ligament is an important mechanical component of the knee, it is also

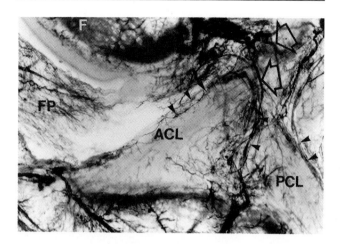

Fig. 6 A sagittal section, 5 mm thick, of a human knee joint showing the vascularity of the anterior cruciate ligament (Spalteholz technique). The ligamentous branch of the middle genicular artery and its divisions (open arrows) can be seen supplying the periligamentous branches (black arrows) of the synovial covering of the anterior cruciate ligament (ACL). F, femur; FP, fat pad; PCL, posterior cruciate ligament. (Reproduced with permission from Arnoczky SP: Anatomy of the anterior cruciate ligament. *Clin Orthop* 1983;172:19–25.)

a biologic tissue with nutritional requirements. These requirements are fulfilled by way of a unique blood supply that also provides the basis for the inflammatory reaction of ligament injury and repair. The blood supply to the cruciate ligaments arises from the ligamentous branches of the middle genicular artery as well as some terminal branches of the inferior genicular arteries.[7,8]

The cruciate ligaments are covered by a synovial fold that originates at the posterior inlet of the intercondylar notch and extends to the anterior tibial insertion of the ligament, where it joins the synovial tissue of the joint capsule distal to the infrapatellar fat pad.[8,9] This synovial membrane, which forms an envelope about the ligaments, is richly endowed with vessels that originate predominantly from the ligamentous branches of the middle genicular artery (Fig. 6). A few smaller terminal branches of the lateral and medial inferior genicular arteries also contribute some vessels to this synovial plexus through its connection with the infrapatellar fat pad.[8,9] The synovial vessels branch to form a web-like network of periligamentous vessels, which ensheath the entire ligament (Fig. 7). These periligamentous vessels give rise to smaller connecting branches that penetrate the ligament transversely and anastomose with a network of endoligamentous vessels (Fig. 8). These vessels, along with their supporting connective tissues, are oriented longitudinally and parallel the collagen bundles within the ligament.[8,9]

The blood supply to the cruciate ligaments is predominantly of soft-tissue origin. Although the middle genicular artery gives off additional branches to the

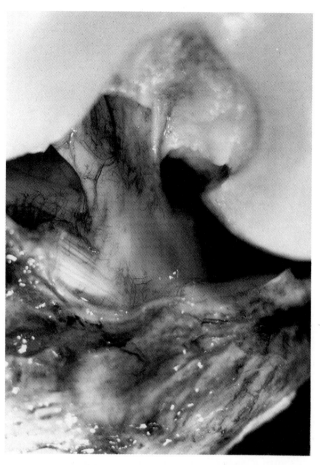

Fig. 7 Photograph of a human knee specimen demonstrating the synovial (periligamentous) vasculature on the surface of the anterior cruciate ligament (india ink injection). (Note that the infrapatellar fat pad has been removed for better visualization.) (Reproduced with permission from Arnoczky SP: Blood supply to the anterior cruciate ligament and supporting structures. *Orthop Clin North Am* 1985;16:15–28.)

distal femoral epiphysis and proximal tibial epiphysis, the ligamentous-osseous junctions of the cruciate ligaments do not contribute significantly to the vascular scheme of the ligaments themselves.[8,9]

Primary Repair of the Anterior Cruciate Ligament

The ability of the anterior cruciate ligament to mount a reparative response has been the focus of several experimental studies.[10-12] One such study demonstrated that, in a dog, a surgically created lesion of the anterior cruciate ligament results in a significant vascular response throughout the ligament (Fig. 9).[10] This vascular response arises from the soft tissues (infrapatellar fat pad and synovium) that surround the ligament. When these vascular soft tissues are removed at the time of injury, the intraligamentous vascular response is minimal and delayed (Fig.

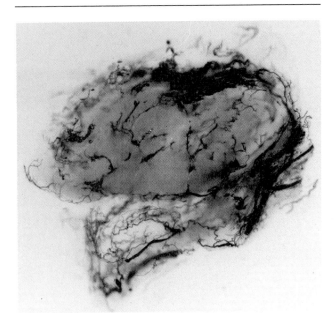

Fig. 8 Cross section of a human anterior cruciate ligament demonstrating the periligamentous as well as endoligamentous vasculature (Spalteholz technique). The fold of the synovial membrane (arrow) can be seen supplying vessels to the synovial covering of the ligament. (Reproduced with permission from Arnoczky SP: Anatomy of the anterior cruciate ligament. *Clin Orthop* 1983;172:19–25).

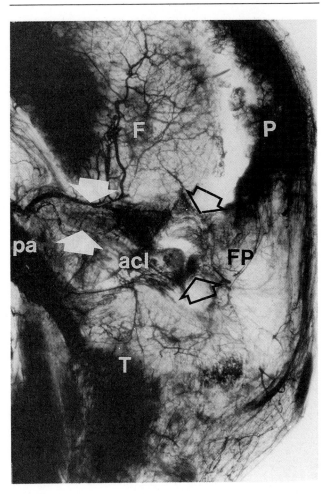

Fig. 9 A section of a dog's knee, 5 mm thick, 2.5 weeks after partial surgical transection of the anterior cruciate ligament (ACL) (Spalteholz technique). Note the rich vascular reaction at the site of the lesion (L) and throughout the entire anterior cruciate ligament. Vessels from the infrapatellar fat pad (open arrows) and branches of the middle genicular artery posteriorly (closed arrows) appear to contribute to the vascular response. PA, popliteal artery; F, femur; T, tibia; P, patella; FP, fat pad. (Reproduced with permission from Arnoczky SP, Rubin RM, Marshall JL: Microvasculature of the cruciate ligaments and its response to injury: An experimental study in dogs. *J Bone Joint Surg* 1979;61A:1221–1229.)

10). These findings suggest that preserving and using the soft tissue of the joint when repairing anterior cruciate ligament lesions optimizes the vascular response of the ligament.

Studies have also shown that, although the anterior cruciate ligament is capable of a vascular response after injury, spontaneous repair (or healing by second intention) does not occur (Fig. 11).[10,11] This may be because the synovial fluid dilution of the hematoma after injury prevents formation of a fibrin clot and thus the initiation of healing mechanism. Another theory suggests that the dynamic nature of the fascicles of the anterior cruciate ligament through the range of motion prohibits the spontaneous union of these fibers.[10]

The observations stated above support the primary repair of certain anterior cruciate ligament lesions. Experimental studies have shown that although surgical apposition of severed anterior cruciate ligaments in dogs and monkeys allows healing through the formation and organization of a vascular scar (Fig. 12), the tensile strength of the repairs at ten and 16 weeks is substantially less than that of normal ligaments.[9,12] These poor results have also been observed in long-term clinical evaluations of primary cruciate ligament repair in humans and may be the result of technical difficulties (suture placement and tension) and prolonged periods of immobilization associated with primary repair.[13]

Anterior Cruciate Ligament Reconstruction

The replacement or reconstruction of the anterior cruciate ligament encompasses several basic science considerations, including graft selection, graft orientation, and graft biology. Successful reconstruction is based, in part, on understanding and using these fundamental concepts.

Graft Materials

The selection of graft material for the reconstruction of the anterior cruciate ligament is largely a matter of personal preference, although some materials have gained wider acceptance than others. The selection criteria have been based, in large part, on the material

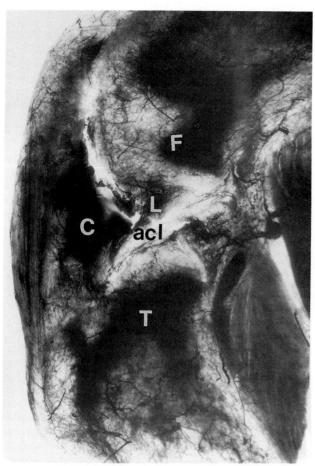

Fig. 10 A sagittal section of a dog's knee, 5 mm thick, 2.5 weeks after partial surgical transection of the anterior cruciate ligament (ACL) and resection of the infrapatellar fat and synovium (Spalteholz technique). Note the abundance of vessels at the site of the lesion (L) and the intraligamentous vascular response seen in the specimen without synovectomy and resection of the fat pad. The clot (C) in the area of the resected fat pad, when dissected out appeared to be densely adherent to the anterior cruciate ligament. F, femur; T, tibia. (Reproduced with permission from Arnoczky SP, Rubin RM, Marshall JL: Microvasculature of the cruciate ligaments and its response to injury: An experimental study in dogs. *J Bone Joint Surg* 1979;61A: 1221–1229.)

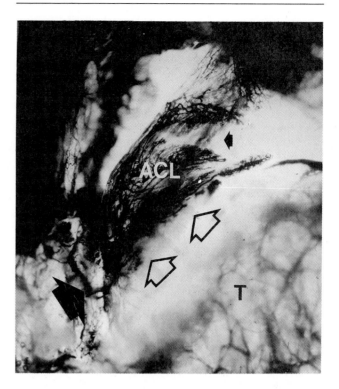

Fig. 11 A sagittal section of a dog's knee, 5 mm thick, eight weeks after partial surgical transection of the anterior cruciate ligament, leaving the infrapatellar fat pad and synovial membrane intact (Spalteholz technique, × 5). A portion of the infrapatellar fat pad has been dissected to permit better visualization of the anterior cruciate ligament. The incision in the anterior cruciate ligament can be seen as a defect (small arrow) that, even at eight weeks, has not filled in. The vigorous and extensive intraligamentous vasculature of the anterior cruciate ligament outlines the borders of the lesion. The intraligamentous vessels appear to be derived from the soft tissues (infrapatellar fat pad and synovial tissue). Several so-called "feeder vessels" (larger closed arrows) are visible at the base of the ligament. No reactive vessels cross the ligamentous-osseous attachment site (open arrows) on the tibia (T) at the anterior cruciate ligament. (Reproduced with permission from Arnoczky SP, Rubin RM, Marshall J: Microvasculature of the cruciate ligaments and its response to injury: An experimental study in dogs. *J Bone Joint Surg* 1979;61A: 1221–1229.)

characteristics of the individual tissues, following the theory that the replacement material should be at least as strong as the normal anterior cruciate ligament. In a classic study, Noyes and associates[14] provided a material analysis of biologic tissues commonly used to replace the anterior cruciate ligament and compared the results to those of the anterior cruciate ligament (Table 1). The results demonstrated that bone-patellar tendon-bone preparations had maximum loads in excess of that of a normal anterior cruciate ligament, while loads for semitendinosus and gracilis specimens were somewhat less.[14,15] However, it should be noted that the bone-patellar tendon-bone specimens were somewhat larger than those normally used for reconstructive procedures. This point notwithstanding, the bone-patellar

tendon-bone preparation was still the strongest of the biologic tissues tested.

Graft Orientation

The complexities of the anterior cruciate ligament, which allow its unique function within the knee, make it a most difficult structure to duplicate. This is because most reconstruction techniques use a single (or in some cases a double) strand of material to replace the original multifascicular ligament. In addition, bony attachment of such a reconstruction is accomplished through a single femoral and tibial drill hole as opposed to the broad individual attachments of the normal ligament. Therefore, for the reconstruction to maintain functional stability throughout the range of motion, the bony attachments must be located at points on the tibia and

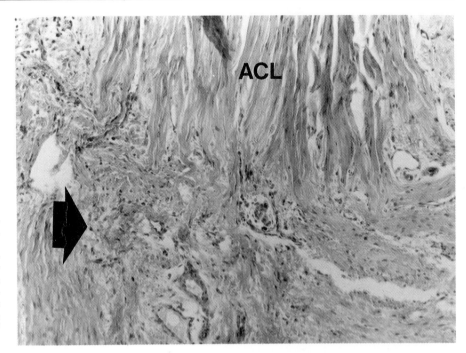

Fig. 12 Photomicrograph showing the repair site of an anterior cruciate ligament of a dog six weeks after transection and primary repair. Note the fibrovascular scar tissue present at the repair site (arrow) and the adjacent normal ligamentous tissue of the anterior cruciate ligament (ACL) (hematoxylin-eosin, × 100). (Reproduced with permission from Arnoczky SP: The vascularity of the anterior cruciate ligament and associated structures: Its role in repair and reconstruction, in Jackson DW, Drez D Jr (eds): *The Anterior Cruciate Deficient Knee: New Concepts in Ligament Repair.* St. Louis, CV Mosby, 1987, pp 27–54.)

Table 1
Maximum loads for the human anterior cruciate ligament and its replacements*

Tissue	Maximum Load (Mean ± SE)	% of Anterior Cruciate Ligament
Anterior cruciate ligament	1725 ± 269	100
Bone-patella-bone		
Central third	2900 ± 260	168
Medial third	2734 ± 298	159
Semitendinosus	1216 ± 50	70
Gracilis	838 ± 30	49
Distal iliotibial tract (18 mm width)	769 ± 99	44
Fascia lata	628 ± 35	36

*Reproduced with permission from Noyes FR, Butler DL, Grood ES, et al; Biomechanical analysis of human ligament grafts used in knee-ligament repairs and reconstructions. *J Bone Joint Surg* 1984;66A: 344–352.

femur at which length changes are minimal. This has been termed the isometric point, but this is actually a misnomer, because through the functional range of motion there is no one point on the femur that maintains the same distance (is isometric) from a point on the tibia.[16] At best, the surgeon will locate an area within the normal attachments of the anterior cruciate ligament that undergoes minimal length changes through the range of motion.[16] An experimental study using a computer-generated knee model identified an area of minimal length change (less than 1%) through the range of motion (0 to 110 degrees of flexion).[17]

This area, less than 2 mm square, is located in the posterior superior aspect of the femoral attachment. It should be noted that for this condition to occur, the tibial insertion site must be located in the anterior aspect of the normal attachment site. Variation of the tibial site directly affects the area of least length change on the femur, with a posterior tibial site being the least desirable.[17]

The over-the-top position (using an anteriorly placed tibial insertion) demonstrated a relatively large area of minimal length change.[17] However, this only occurred through a limited range of motion (0 to 30 degrees of flexion). With increasing angles of knee flexion, the length patterns indicated that graft laxity would occur.[17]

Physiology of Biologic Replacement Grafts for the Anterior Cruciate Ligament

Intra-articular transplantation of biologic tissues has long been advocated as a method for replacement of the anterior cruciate ligament.[18-22] The success of these transplants depends, in large part, on the ability of these tissues to survive and function in the intra-articular environment of the knee. Several experimental and clinical studies have demonstrated that biologic grafts undergo a physiologic and biomechanical remodeling process after transplantation.[23-28]

Autografts Autogenous grafts are defined as tissues taken from one part of the body and transplanted to another location in the same individual. Several studies

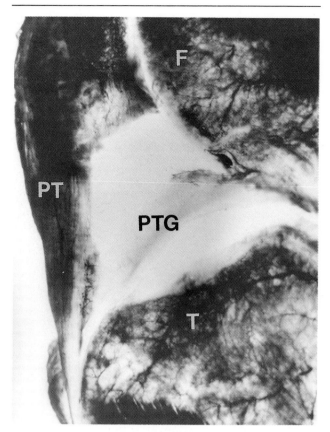

Fig. 13 A sagittal section of a dog's knee, 5 mm thick, two weeks after replacement with a patellar tendon graft (Spalteholz technique, × 2). The patellar tendon graft (PTG) shows no evidence of perfused vessels. Note the absence of vessels crossing the tibial attachment of the graft (arrow). (The infrapatellar fat pad and the posterior cruciate ligament were removed after clearing to permit better visualization.) F, femur; T, tibia; PT, patellar tendon. (Reproduced with permission from Arnoczky SP, Tarvin GB, Marshall JL: Anterior cruciate ligament replacement using patellar tendon: An evaluation of graft revascularization in the dog. *J Bone Joint Surg* 1982;64A:217–224.)

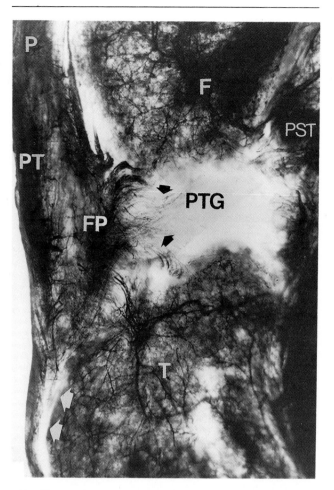

Fig. 14 A sagittal section of a dog's knee, 5 mm thick, six weeks after replacement of the anterior cruciate ligament with a patellar tendon graft (PTG). Note the vascular response of the infrapatellar fat pad (FP) and posterior soft tissues (PST). Vessels from the fat pad can be seen extending over the surface of the patellar tendon graft (black arrows) and are part of the vascular synovial envelope. Note that the tibial attachment of the graft (white arrows) does not contribute any vessels to the graft. F, femur; T, tibia; PT, patellar tendon; P, patella. (Reproduced with permission from Arnoczky SP, Tarvin GB, Marshall JL: Anterior cruciate ligament replacement using patellar tendon: An evaluation of graft revascularization in the dog. *J Bone Joint Surg* 1982;64A:217–224.)

have shown that patellar tendon autografts used to replace the anterior cruciate ligament are essentially avascular at the time of transplantation (Fig. 13).[24-26] If these tissues are to remain viable within the joint, they must be revascularized. Experimental studies have shown that, after transplantation, patellar tendon grafts are initially enveloped with a vascular synovial tissue that originated from the soft tissues of the knee (infrapatellar fat pad and synovium) (Fig. 14).[25] This synovialization process occurs during the first four to six weeks after transplantation. During that time, the central avascular core of the graft undergoes a process of ischemic necrosis.[25] Thus, the graft plays an innocent role in a race between avascular necrosis and revascularization. Fortunately, the soft tissues that initiated the synovialization of the graft also provide the source for an intrinsic revascularization response in which vessels from the infrapatellar fat pad and synovium penetrate the connective tissue that makes up the graft and revascularize the transplanted tissue (Fig. 15). This re-

vascularization response is accompanied by a cellular proliferation that eventually repopulates the graft with new cells (Fig. 16).[25] Although the complete revascularization of the patellar tendon grafts can take as long as 20 weeks, even more time is required for the graft to remodel and take on the structural and mechanical characteristics of a ligament (Fig. 17).[25]

Along with the process of revascularization, the transplanted patellar tendon undergoes additional morphologic, biochemical, and biomechanical changes. A classic experimental study in rabbits described the ligamentization of patellar tendon autografts transplanted into the intra-articular milieu.[27] This metamorphosis of the patellar tendon graft occurs over a 30-week period and is characterized by a gradual

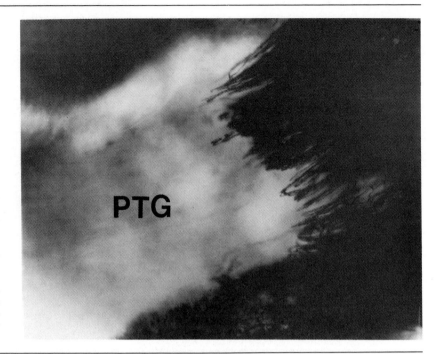

Fig. 15 A sagittal section of a dog's knee, 5 mm thick, ten weeks after replacement of the anterior cruciate ligament with a patellar tendon graft (PTG) (Spalteholz technique, × 20). Note the advancing brushlike border of the intrinsic vascular response. These terminally looped capillaries are migrating within the substance of the avascular patellar tendon. (Reproduced with permission from Arnoczky SP, Tarvin GB, Marshall JL: Anterior cruciate ligament replacement using patellar tendon: An evaluation of graft revascularization in the dog. *J Bone Joint Surg* 1982;64A:217–224.)

Fig. 16 Photomicrograph of a longitudinal section of a patellar tendon graft ten weeks after replacement of the anterior cruciate ligament. There is an invasion of capillary buds (arrows) into the avascular graft. Note the cellular proliferation that accompanies the vascular ingrowth (hematoxylin-eosin, × 100). (Reproduced with permission from Arnoczky SP, Tarvin GB, Marshall JL: Anterior cruciate ligament replacement using patellar tendon: An evaluation of graft revascularization in the dog. *J Bone Joint Surg* 1982;64A:217–224.)

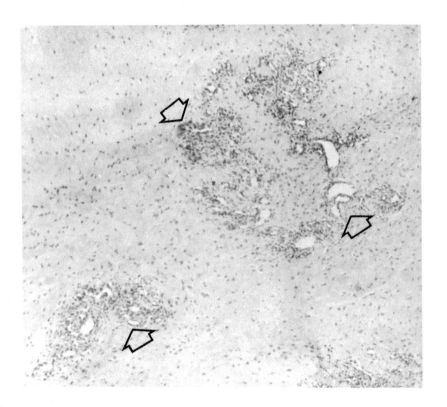

change in cell morphology, collagen profile and crosslinking pattern, and glycosaminoglycan content. These alterations result in a graft with the morphologic and biochemical profile of a normal anterior cruciate ligament.[27]

Although this remodeling process results in a graft

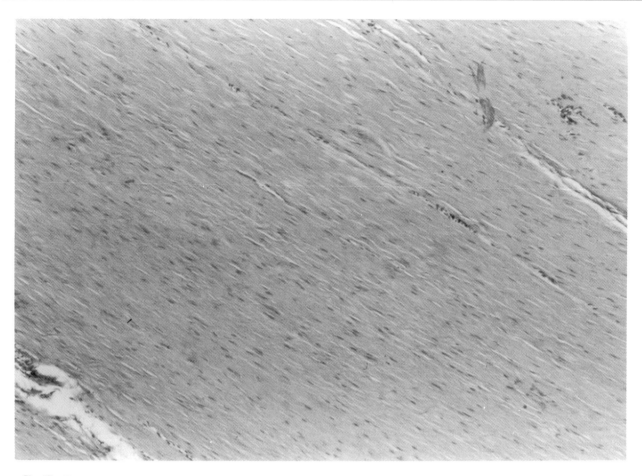

Fig. 17   Photomicrograph of a longitudinal section of a patellar tendon graft 26 weeks after replacement of the anterior cruciate ligament. The cellular proliferation as well as the vascular response has begun to subside (hematoxylin-eosin, × 100). (Reproduced with permission from Arnoczky SP, Tarvin GB, Marshall JL: Anterior cruciate ligament replacement using patellar tendon: An evaluation of graft revascularization in the dog. *J Bone Joint Surg* 1982;64A:217–224.)

that physiologically resembles a normal anterior cruciate ligament, the biomaterial character of the remodeled graft is less comparable. Experimental studies have shown that there is an initial decrease in the ultimate tensile strength of the graft after transportation.[26,29] This is followed by a gradual increase in strength as the graft remodels. Although variations in testing methods, graft materials, postoperative protocols, and data analysis make direct comparisons between studies impossible, in no study has a graft demonstrated a return to 100% of preoperative strength.

The decrease in the ultimate tensile strength of patellar tendon grafts observed after transplantation was thought to occur in association with the aforementioned period of ischemic necrosis and revascularization of the graft.[19,22] In an effort to eliminate the period of ischemic necrosis and revascularization that follows patellar tendon transplantation, surgical procedures have been described that preserve a portion of the graft's blood supply. In one technique, the central third of the patellar ligament, along with its infrapatellar

blood supply, is used as a vascularized graft.[19] Another technique uses the medial third of the patellar ligament, preserving its "vascular leash" within the medial retinacular tissues.[22] It was theorized that preserving the blood supply of the graft would maintain tissue viability throughout the postoperative period, minimizing or avoiding the process of ischemic necrosis and graft revascularization usually associated with patellar tendon grafts. Although the use of vascularized patellar tendon grafts was also thought to enhance the material properties of the graft (over avascular grafts), experimental evidence has demonstrated that maintaining the vascular supply to transplanted patellar tendon grafts does not prevent a significant postoperative reduction in the material properties of the graft, nor does it accelerate the return of graft strength.[30]

A recent experimental study has suggested that the mechanical environment (proper orientation and tensioning) of the graft may be the major factor in determining the ability of a transplanted graft to better maintain its material properties.[31] The results of this study

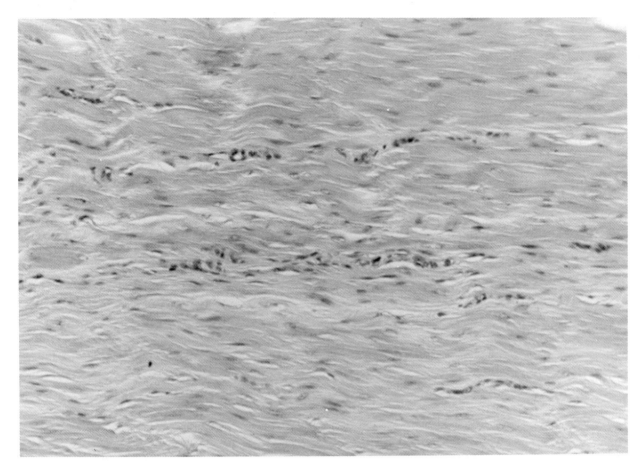

Fig. 18   Photomicrograph of a longitudinal section of a patellar tendon allograft six months after transplantation. The graft resembles a normal ligamentous structure (hematoxylin-eosin, × 100).

demonstrated that maintaining a ligament under normal tension significantly reduces the amount of tensile strength lost during the period of revascularization and cellular changes.[31] The study demonstrated a complete return to normal biomaterial properties at one year. These findings suggest that surgical technique and the creation of appropriate graft tension and orientation may have the most profound effect on the ultimate material properties of the graft.[31]

Allografts   The success of autogenous tissues as anterior cruciate ligament substitutes and the fact that these grafts are avascular at the time of transplantation have led to the concept of using allograft tissues for anterior cruciate ligament replacement.[29,32,33] Allografts are defined as tissues taken from one individual and transplanted into another individual of the same species. As with autogenous tissues, these allografts must be revascularized and revitalized if they are to remain functional within the joint. Because such preservation techniques as freeze-drying or deep-freezing are used to destroy the cellular components of the graft and thus

make them less immunogenic, the allografts are essentially inert collagen scaffolds that must be revascularized and remodeled with host tissue.[32] Several experimental studies have examined the biology of allograft tissues used to replace the anterior cruciate ligament.[29,32,33] It has been shown that deep-frozen patellar tendon allografts undergo a revascularization process after transplantation that is similar to that observed in patellar tendon autografts.[32] The vascular tissues of the infrapatellar fat pad and synovium that provide a vascular synovial envelope around the graft supply the origin for the intrinsic revascularization and cellular proliferation within the allograft. As in the autogenous patellar tendon grafts, this revascularization process was complete at five months, and by six months the allograft resembled a normal ligament (Fig. 18).[32]

Biomechanical evaluation of allografts used to reconstruct the anterior cruciate ligament in animals demonstrates a pattern similar to that observed with autografts.[29,33] There is an initial decrease in the ultimate tensile strength of the graft followed by a gradual increase in this value. As in the autografts, however, this value has never been shown to return to normal.[29]

Rehabilitation

Several studies have shown that normal ligaments respond to changes in stress patterns such as those that occur in both training (increased stress)[34-39] and immobilization (decreased stress).[38,40] After nine weeks of immobilization, a loss of the parallel organization of the collagen fibers and a decrease in the number and size of the collagen bundles were noted.[41] These morphologic changes are reflected, biomechanically, by a decrease in the ultimate load, linear stiffness, and energy-absorbing capacity of the ligament.[41]

The effect of training (increased stress) on the material properties of normal ligaments appears to be somewhat less profound than that observed with exercise after immobilization.[34-36] However, experimental studies have shown an increase in the size of collagen bundles and an accompanying increase in material properties after certain exercise regimes.[34,36]

Although no scientific data have demonstrated any alteration in the return to strength of biologic grafts after immobilization or exercise, it is reasonable to assume that prolonged immobilization is detrimental to the material properties of any biologic tissue. However, the extent and timing of an exercise program that would beneficially affect the biomaterial remodeling of such a graft has yet to be determined. The most that can be said is that, on the basis of current knowledge, these grafts are strongest the day they are placed inside the knee. After this placement, the graft undergoes a biologic and biomechanical remodeling process that alters its biomaterial properties. Experimental studies have yet to demonstrate a complete return to original graft strength. Further investigations are needed to examine the basic science effects of rehabilitation on the biologic and biomaterial character of these grafts.

Summary

The anterior cruciate ligament is a complex structure. Its design and orientation relate directly to its function in constraining joint motion. Successful repair or replacement of this structure requires not only a precise surgical technique but also a fundamental understanding of the basic science principles of graft biology.

References

1. Palmer I: On the injuries to the ligaments of the knee joint: A clinical study. *Acta Chir Scand* 1938;81(suppl 53):3–282.

2. Johnson RJ: The anterior cruciate ligament problem. *Clin Orthop* 1983;172:14–18.

3. Kennedy JC, Weinberg HW, Wilson AS: The anatomy and function of the anterior cruciate ligament: As determined by clinical and morphological studies. *J Bone Joint Surg* 1974;56A:223–235.

4. Girgis FG, Marshall JL, Al Monajem ARS: The cruciate ligaments of the knee joint: Anatomical, functional, and experimental analysis. *Clin Orthop* 1975;106:216–231.

5. Cabaud HE: Biomechanics of the anterior cruciate ligament. *Clin Orthop* 1983;172:26–31.

6. Arnoczky SP: Anatomy of the anterior cruciate ligament. *Clin Orthop* 1983;172:19–25.

7. Arnoczky SP: Blood supply to the anterior cruciate ligament and supporting structures. *Orthop Clin North Am* 1985;16:15–28.

8. Scapinelli R: Studies on the vasculature of the human knee joint. *Acta Anat* 1968;70:305–331.

9. Arnoczky SP: The vascularity of the anterior cruciate ligament and associated structures: Its role in repair and reconstruction, in Jackson DW, Drez D Jr (eds): *The Anterior Cruciate Deficient Knee: New Concepts in Ligament Repair.* St. Louis, CV Mosby, 1988, pp 27–54.

10. Arnoczky SP, Rubin RM, Marshall JL: Microvasculature of the cruciate ligaments and its response to injury: An experimental study in dogs. *J Bone Joint Surg* 1979;61A:1221–1229.

11. O'Donoghue DH, Rockwood CA Jr, Frank GR, et al: Repair of the anterior cruciate ligament in dogs. *J Bone Joint Surg* 1966;48A:503–519.

12. Cabaud HE, Rodkey WG, Feagin JA: Experimental studies of acute anterior cruciate ligament injury and repair. *Am J Sports Med* 1979;7:18–22.

13. Feagin JA Jr, Curl WW: Isolated tear of the anterior cruciate ligament: 5-year follow-up study. *Am J Sports Med* 1976;4:95–100.

14. Noyes FR, Butler DL, Grood ES, et al: Biomechanical analysis of human ligament grafts used in knee-ligament repairs and reconstructions. *J Bone Joint Surg* 1984;66A:344–352.

15. Butler DL, Grood ES, Noyes FR, et al: On the interpretation of our anterior cruciate ligament data. *Clin Orthop* 1985;196:26–34.

16. Sapega AA, Moyer RA, Schneck C, et al: Testing for isometry during reconstruction of the anterior cruciate ligament: Anatomical and biomechanical considerations. *J Bone Joint Surg* 1990;72A:259–267.

17. Sidles JA, Larson RV, Garbini JL, et al: III. Ligament length relationships in the moving knee. *J Orthop Res* 1988;6:593–610.

18. Alm A: Survival of part of patellar tendon transposed for reconstruction of anterior cruciate ligament. *Acta Chir Scand* 1973;139:443–447.

19. Clancy WG Jr: Anterior cruciate ligament functional instability: A static intra-articular and dynamic extra-articular procedure. *Clin Orthop* 1983;172:102–106.

20. Kennedy JC, Roth JH, Mendenhall HV, et al: Presidential address: Intra-articular replacement in the anterior cruciate ligament-deficient knee. *Am J Sports Med* 1980;8:1–8.

21. O'Donoghue DH: A method of replacement of the anterior cruciate ligament of the knee: Report of twenty cases. *J Bone Joint Surg* 1963;45A:905–924.

22. Paulos LE, Butler DL, Noyes FR, et al: Intra-articular cruciate reconstruction: II. Replacement with vascularized patellar tendon. *Clin Orthop* 1983;172:78–84.

23. Alm A, Liljedahl SO, Strömberg B: Clinical and experimental experience in reconstruction of the anterior cruciate ligament. *Orthop Clin North Am* 1976;7:181–189.

24. Alm A, Strömberg B: Transposed medial third of patellar ligament in reconstruction of the anterior cruciate ligament: A surgical and morophologic study in dogs. *Acta Chir Scand* 1974;445(suppl):37–49.

25. Arnoczky SP, Tarvin GB, Marshall JL: Anterior cruciate ligament

replacement using patellar tendon: An evaluation of graft revascularization in the dog. *J Bone Joint Surg* 1982;64A:217–224.

26. Clancy WG Jr, Narechania RG, Rosenberg TD, et al: Anterior and posterior cruciate ligament reconstruction in rhesus monkeys: A histological, microangiographic, and biomechanical analysis. *J Bone Joint Surg* 1981;63A:1270–1284.

27. Amiel D, Keiner JB, Roux RD, et al: The phenomenon of "ligamentization": Anterior cruciate ligament reconstruction with autogenous patellar tendon. *J Orthop Res* 1986;4:162–172.

28. O'Donoghue DH, Frank GR, Jeter GL, et al: Repair and reconstruction of the anterior cruciate ligament in dogs: Factors influencing long-term results. *J Bone Joint Surg* 1971;53A:710–718.

29. Shino K, Kawasaki T, Hirose H, et al: Replacement of the anterior cruciate ligament by an allogeneic tendon graft: An experimental study in the dog. *J Bone Joint Surg* 1984;66B:672–681.

30. Butler DL, Grood ES, Noyes FR, et al: Mechanical properties of primate vascularized vs. nonvascularized patellar tendon grafts: Changes over time. *J Orthop Res* 1989;7:68–79.

31. Jackson DW, Grood ES, Cohn BT, et al: The effects of in situ freezing on the anterior cruciate ligament. *Trans Orthop Res Soc* 1989;14:321.

32. Arnoczky SP, Warren RF, Ashlock MA: Replacement of the anterior cruciate ligament using a patellar tendon allograft: An experimental study. *J Bone Joint Surg* 1986;68A:376–385.

33. Curtis RJ, Delee JC, Drez DJ Jr: Reconstruction of the anterior cruciate ligament with freeze dried fascia lata allografts in dogs: A preliminary report. *Am J Sports Med* 1985;13:408–414.

34. Cabaud HE, Chatty A, Gildengorin V, et al: Exercise effects on the strength of the rat anterior cruciate ligament. *Am J Sports Med* 1980;8:79–86.

35. Laros GS, Tipton CM, Cooper RR: Influence of physical activity on ligament insertions in the knees of dogs. *J Bone Joint Surg* 1971;53A:275–286.

36. Tipton CM, Schild RJ, Tomanek RJ: Influence of physical activity on the strength of knee ligaments in rats. *Am J Physiol* 1967;212:783–787.

37. Viidik A: Elasticity and tensile strength of the anterior cruciate ligament in rabbits as influenced by training. *Acta Physiol Scand* 1968;74:372–380.

38. Woo SL-Y, Gomez MA, Woo Y-K, et al: Mechanical properties of tendons and ligaments: II. The relationships of immobilization and exercise on tissue remodeling. *Biorheology* 1982;19:397–408.

39. Zuckerman J, Stull GA: Effects of exercise on knee ligament separation force in rats. *J Appl Physiol* 1969;26:716–719.

40. Noyes FR: Functional properties of knee ligaments and alterations induced by immobilization: A correlative biomechanical and histological study in primates. *Clin Orthop* 1977;123:210–242.

41. Amiel D, Akeson WH, Harwood FL, et al: Stress deprivation effect on metabolic turnover of the medial collateral ligament collagen: A comparison between nine- and 12-week immobilization. *Clin Orthop* 1983;172:265–270.

Prosthetic Replacement of the Anterior Cruciate Ligament With Expanded Polytetrafluoroethylene

Scott R. Grewe, MD

Lonnie E. Paulos, MD

Introduction

Anterior cruciate ligament rupture is a serious injury. Various methods of reconstruction have been used to address the resultant instability and disability. Prosthetic replacement of the anterior cruciate ligament is advocated to avoid the disadvantages of autogenous and allograft materials. Synthetic materials have the advantage of avoiding autograft harvest. Because they do not need to undergo reorganization and revascularization to achieve strength, rehabilitation can be started more quickly. This can help avoid such undesirable effects of immobilization and nonweightbearing as atrophy and adhesions.[1] Also, the strength of biologic materials decreases after initial implantation,[2] whereas prosthetic implants provide immediate strength without biologic ingrowth.

Our experience with prosthetic anterior cruciate ligament reconstruction includes 268 Gore-Tex implants. Of the patients who received the implants, 188 (70%) were followed up for an average of 48 months (range, 24 to 68 months). Evaluation included questionnaires, physical examination, radiographs, KT-1000 arthrometer testing, and activity scoring. Our results and opinions are based on our experience with this patient population.[3]

The Gore-Tex prosthesis is made of expanded polytetrafluoroethylene.[4] This multifilament prosthesis is constructed of a single continuous fiber of expanded polytetrafluoroethylene. Bundles of the fibers are arranged in a braided configuration with eyelets at each end to provide secure internal fixation (Fig. 1). The prosthesis is intended as a permanent implant for correction of anterior cruciate ligament instability.

In 1986 the United States Food and Drug Administration approved the Gore-Tex ligament for commercial use in patients who had undergone previous intra-articular reconstruction. Before approval of the prosthesis, we took part in a clinical trial that used the Gore-Tex prosthesis for anterior cruciate ligament reconstruction.

Technique

The Gore-Tex synthetic ligaments were implanted by means of an arthroscopic technique. The implant was passed through anatomic bone tunnels in the tibia, the over-the-top route was used in the femur. A notchplasty was performed in every case, along with tunnel chamfering to avoid graft abrasion. The grafts were tensioned in extension and fixed through the eyelets to bone with bicortical screws in accordance with the manufacturer's suggested guidelines (Fig. 2).

Rehabilitation

The rehabilitation protocol for anterior cruciate ligament reconstruction with a prosthesis consisted of immobilizing the limb with a splint and keeping it nonweightbearing with crutches for the first week after implantation. Exercises during this period included straight leg raises, quadriceps setting, and ankle pumping exercises. Beginning with the second week, patellar mobilization was started, with patellar tilts and glides. Active and passive motion was also begun, and full range of motion was obtained as soon as possible. Resistance exercises were added as tolerated. Biking was begun, and swimming with straight leg kicks was started

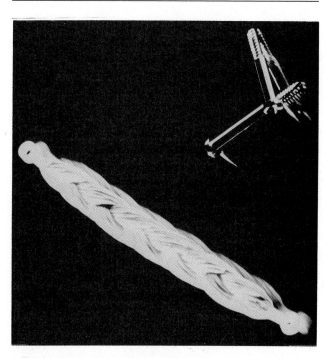

Fig. 1 The Gore-Tex prosthetic ligament.

as soon as the wound had healed. Full weightbearing was allowed as soon as the patient was able to perform a straight leg raise with 5 lb of weight. High-speed iso-kinetics in the 10- to 90-degree extension range were begun on the third week. Other exercises were continued. Sporting activities were started after three months.

Our patient population was typical of the young, active people who are susceptible to anterior cruciate ligament injury. The average age was 27.6 years (SD= 8.44), and the average activity score rated with the Tegner scale[5] was 6.05 (SD=1.53). Prior procedures had been performed in 56% of the patients, and 30% had had previous anterior cruciate ligament surgery. We performed concomitant procedures in 73%, including iliotibial band tenodesis in 65%, partial meniscectomy in 36%, meniscal repairs in 27%, and posterior oblique ligament reefing in 5%. Miscellaneous procedures, including medial collateral ligament repair, high tibial osteotomy, and lateral release, were performed in 6%.

Before implantation, this series showed marked instability. The preoperative pivot shift averaged 2.9 and the KT-1000 arthrometer manual maximum measurement ranged from 10 to 30. The average difference between injured and uninjured limbs was 8.8 mm (range, 3 to 17.5 mm).

Evaluation

Evaluation included both subjective and objective testing. Often, the patients' subjective evaluation failed to correlate with the objective findings. Results were graded by the following criteria. Results were considered excellent if there was no loosening, effusions, instability, or complaints. Results were good if loosening was less than 6 mm, there were fewer than three effusions, and there was a 1+ pivot shift. Results were fair if loosening was no more than 8 mm, there were no more than three effusions, the pivot shift was no more than 1+, and the patient had a sensation of instability and a subjective impression that there had been no change from the preoperative condition. Poor results included any of the following: loosening of more than 8 mm, more than three recurrent effusions, a pivot shift of 2+ or more, actual instability, or a subjective evaluation of being worse.

Complications

Effusions

Effusions occurred in 63 of the patients (34%). A typical effusion was a large accumulation of cloudy white fluid. Laboratory analysis revealed leukocyte counts averaging 70,000/mm³ (range, 51,000 to 80,000/mm³). The majority of the cells (88%) were polymorphonuclear leukocytes. In knees with effusions

examined arthroscopically, the synovium underwent biopsy. Histologic studies of these biopsy specimens revealed evidence of acute and chronic inflammation (Fig. 3). The majority of the cells seen were mononuclear inflammatory cells, but there were some polymorphonuclear leukocytes. Fibrous tissue, with multinucleated giant cells and amorphous birefringent foreign body particles, was also seen. There was capillary synovial formation with prominent vascular congestion. Subpopulations included multinucleated giant cells, both with and without foreign body particulates, histiocytes, and deep inflammatory polymorphonuclear cells. Effusions, first seen at four months after implantation, continued throughout the follow-up period (average, 20 months) (Fig. 4).

In the typical patient with effusion, there was a spontaneous accumulation of fluid, frequently accompanied by fever. Some patients reported antecedent trauma or overuse, but many could not identify a contributing cause. Patients were treated with aspiration (aspired fluid was cultured), nonsteroidal anti-inflammatory medication such as indomethacin, and inactivity.

We considered as failures those cases in which three or more recurrent effusions developed and those in which prostheses were removed because of persistent or recurrent malignant effusions. Explants were performed in eight cases (4%) and 22 cases (12%) were rated as failures on the basis of effusion.

Effusions often occurred with partial graft rupture. Of 15 patients who underwent arthroscopy when an effusion developed, ten (67%) had ruptured grafts. The extent of these ruptures ranged from several fibers to as much as one third of the prosthesis (Fig. 5). Patients with effusions also had a higher rate of later mechanical failure.

Failure

Mechanical failure included breakage and loosening. Breakage occurred in 23 patients (12%) (Fig. 6). Breakage occurred primarily at the posterior notch on the femoral side (70%). Some ruptures were also seen in the midsubstance (13%), and at the tibial tunnel (8%). Prostheses were more likely to break in patients who were more active, were younger, and who had high rates of previous effusions and loosening. Of the patients whose implants eventually broke, 48% had had an effusion and 26% had had documented loosening on KT-1000 evaluation. Rupture occurred at an average of 26.2 months (range, five to 61 months) and continued to be seen throughout the follow-up period (Fig. 7).

Loosening

Loosening was evaluated with KT-1000 manual maximum values. The final value was compared with previously obtained postoperative base-line values and with values for the opposite normal knee. It has been re-

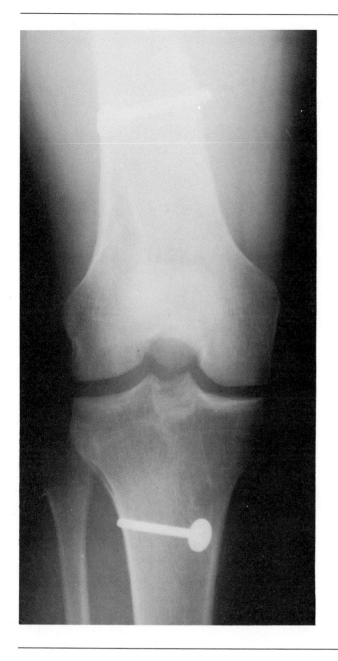

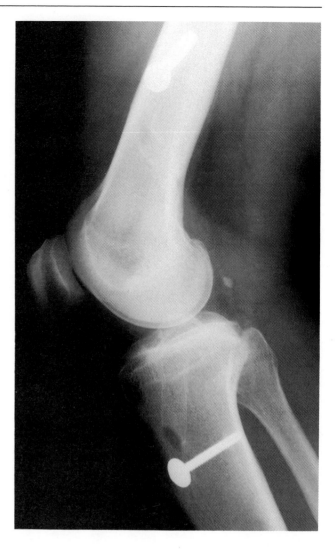

Fig. 2 Radiographs showing placement of ligament with bicortical screw fixation. **Left**, Anteroposterior. **Right**, Lateral.

ported that a difference of 2 to 3 mm on KT testing can be physiologically normal.[6] The difference in manual maximum KT values was therefore considered to be normal in our patients if the difference between injured and uninjured knees was 3 mm or less.

Loosening was not by itself necessarily a criterion for failure. For the prostheses to be considered a failure, the patients had to have a pivot shift of more than 1+, a functional instability, or a subjective evaluation of being worse. Loosening of 3 to 5 mm occurred in 27 patients, but only five cases were considered failures.

Intermediate loosening of 5 to 8 mm occurred in 23 prostheses in which total preoperative laxity averaged 19.7 mm. Of prostheses with this amount of loosening, 14 (60%) were failures. These failures had a higher total

laxity, averaging 17.1 mm, than prostheses not considered failures, in which laxity averaged 14.5 mm, but loosening was the same. Instability was reported in 26% of this subgroup of failures. It is not only the amount of loosening, but also the total measured laxity that is important in determining instability.

Loosening in excess of 8 mm occurred in ten patients. All these patients had a pivot shift, and the average pivot shift was 2+. Average total laxity was 17.9 mm. When questioned regarding instability, 60% were symptomatic.

Infection

Infection is always a concern in orthopaedic surgery. This is especially true when a prosthesis is implanted.

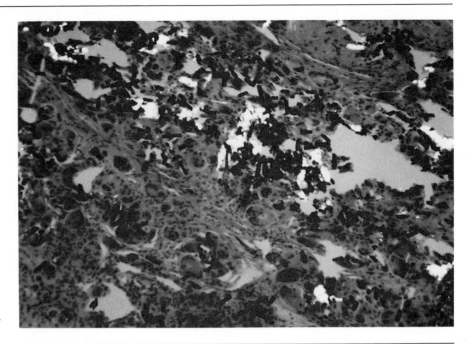

Fig. 3 Histologic specimen from synovial biopsy.

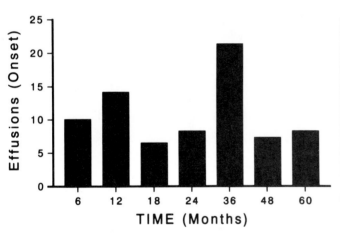

Fig. 4 Effusions occurring with time.

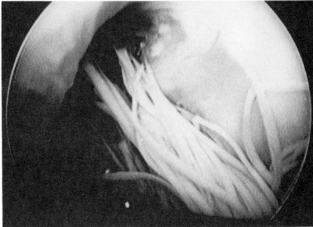

Fig. 5 Arthroscopic finding of partial graft rupture.

Infection occurred in five patients (2.7%). There was one acute postoperative infection and four delayed infections that occurred at an average of 32 months (range, 24 to 43 months). The late infections developed in patients with other systemic problems, such as ulcerative colitis, pneumonia, and asplenia. Infection was also seen after local wound problems from underlying hardware and after hardware removal. Organisms isolated from culture included *Staphylococcus aureus* and *Staphylococcus epidermidis*. The one acute postoperative infection was resolved with antibiotic therapy. All delayed infections required prosthesis removal for resolution. Infection continues to be a concern throughout the life of the prosthesis. Despite synovialization, the prosthesis continues to be a nonviable substance with the concomitant risks of developing a late infection. Patients should receive prophylaxis whenever there is a risk of seeding the joint with bacteria.

Results

Prosthetic replacement of the anterior cruciate ligament allowed rapid return of function. Activity level, as rated by the Tegner score, remained the same in 89% of the patients (Fig. 8). Only 1% of patients improved

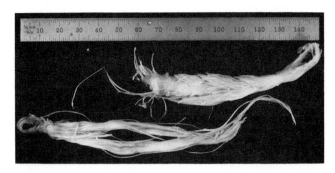

Fig. 6   Ruptured prosthesis.

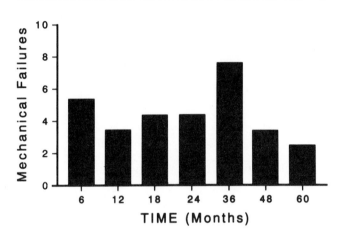

Fig. 7   Mechanical failures occurring with time.

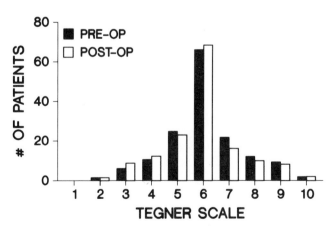

Fig. 8   Preoperative and postoperative activity levels.

above their preinjury level. A decrease in activity level was seen in 19 patients (10%).

Subsequent procedures were performed in 45% of the patients. Procedures included arthroscopy, hardware removal, and manipulations.

Patients with excellent results were analyzed as a group. It was found that they were significantly (P = .045) older (average, 29.5 years) and had significantly (P = .012) lower activity levels (Tegner score, 5.8). This subgroup also included a higher percentage of females (57%).

Previous intra-articular anterior cruciate ligament reconstructions were evaluated as a separate group. Complications, which developed in 76% of this group, included loosening in 33%, effusions in 29%, and rupture in 14%. Failures occurred in 42%.

Most patients in our series were happy with their outcome. Subjective improvement was indicated by 89% of the patients. Unfortunately, objective evaluation revealed an excellent or good result in only 43%. Although this discrepancy between subjective and objective results has not been fully explained, we believe it is the result of the extra-articular surgery and the fact that other problems, such as meniscal lesions, were also addressed. We are continuing to see an increase in the complications with time. Longer follow-up will allow further delineation of the natural history of prosthetic replacement of the anterior cruciate ligament. It appears the indications for using the polytetrafluoroethylene prosthesis in its present form are extremely limited. It is possible that the present FDA recommendations for use of the device in previously failed intra-articular procedures are inappropriate.

References

1. Bruchman WC, Bain JR, Bolton CW: Prosthetic replacement of the cruciate ligaments with expanded polytetrafluoroethylene, in Feagin JA Jr (ed): *The Crucial Ligaments*. New York, Churchill Livingstone, 1988, pp 507–515.
2. Noyes FR, Butler DL, Grood ES, et al: Biomechanical analysis of human ligament grafts used in knee-ligament repairs and reconstructions. *J Bone Joint Surg* 1984;66A:344–352.
3. Paulos LE, Rosenberg TD, Tearse DS, et al: Gore-Tex prosthetic anterior cruciate ligament reconstruction: A long-term follow-up. Presented at the 57th Annual Meeting of the American Academy of Orthopaedic Surgeons, New Orleans, Feb 8–13, 1990.
4. Bolton CW, Bruchman WC: The Gore-Tex expanded polytetrafluoroethylene prosthetic ligament: An in vitro and in vivo evaluation. *Clin Orthop* 1985;196:202–213.
5. Tegner Y, Lysholm J: Rating systems in the evaluation of knee ligament injuries. *Clin Orthop* 1985;198:43–49.
6. Daniel DM. Malcom LL, Losse G, et al: Instrumented measurement of anterior laxity of the knee. *J Bone Joint Surg* 1985;67A:720–726.

Management of Acute Anterior Cruciate Ligament Injury

Jon J. P. Warner, MD

Russell F. Warren, MD

Daniel E. Cooper, MD

Significance of the Anterior Cruciate Ligament

Function of the Anterior Cruciate Ligament

Diagnosis and treatment of acute anterior cruciate ligament (ACL) injuries requires a firm knowledge of how these injuries have been viewed historically. In the past, there was great uncertainty as to the role of the ACL in stability of the knee joint. Because of this uncertainty, the need for repair of this structure remained in question. Moreover, clinical recognition of acute injury was inconsistent. With the descriptions and recent refinements of the Lachman[1] and pivot shift[2] tests, and the development of instrumented testing devices, diagnosis is no longer the central issue. The controversy is whether all acute ACL injuries should be repaired and, if so, what technique is the best.

Although Groves[3] was the first to perform ACL reconstruction, Palmer,[4] in 1938, was the first surgeon to provide a rationale for early repair based on both clinical and experimental studies. In 1941, Brantigan and Voshell[5] published their classic work on the mechanics of the ligaments and menisci of the knee joint. The clinical work of O'Donoghue and associates[6-11] in the 1950s and 1960s presaged a new age of aggressive surgical management of ACL injuries in the United States. However, in 1976, Feagin and Curl[12] reported late deterioration of early encouraging results of acute ACL repair. This led to a more cautious attitude toward early surgical repair of the ACL injury.

In the late 1970s and early 1980s Marshall and associates[13-18] carried out a series of clinical and experimental studies that renewed interest in acute surgical repair of the ACL. Furman and associates[19] and Girgis and associates[20] were the first to elucidate the central role of the ACL in the control of anterior tibial translation and hyperextension, as well as its secondary role in the control of varus-valgus and rotational stability. Marshall and associates drew anatomic and functional distinctions between two portions of the ACL, but Odensten and Gillquist[21] subsequently observed only functional differences between the anteromedial and the posterolateral portions of the ACL.

Since Marshall and associates' work, there have been many functional and anatomic studies building on the foundation provided by their observations.[3,5,22-26] Recent studies have sought to measure anteroposterior displacement with externally applied loads simulating clinical drawer tests,[22,23,25,27-29] and a few studies have focused on three-dimensional measurements of knee

motion in vitro.[30] We now know that the absence of the ACL causes multiplanar instability of the knee.[20,31,32]

Butler and associates[22] reintroduced the concept of primary and secondary restraints to clinical anterior drawer testing, and they identified the ACL as the primary restraint. The iliotibial band, medial collateral ligament, lateral collateral ligament, and medial and lateral capsules were considered secondary restraints to anterior tibial translation. These researchers further distinguished between low clinical testing anteroposterior loads and higher anteroposterior loads that result in functional instability. Fukubayashi and associates[23] confirmed the primary role of the ACL and observed that absence of the ACL resulted in anterior displacement that was greatest at 30 degrees of flexion.

On the basis of these studies, the ACL has been defined as the main stabilizer in the knee controlling anterior tibial translation, and its absence is most apparent when the knee is at 20 to 30 degrees of flexion. The ACL has an additional primary role in control of hyperextension and secondary roles in controlling varus-valgus and rotational stability of the knee.[33]

Protection of the Meniscus and Role in Osteoarthritis

The menisci play an important role in stability and load transmission in the normal knee, and the ACL apparently protects the menisci.[34-36] There is a high incidence of meniscal injury at the time of an initial ACL injury and meniscal injury is common as a late sequella of ACL deficiency.[37-47] Moreover, the presence of a meniscal lesion may decrease stability,[34,48] alter load transmission,[24,36] and contribute to the development of osteoarthritis in the ACL-deficient knee.[49] Marked increases in stress to the knee cartilage have been shown experimentally after total meniscectomy.[50-53]

Loss of the ACL allows increased anterior tibial slide near full extension and excessive roll in flexion, which place the menisci at risk. Palmer[4] noted a propensity for lateral meniscal injury at the time of ACL disruption and Smillie[54] suggested that the lateral meniscus may be more susceptible to radial tears because of its increased concavity and lack of collateral attachment. Brantigan and Voshell[5] also suggested that the lateral meniscus was more vulnerable to radial and axial loading injury between the tibia and femur because of its increased mobility. Because the medial meniscus is larger in radial diameter and is more intimately connected to the peripheral capsule, it is less mobile and therefore has a higher risk for peripheral, longitudinal tears with valgus injury.[37] An understanding of these patterns of injury is of prognostic value in light of the experimental and clinical evidence in support of acute meniscal repair.[39,55-60] Furthermore, it has been shown that concomitant repair of an ACL injury improves the results of meniscal repair.[38,61,62]

Menisci, by virtue of their function as tensile hoops, help stabilize the knee. Levy and associates[34] demonstrated the importance of the menisci, particularly the medial side, in providing anteroposterior stability, and clinical studies have documented increased anterior laxity after total meniscectomy.[63-65] Even in the ACL-deficient knee, if the posterior horn of the medial meniscus is preserved, a significant amount of anterior resistive forces can be retained.[66,67]

The Natural History of the ACL-Deficient Knee

Our developing understanding of the anatomy, physiology, and function of the ACL, and appreciation of the instability and functional disability that result from its injury, have led to the definition of the syndrome of the ACL-deficient knee.[68-70] The hallmarks of this syndrome are unpredictable instability that occurs with jumping, cutting, and deceleration maneuvers.[71]

In 1978, Marshall and associates[16] proposed that the natural history of this syndrome is marked by progressive functional and anatomic deterioration of the knee. These researchers observed that, in the dog, loss of the ACL resulted in a predictable process of synovial hypertrophy and fibrosis, early periarticular osteophytes, degenerative meniscal tears, and late degenerative osteoarthritis.[13,14] Subsequent studies provided mounting evidence of progressive deterioration of knee function,[72] meniscal deterioration[14,34,73-75] stretching of secondary ligamentous restraints,[70] and eventual osteoarthritis.[13,14,76-78]

Nevertheless, numerous clinical studies have suggested a benign course for the knee after complete ACL disruption (Table 1). McDaniel and Dameron,[73,74] Balkfors,[79] Noyes and associates,[75] and others[60,80-83] suggested that conservative management with a directed rehabilitation program can compensate for the loss of the ACL in the young athlete. In contrast, Hawkins and associates,[69] Odensten and associates,[84] Kannus and Järvenin,[85] and others[42,65,86,87] observed a high rate of failure with the nonsurgical approach in the active, young athlete. Critical review of these studies reveals that the controversy regarding indications for nonsurgical treatment is the result of the wide diversity of study populations, assessment techniques, compliance with rehabilitation programs, and definitions of a successful outcome. Moreover, it is important to consider all retrospective studies within the framework of the selection bias that automatically defines them. An accurate natural history of the ACL-deficient knee may never be known, because few studies have been prospective and unselected.

In our experience, a study of 52 nonathletic patients, who received follow-up examinations for a minimum of two years, showed that patients with acute ACL injuries, even those with low athletic expectations, run a significant risk (49%) of having an undependable knee with conservative treatment.[88] Of these, 15% required late reconstruction with the mid-third patellar tendon.

Partial ACL Injury

Partial injury to the ACL represents 10% to 28% of all ACL injuries.[40,44,74,89] Fifty years after Darrach[90] first commented on the occurrence of this injury, there is still no consensus as to the best approach to its management.[91,92] Palmer,[4] Liljedahl and associates,[89] and O'Donoghue[7] recommended surgery for all partial ACL injuries, although McDaniel,[93] Sandberg and Balkfors,[94] and other researchers[84,95] observed a favorable course after conservative treatment of partial ACL injuries (Table 2).

Because failure of the ACL occurs first by plastic deformation with loss of collagen cross-linking, rupture usually occurs as a single fiber-mass failure rather than sequential fiber failure.[42,96] This probably explains why partial ACL injury is less common than complete rupture. In reality, subclinical partial ACL rupture involving a subsynovial rupture with absent or small hemarthrosis is probably more common than is generally recognized.[95]

Although several studies [94,95] proposed minimal fiber disruption of the ACL as a favorable prognostic factor, others[97] suggested that the percentage of the tear is not a useful clinical observation. Both Kennedy and associates[98] and Noyes and associates[99] emphasized that the macroscopic appearance of the ACL may not accurately represent its functional capacity, because plastic deformation has occurred in the remaining fibers. Most studies concluded that, although partial ACL injury produces a functionally symptomatic knee in most cases, the degree of functional instability over time does not warrant early surgical repair or reconstruction of the ligament.[84,94,97]

Our approach is to carry out arthroscopy and examination with the patient under anesthesia and then consider the findings in the context of the athletic demands of each patient. A 25% tear of the ACL with a negative pivot shift would be treated conservatively, whereas a 25% tear with a strongly positive pivot shift in an active athlete would be treated with augmentation using semitendinosus and gracilis tendons as described below.

Table 1
Conservative treatment of acute (total) anterior cruciate ligament tears

Study	Type of Study	Follow-up (yrs)	No. of Patients	% Meniscal Tears	% Osteoarthritis by Radiograph	% Functional Instability	% Objective Instability	% Requiring ACL Reconstruction
Jacobsen[77]	Retrospective	0.5 to 5	43	50	40	100	—	100
Chick and Jackson[80]	Retrospective	2.6	30	100	50	33	20	—
McDaniel and Dameron[74]	Retrospective	10.0	55	18	56	76	83	16
Balkfors[79]	Retrospective	10.0	87	—	40	40	80	—
Giove et al[60]	Retrospective	—	24	—	59	88	96	—
Noyes et al[75]	Retrospective	5.5	103	—	21	81	—	—
Noyes et al[87]	Retrospective	8.0	84	—	—	43	99	22
Jokl et al[82]	Retrospective	3.0	28	—	—	14	—	14
Indelicato and Bittar[86]	Retrospective	—	56	94	54	—	100	—
Odensten et al[84]	Prospective	1.5	45	—	—	28	90	11
Hawkins et al[69]	Retrospective	4.0	40	10	—	86	100	30
Kannus and Järvinen[85]	Retrospective	8.0	49	19	70	80	95	35
Aglietti et al[63]	Retrospective	3.5	100	—	—	53	86	—
Clancy et al[106]	Prospective	4.0	22	—	—	—	—	18
Pattee et al[83]	Retrospective	4 to 10	40	5	65	38	87	0
Andersson et al[155]	Prospective	4.75	100	33	—	35	95	35

Table 2
Conservative treatment of acute (partial) anterior cruciate ligament tears

Study	Type of Study	Follow-up (yrs)	No. of Patients	% Meniscal Tears	% Osteoarthritis by Radiograph	% Functional Instability	% Objective Instability	% Requiring ACL Reconstruction
McDaniel[93]	Retrospective	4.25	9	33	—	11	—	0
Odensten et al[156]	Prospective	6.0	21	0	—	10	10	0
Sandberg and Balkfors[94]	Prospective	1 to 5	29	—	—	13	61	0
Kannus and Järvinen[85]	Retrospective	8.0	41	10	15	24	73	0
Noyes et al[95]	Prospective	7.0	32	—	—	38	61	—
Buckley et al[97]	Retrospective	1.5	25	8	—	52	—	8

Historical and Current Perspectives in Treatment

Indications for Surgery

In 1983, Noyes and associates,[87] on the basis of an eight-year follow-up study of the effect of rehabilitation and activity modification on functional disability, concluded that an initial nonsurgical approach to the acute ACL injury was appropriate because it was impossible to predict which knees would respond to such a program. These recommendations were made in the context of their judgment that no predictable reconstructive procedures for the ACL were available at that time. More recently, growing success with a number of surgical techniques has led to a more aggressive approach to these injuries.[38,45,100] Most surgeons agree that treatment should be individualized, and that acute ACL reconstruction is recommended only for carefully selected patients.[49,101]

A variety of high and low risk factors can be identified for poor results with conservative approach. A physiologically young patient with a high activity level that places deceleration and rotational demands on the knee would have a high risk profile. Such individuals are rarely willing to modify or change their life style. Other high risk factors include the presence of associated grade III collateral ligament injuries, the presence of associated repairable meniscus tears, and generalized ligamentous laxity. Patients with the psychosocial and economic ability to comply with a vigorous postoperative rehabilitation program are also better candidates for surgery than for conservative treatment.[38,68–70,89,102–105]

A low risk profile for conservative treatment characterizes an individual who is physiologically older, with a modest to low activity level, without associated grade III collateral ligament injuries or repairable meniscal tears, mild to moderate objective knee laxity, and an unfavorable profile with regard to the psychosocial and economic factors necessary for compliance with postoperative rehabilitation.

Role of Examination With the Patient Under Anesthesia and Arthroscopy

Several authors have suggested that a minimally positive pivot shift test on examination with the patient under anesthesia is a favorable predictor of a successful conservative approach to complete ACL tear.[63,64,106] Our experience has been that complete acute ACL disruption in the young and active individual often progresses to functional instability regardless of the grade of the pivot shift test.

Several authors have recommended arthroscopy for all cases of acute hemarthrosis.[38,40,41,44,107,108] We have found, however, that most ACL injuries can be confirmed by Lachman testing and KT-1000 arthrometer measurement in the awake patient. Arthroscopy can be reserved for proven ACL tears requiring reconstruction, or for management of associated meniscal or chondral damage.[38,40,44] It is important to appreciate that tense hemarthrosis of the knee can reflect intraarticular injury alone, while a knee with marked instability and no effusion can indicate extensive capsular disruption along with cruciate injury. This latter situation can present a problem for arthroscopic evaluation, because fluid extravasation into the compartments of the leg can create a risk.

Our recommendations for arthroscopy and examination with the patient under anesthesia include all young, active, athletic patients with clinical evidence of ACL disruption with or without associated collateral ligament and meniscal injuries. During arthroscopy, the ACL may appear to be intact because the proximal stump has remained within the notch, adherent to the posterior cruciate ligament. To avoid error, look for the empty lateral wall and vertical strut signs, which are most easily recognized with the knee in the figure-of-four position.[109] These findings result from the ACL rupture adhering to the posterior cruciate ligament with a vertical orientation in the several weeks after injury.

In general, we recommend aggressive treatment for young athletes with partial disruption of the ACL. If disruption is 25% or more, and a distinctly positive pivot shift is noted during examination with the patient under anesthesia, we use augmentation in treating these injuries. If disruption is 25% or less, and a pivot shift is negative, we will treat these individuals conservatively, with protection followed by rehabilitation for eight to ten weeks.

Timing of Surgery (Acute Versus Chronic)

Use of the mid-third patellar tendon for reconstruction of the chronic ACL-deficient knee has been favorable in our experience, with an overall good to excellent result in more than 90% of cases with both arthroscopic and open techniques. Nevertheless, there are several advantages to an initial surgical approach to this injury. With acute reconstruction it is possible to manage both the ACL deficiency and concomitant meniscal abnormalities from the start, requiring only a single period of rehabilitation and eliminating subsequent need for bracing. We believe that such management also reduces the risk of late meniscal injury and resulting arthritis. Also, the competitive athlete can avoid the possibility of missing two seasons of play. Disadvantages of this approach include the usual risks that accompany surgery and the use of anesthesia, as well as the possibility of overtreating a select group of patients who may continue to function well without an ACL.

Primary Repair of the ACL

Robson[110] reported the first ACL repair in 1903. This was followed by similar reports from Battle,[111] Pringle,[112] and Jones and Smith.[113] Palmer[4] in the 1930s and O'Donoghue and associates[6-11] in the 1950s and 1960s stressed the need for early repair by suture approximation. In the 1970s Marshall and Rubin[15] described management of the acute ACL injury as "a golden opportunity for primary repair."

Early rationale for acute suture repair was based on experimental studies that showed that transected ligaments will heal after suture approximation.[11,96] However, Cabaud and associates[96,114] observed that repair was attended by decreased ligament tensile strength eight months after surgery.

Feagin and Curl,[12] in 1976, were the first to report poor five-year results after isolated figure-of-eight suture repair of acute ACL injuries in active men. Others have since reported poor outcomes following suture repair.[79,115-118]

Marshall and associates'[17] original follow-up study, in 1982, reported encouraging results in recreational athletes after more than two years of follow-up examinations. This study provided the rationale for acute ACL management at The Hospital for Special Surgery in the late 1970s and early 1980s. More recently, a six-year follow-up of 52 of the original 70 patients in that study disclosed an overall failure rate of 29% based on objective clinical findings.[119] However, 71% had a 0 pivot shift test and were able to return to sports participation, and none required meniscectomy. Fifteen percent had a 1+ pivot shift test, and 14% had a 2+ or 3+ pivot shift test.

The difference between the relatively favorable long-term results of Marshall and associates[17] and the poor results of Feagin and Curl[12] may be partly attributable to technical differences in the procedure used. Marshall and associates emphasized multiple depth sutures through the ligament; the other team used a single figure-of-eight suture to repair the ligament.

Several authors continue to report acceptable results using suture repair alone.[49,89,120-124] In 1987, Higgins and Steadman[49] reported excellent results in 30 U.S. Ski Team members who underwent primary suture repair of the ACL and other ligament injuries and iliotibial band extra-articular tenodesis. A number of factors may be responsible for the success of this approach. More than 80% of their patients had proximal disruption of the ACL, which is more amenable to suture repair. In most other series, this location of the tear accounted for only 25% of the cases, and the more common midsubstance disruption of the ligament is usually more difficult to repair.[17,18,68] Aggressive notchplasty, placement of multiple sutures distal to the over-the-top position, and extra-articular lateral augmentation with the iliotibial band are other factors that may account for their excellent results. Cross and associates[120] also reported excellent results when acute repair was combined with lateral extra-articular augmentation.

Although primary repair of the ACL works in some patients, the results are unpredictable.[119] On the basis of our experience of a 29% failure rate with primary repair in active, young patients, our current recommendation is for routine intra-articular augmentation with semitendinosus and gracilis tendons.

Primary Repair of the ACL With Augmentation

The inconsistency of clinical results with primary repair alone led to the concept of augmentation of acute ACL repairs. This approach was supported by the experimental work of Cabaud and associates,[96,114] who used histologic and biomechanical testing to demonstrate the superiority of augmentation over primary repair alone.

In 1950, Lindemann[125] performed intra-articular transfer of the gracilis tendon through a posterior approach, and, in 1968, Lange[126] reported on the use of the semitendinosus tendon with this approach. Slocum and Larson,[127] in the late 1960s, described medial and proximal transplantation of the pes anserinus insertion to control rotatory instability. Cho,[128] in 1975, was the first to describe clearly a technique using the semitendinosus intra-articularly. He used a medial parapatellar arthrotomy, harvested only the semitendinosus, passed the tendon through both tibial and femoral tunnels, and applied cast immobilization in 30 degrees of flexion for six weeks. The reported short-term results were good in five of seven patients.[128] In 1986, Lipscomb and Anderson[62] reported good results in 23 of 24 adolescent athletes using both semitendinosus and gracilis tendons through an arthrotomy and in combination with either an Ellison[129] or Losee and associates[130] extra-articular procedure.

In the early 1980s we began routinely augmenting primary ACL repairs using the semitendinosus tendon passed over the top.[101] This technique was based on the original suture repair of Marshall and Rubin[15] and Marshall and associates[18] with the addition of a distally based semitendinosus tendon transferred intra-articu-

larly as originally described by Cho.[128] A total of 220 athletically active individuals underwent this procedure within three weeks of acute disruption of the ACL. In 71% of cases an extra-articular lateral sling of distally based iliotibial band was employed as well. Critical review of results, at an average follow-up of 39 months, demonstrated that, contrary to the observations of Lipscomb and Anderson,[62] extra-articular augmentation did not improve the results of the procedure. Overall, 82% had good to excellent objective results, 93% had a KT-1000 arthrometer side-to-side measurement of 3 mm or less at 30 degrees of flexion and a load of 89 N, and 86% had a negative pivot shift.

A criticism of this technique has been that loss of terminal extension or loosening of the graft can occur, because the over-the-top position can lengthen the graft by as much as 10 mm during knee extension.[21] In the above series, loss of flexion was believed to be attributable to postoperative cast immobilization rather than to graft position.

Various factors must be considered when comparing the augmentation technique with acute reconstruction using the mid-third of the patellar tendon. These factors include the need for adequate initial mechanical properties of the graft, graft viability, graft accessibility, the desirability of bone-bone fixation, proper placement and tensioning of the graft, and minimal surgical morbidity from harvesting and placement of the graft.[131] In addition, it must be kept in mind that no chosen graft can duplicate the complex fiber geometry of the ACL.[19-22,33] Even an ideal graft is probably little more than a checkrein to excessive joint displacements.

In managing acute ACL disruption, replacement of the ligament and the facilitation of early motion and rehabilitation are the basic goals. Clancy and associates[106,132,133] documented excellent results with a mid-third patellar tendon reconstruction in cases of chronic insufficiency, and other researchers confirmed these observations.[119] In managing acute ACL disruption, proponents of the mid-third patellar tendon graft point out that it provides reproducibly excellent results.[106,131] Noyes and associates[134] suggested that even under the most strenuous conditions, the ACL is never subjected to more than 50% of its maximum load potential. On the basis of their experimental data for mid-third patellar tendon (maximum load per unit width = 208 N), a 10-mm graft would have a maximum strength of 1800 N or 104% of the ACL strength.[134,135] Semitendinosus and gracilis tendons have 70% and 49% of ACL strength, respectively. The combined strength of the two has never been determined. Moreover, the semitendinosus and gracilis tendons have about the same stiffness as the ACL, whereas the mid-third patellar tendon is significantly stiffer.[134]

Additional advantages of the semitendinosus-gracilis graft over the mid-third patellar tendon are that it avoids the extensor mechanism and the risk of patellar fracture and does not disrupt the patellar tendon.[136-138] It is technically easier to harvest and prepare the semitendinosus-gracilis graft, and there is minimal loss of hamstring strength.[139,140] In addition, Sachs and associates[139] found significantly stronger quadriceps function one year after use of semitendinosus-gracilis than with the mid-third patellar tendon, and this result was independent of any flexion contracture. Since 1986, we have been routinely using arthroscopically directed primary repair with intra-articular augmentation using semitendinosus-gracilis tendon within three weeks of injury in patients with acute ACL injuries. Although it is our impression that this technique is easier and provides results comparable to reconstruction with mid-third patellar tendon, we are currently evaluating this technique by randomization.

Surgical Technique of Primary Repair and Augmentation

Currently we prefer to perform primary repair with semitendinosus-gracilis by an arthroscopic technique no more than three weeks after an acute ACL disruption. The patient is placed supine on the operating table and a lateral post is used against the proximal thigh. A tourniquet is applied, but is usually not used, because one ampule of epinephrine in each 3-L inflow bag generally allows excellent arthroscopic visualization. Examination with the patient under anesthesia confirms the diagnosis in more than 98% of cases.[141] Arthroscopy is then performed, and any associated meniscal lesions are either repaired or excised. We do not routinely perform a notchplasty in these acute cases, but we are careful to confirm that there is no impingement of the repair and graft against the lateral condyle or the roof of the notch in full extension. In some cases the notch is cathedral- or trephine-shaped and requires extensive widening. This is usually a more serious concern in chronic cases, in which osteophytes may have narrowed the notch.[142]

If the ligament is disrupted proximally, we place a series of sutures through it arthroscopically with the Schutte suture passer. With most midsubstance tears, no attempt at repair is made.

In cases of distal avulsion of the ACL with a small wedge of bony insertion, we have been able to perform arthroscopic repair with transosseous sutures. We generally do not use augmentation with these injuries.

It is essential to appreciate the relevant anatomy of the pes anserinus if the semitendinosus-gracilis tendons are to be harvested successfully (Fig. 1). Placing the leg in the figure-of-four position facilitates both dissection and harvesting (Fig. 1, A). The semitendinosus-gracilis tendons course distally on the undersurface of layer I, beneath the sartorius (Fig. 1, B). They insert as a common tendon on the anteromedial tibial surface, approximately 2 cm distal and 1 cm medial to the tibial

tubercle (Figs. 1, C, and 2). A small longitudinal skin incision is made at this location and layer I is identified. The tendons can usually be palpated underneath this layer, and division of layer I should be just above the palpable gracilis tendon and in line with its fibers. Each tendon can then be identified and elevated with the aid of a right angle clamp (Fig. 1, D). Care must be taken not to injure the medial collateral ligament, which courses deep to these structures. Each tendon can have a significant fascial expansion posteriorly and distally into the gastrocnemius fascia, and proximally there is often a thick band forming a tight tunnel around the tendons at the level of the semimembranous insertion (Fig. 2). Both sharp and blunt dissection are necessary to mobilize each tendon prior to stripping. We use a specially designed tendon stripper and can usually harvest 23 mm of usable tendon length (Fig. 3). A rule of thumb for usable tendon length is that the length of the harvested tendons should reach about 2 inches proximal to the superior pole of the patella when held against the leg.

Two potential pitfalls are injury to the saphenous vein or nerve during dissection and stripping of the tendons. Injury to the former may occur if the scissors are permitted to stray too far posteriorly and external to layer I when fascial connections are divided from either tendon. This can be avoided by maintaining firm countertraction on the tendons and dissecting with clear visualization. In our early experience with harvesting the semitendinosus, we observed a 37.5% incidence of residual numbness in the sensory distribution of the infrapatellar branch of the saphenous nerve.[101] Although only one individual found this bothersome, patients should be informed of this possibility. The problem of numbness has become less serious since we began to use the figure-of-four position and the tendon stripper to harvest the graft.

The tendons are prepared carefully in order to allow ease of passage through the knee. A series of Thompson and Bunnell sutures are placed through the tendons, and a whip stitch is used at the terminal portion of the graft (Fig. 1, E).

The over-the-top position is developed through a lateral incision 3 cm long over the flare of the distal femur. The lateral intermuscular septum is dissected posteriorly down to the flare of the lateral condyle, and a curved Cobb gauge is used to cut a notch in the posterolateral cortex down to the over-the-top position (Fig. 4). It is useful to palpate this location bimanually with two small periosteal elevators, while looking through the arthroscope, in order to determine the orientation of this notch. Though Odensten and Gillquist[21] observed that the over-the-top position produced a 10-mm elongation of the graft in full extension, we have found that cutting this notch positions the graft closer to the isometric position, and graft elongation

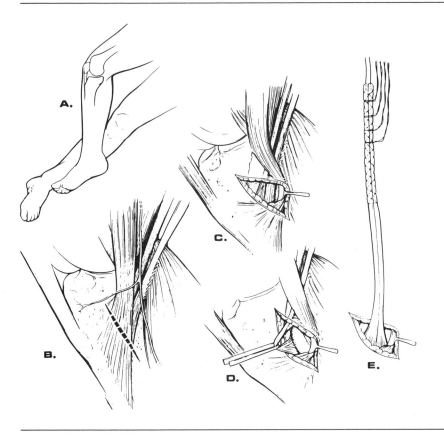

Fig. 1 **A**, Figure-of-four position used to facilitate harvesting of the semitendinosus and gracilis tendons. **B**, Regional surgical anatomy for harvesting of semitendinosus and gracilis tendons. **C**, Sartorius is retracted medially and posteriorly after layer I is divided in line with its fibers. **D**, The gracilis and semitendinosus tendons are elevated and traction is applied through a Penrose drain while fascial expansions into layer I distally and proximally are divided. **E**, The tendon graft is prepared by placing a series of Thompson and Bunnell sutures through the distal half. A whip-stitch is used to tubulate the end of the graft in order to permit easier passage of the graft through the knee.

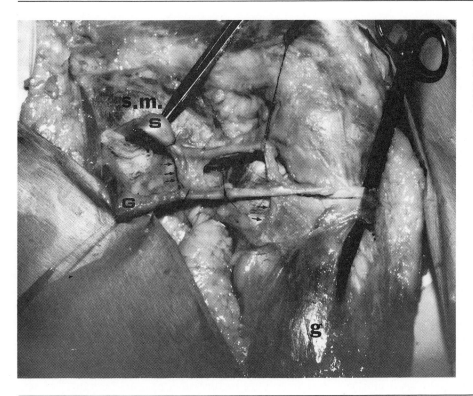

Fig. 2 Anatomic dissection showing fascial bands (arrows) from both semitendinosus (S) and gracilis (G) tendons. Semimembranosus (s.m.) and gastrocnemius (g) are marked and the scissors have been placed underneath the combined insertion of the semitendinosus and gracilis. The sartorius has been removed.

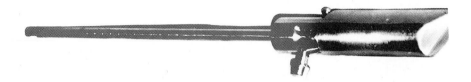

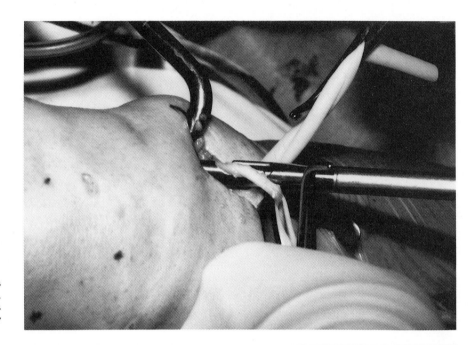

Fig. 3 **Top**, The tendon stripper allows easy harvesting of each tendon. **Bottom**, Traction is maintained on the tendon as the tendon stripper is pushed proximally to 20 mm.

in extension is usually limited to 2 to 3 mm (Fig. 4, *bottom left*).

A tibial tunnel is drilled from the anteromedial tibial cortex, just above the common insertion of the semitendinosus-gracilis. Drilling is done with a 7- to 8-mm cannulated reamer placed over a wire that enters the center of the tibial insertion of the ACL. Care is taken to avoid injury to the peripheral ACL insertion. Thus, the graft will be housed within the remnant of the ACL as it passes through the knee (Fig. 4, *top right*).

A special, curved cannula is then passed into the knee from the over-the-top position, and the prepared graft, along with the sutures through the ACL, is passed back out of the knee using this device (Fig. 4, *top left*). A Sitinsky clamp may be used if this cannula is not available.

We have found it useful to measure excursion of the graft by marking it with methylene blue at the level of the posterior femoral cortex and then flexing and extending the knee while maintaining tension on the graft. This allows us to confirm minimal lengthening of the graft in full extension, indicated if the mark moves only 2 to 3 mm. If excursion is greater, further rasping of the posterolateral notch will move the graft closer

to the isometric point. With the knee at about 30 degrees of flexion, the graft is fixed to the lateral cortex of the femur using two ligament staples, and the sutures through the ACL are tied around a staple (Fig. 4, *top right* and *bottom right*). The incisions are closed over a drain, the knee is placed into a hinged brace, and motion is begun in the recovery room on the continuous passive motion machine in an arc from 0 to 90 degrees.

If the semitendinosus-gracilis is damaged during harvesting or if the ACL injury appears to be the result of chronic insufficiency, we use the mid-third patellar tendon instead. It should be emphasized that the semitendinosus-gracilis has not been used by us for reconstruction to correct chronic insufficiency.

Postoperative Rehabilitation Program

A physiologic and practical rehabilitation program must rely on basic research data regarding biomechanical principles, soft-tissue healing, and effects of immobilization.[134,143-145] Criteria that influence the approach to rehabilitation include the type of surgery (repair versus reconstruction), concomitant ligamentous or meniscal repairs, the strength of the graft used, and graft placement.

Although several surgeons had previously described a general approach to the postoperative rehabilitation program for an ACL reconstructed knee, Paulos and associates,[146] in 1981, were the first to present a comprehensive rationale for postoperative rehabilitation. After conducting an international survey of 50 knee experts, Paulos and associates proposed a graduated five-phase rehabilitation program. The earliest phase consisted of four to six weeks of immobilization of the leg in a cast at 30 to 60 degrees of flexion, followed by a gradual, controlled increase of motion in a cast brace over six weeks. About 60% of the international knee surgeons polled at that time used a long leg cast or cast brace with the knee flexed to 30 to 60 degrees, although most allowed early range of motion within the first three weeks. Thirty percent began isotonic knee extension exercises within two months. The rationale for limiting motion was to allow ligament healing and collagen maturation.[146]

A more recent prospective study by Noyes and associates[147] strongly recommended early postoperative range of motion and found that ligament repairs did not stretch out. This has been our experience as well, and although we currently use continuous passive motion in the range of 0 to 90 degrees immediately after surgery, we emphasize the importance of continuing passive, assisted range-of-motion exercise. In cases of repair of an ACL avulsion, we limit the terminal extension to 10 degrees of flexion. Advantages of an early motion program include decreased effects of disuse, reduced problems with capsular contracture, maintenance of articular nutrition, and control of forces on healing collagen tissue.[134,148,149]

Noyes and associates[134] reported that eight weeks of immobilization in a plaster cast decreased ACL strength by 39% and ligament stiffness by 36%, requiring as long as one year for ligament properties to return to normal.

Traditional postoperative care usually delayed walking and weightbearing for as long as 16 weeks.[146] This delay was prescribed on the basis of studies that showed that walking creates large ACL forces at a time when healing strength is still low and neuromuscular control of the knee is still compromised.[26,131,148,150] A survey of 50 international knee surgeons in 1981 found that the average time before full weightbearing was permitted was 7.7 weeks, and that 40% of the surgeons did not restrict range of motion for isometric exercises.[146] Most of these surgeons attempted to obtain full range of motion by the sixth month after surgery.

Our current approach is to permit full passive extension and active flexion through an arc of 0 to 120 degrees, beginning on the second day after surgery. Passive extension is encouraged with the leg on the bed. Patients are generally discharged on the third day after surgery, wearing a hinged brace and nonweightbearing.

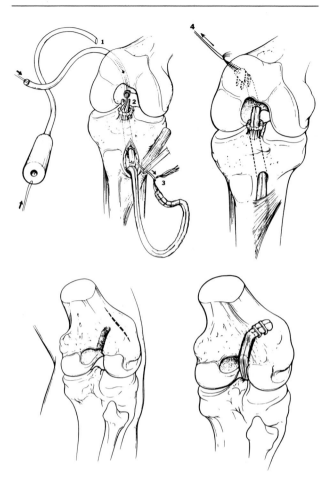

Fig. 4 **Top left**, Tendon passing sequence: (1) A special curved tendon passer facilitates over-the-top passage of the graft. (2) An arthroscopic grasping instrument pulls the wire loop through the tibial hole. (3) The sutures and tendon are passed through the tibial tunnel and over the top. The graft is well housed in the ACL remnant. **Top right**, The graft is well housed in the ACL stump. **Bottom left**, A notch is cut with a Cobb gauge from the posterolateral femur cortex to the over-the-top position. The graft is more isometric in this position. **Bottom right,** The graft is passed over the top and fixed with two staples. The graft is usually doubled over itself after the first staple and then fixed with a second larger staple (not shown).

An exercise bike is added to their program after one to two weeks. Patients begin partial weightbearing with their braces locked in full extension during week 2; in week 6 crutch use is discontinued. The long leg brace is also discontinued at this time, and a shorter derotational brace is worn only while walking. We permit isometric quadriceps contraction with the knee at 90 degrees of flexion, because a posterior vector of force is produced with the knee in this position.[151] Kain and associates[152] and others[26,30,146,150,153,154] found that isolated quadriceps contraction with the knee at 30 to 45 degrees of flexion develops a strong anterior vector at the tibia and that this vector is resisted by the ACL or graft. However, Jurist and Otis[151] demonstrated that tibiofemoral displacements depend both on the location of the resistance force (whether placed proximally

Table 3
Incidence of extensor mechanism problems at The Hospital for Special Surgery

Type of Reconstruction	Early Treatment	Patellofemoral Pain (% of Patients)	Flexion Contracture	
			% of Patients	Average Amount (Degrees)
Chronic ACL reconstruction with mid-third patellar tendon				
Via arthrotomy	Casting in 30°	37	19	9.0
Via arthroscopy	Continuous passive motion	26	20	—
Acute primary				
Via arthrotomy	Casting in 30°	57	25	4.2
With semitendinosus augmentation	Casting in 30°	27	35	9.6
			6*	16.0
Conservatively treated acute ACL	Early motion	22	0	—

*This group had limited flexion as well as extension.

or distally on the leg) and on the flexion angle of the knee. On the basis of their observations, we begin isotonic quadriceps exercises at six weeks, limiting extension to 40 degrees, with the resistance pad placed proximally. At the same time hamstring exercises are begun from 0 to 90 degrees.

The group of international knee experts surveyed in 1981 indicated that the majority of them permitted running within the first six months after surgery. We initiate straight-ahead running combined with figures-of-eight and jumping rope at the fifth month, racket sports during the sixth month, and contact sports in the seventh month. Bracing, omitted for daily activities, is used during running and participation in sports. Bracing can be discontinued when the athlete has gained confidence and the repaired knee is stronger, provided that a stable knee has been obtained.

Consideration of Patellofemoral Pain

Recently, Sachs and associates[139] found, in a prospective study of 126 patients, an 11-year literature review, and a poll of 50 prominent knee surgeons, that quadriceps weakness (23% to 65%), flexion contracture (24% to 32%), and patellofemoral pain (12% to 32%) were the most common complications after ACL surgery. These problems correlated positively with the choice of graft (mid-third patellar tendon had a higher incidence of problems than did the semitendinosus-gracilis graft) and increased age. The type of rehabilitation program employed also affected the incidence of these complications. They postulated that patellar irritability, flexion contracture, and patellar graft source diminished quadriceps strength in an additive fashion, and they concluded that the best approach is an aggressive rehabilitation program that emphasizes avoidance of flexion contracture.

A critical review of our experience at The Hospital for Special Surgery is shown in Table 3. Our impression is that early motion and avoidance of arthrotomy and cast immobilization will decrease the incidence of extensor mechanism problems. This continues to be our experience with our current approach, which uses arthroscopically directed repair and augmentation with semitendinosus-gracilis tendons. To avoid flexion contracture, we recommend locking the patient's brace in full extension at night. During the day, we recommend the use of continuous passive motion, with active work on motion. We have not, however, observed a consistent relationship between patellofemoral pain and the incidence of flexion contracture.

References

1. Torg JS, Conrad W, Kalen V: Clinical diagnosis of anterior cruciate ligament instability in the athlete. *Am J Sports Med* 1976;4:84–93.
2. Bach BR Jr, Warren RF, Wickiewicz TL: The pivot shift phenomenon: Results and description of a modified clinical test for anterior cruciate ligament insufficiency. *Am J Sports Med* 1988;16:571–576.
3. Groves EWH: The crucial ligaments of the knee-joint: Their function, rupture, and the operative treatment of the same. *Br J Surg* 1919–20;7:505–515.
4. Palmer I: On the injuries to the ligaments of the knee joint: A clinical study. *Acta Chir Scand* 1938;81(suppl 53):1–282.
5. Brantigan OC, Voshell AF: The mechanics of the ligaments and menisci of the knee joint. *J Bone Joint Surg* 1941;23:44–66.
6. O'Donoghue DH: An analysis of end results of surgical treatment of major injuries to the ligaments of the knee. *J Bone Joint Surg* 1955;37A:1–13.
7. O'Donoghue DH: Treatment of acute ligamentous injuries of the knee. *Orthop Clin North Am* 1973;4:617–645.
8. O'Donoghue DH: Surgical treatment of injuries to the knee. *Clin Orthop* 1960;18:11–36.
9. O'Donoghue DH: Surgical treatment of fresh injuries to the major ligaments of the knee. *J Bone Joint Surg* 1950;32A:721–738.
10. O'Donoghue DH, Frank GR, Jeter GL, et al: Repair and reconstruction of the anterior cruciate ligament in dogs: Factors influencing long-term results. *J Bone Joint Surg* 1971;53A:710–718.
11. O'Donoghue DH, Rockwood CA Jr, Frank GR, et al: Repair of the anterior cruciate ligament in dogs. *J Bone Joint Surg* 1966;48A:503–519.
12. Feagin JA Jr, Curl WW: Isolated tear of the anterior cruciate

ligament: 5-year follow-up study. *Am J Sports Med* 1976;4:95–100.

13. Marshall JL: Periarticular osteophytes: Initiation and formation in the knee of the dog. *Clin Orthop* 1969;62:37–47.

14. Marshall JL, Olsson S-E: Instability of the knee: A long-term experimental study in dogs. *J Bone Joint Surg* 1971;53A:1561–1570.

15. Marshall JL, Rubin RM: Knee ligament injuries: A diagnostic and therapeutic approach. *Orthop Clin North Am* 1977;8:641–668.

16. Marshall JL, Rubin RM, Wang JB, et al: The anterior cruciate ligament: The diagnosis and treatment of its injuries and their serious prognostic implications. *Orthop Rev* 1978;7(10):35–46.

17. Marshall JL, Warren RF, Wickiewicz TL: Primary surgical treatment of anterior cruciate ligament lesions. *Am J Sports Med* 1982;10:103–107.

18. Marshall JL, Warren RF, Wickiewicz TL, et al: The anterior cruciate ligament: A technique of repair and reconstruction. *Clin Orthop* 1979;143:97–106.

19. Furman W, Marshall JL, Girgis FG: The anterior cruciate ligament: A functional analysis based on postmortem studies. *J Bone Joint Surg* 1976;58A:179–185.

20. Girgis FG, Marshall JL, Al Monajem ARS: The cruciate ligaments of the knee joint: Anatomical, functional and experimental analysis. *Clin Orthop* 1975;106:216–231.

21. Odensten M, Gillquist J: Functional anatomy of the anterior cruciate ligament and a rationale for reconstruction. *J Bone Joint Surg* 1985;67A:257–262.

22. Butler DL, Noyes FR, Grood ES: Ligamentous restraints to anterior-posterior drawer in the human knee: A biomechanical study. *J Bone Joint Surg* 1980;62A:259–270.

23. Fukubayashi T, Torzilli PA, Sherman MF, et al: An in vitro biomechanical evaluation of anterior-posterior motion of the knee: Tibial displacement, rotation, and torque. *J Bone Joint Surg* 1982;64A:258–264.

24. Hsieh HH, Walker PS: Stabilizing mechanisms of the loaded and unloaded knee joint. *J Bone Joint Surg* 1976;58A:87–93.

25. Markolf KL, Mensch JS, Amstutz HC: Stiffness and laxity of the knee: The contributions of the supporting structures. A quantitative in vitro study. *J Bone Joint Surg* 1976;58A:583–594.

26. Morrison JB: The mechanics of the knee joint in relation to normal walking. *J Biomech* 1970;3:51–61.

27. Kennedy JC, Fowler PJ: Medial and anterior instability of the knee: An anatomical and clinical study using stress machines. *J Bone Joint Surg* 1971;53A:1257–1270.

28. Markolf KL, Graff-Radford A, Amstutz HC: In vivo knee stability: A quantitative assessment using an instrumented clinical testing apparatus. *J Bone Joint Surg* 1978;60A:664–674.

29. Torzilli PA, Greenberg RL, Insall J: An in vivo biomechanical evaluation of anterior-posterior motion of the knee: Roentgenographic measurement technique, stress machine, and stable population. *J Bone Joint Surg* 1981;63A:960–968.

30. Grood ES, Suntay WJ, Noyes FR, et al: Biomechanics of the knee-extension exercise: Effect of cutting the anterior cruciate ligament. *J Bone Joint Surg* 1984;66A:725–734.

31. Bryant JT, Cooke TDV: A biomechanical function of the ACL: Prevention of medial translation of the tibia, in Feagin JA Jr (ed): *The Crucial Ligaments: Diagnosis and Treatment of Ligamentous Injuries About the Knee.* New York, Churchill Livingstone, 1988, pp 235–242.

32. Karrholm J, Elmqvist LG, Selvik G, et al: Chronic anterolateral instability of the knee: A roentgen stereophotogrammetric evaluation. *Am J Sports Med* 1989;17:555–563.

33. Grood ES, Noyes FR, Butler DL, et al: Ligamentous and capsular restraints preventing straight medial and lateral laxity in intact human cadaver knees. *J Bone Joint Surg* 1981;63A:1257–1269.

34. Levy IM, Torzilli PA, Warren RF: The effect of medial meniscectomy on anterior-posterior motion of the knee. *J Bone Joint Surg* 1982;64A:883–888.

35. Tapper EM, Hoover NW: Late results after meniscectomy. *J Bone Joint Surg* 1969;51A:517–526.

36. Walker PS, Erkman MJ: The role of the menisci in force transmission across the knee. *Clin Orthop* 1975;109:184–192.

37. Cerabona F, Sherman MF, Bonamo JR, et al: Patterns of meniscal injury with acute anterior cruciate ligament tears. *Am J Sports Med* 1988;16:603–609.

38. DeHaven KE: Decision-making in acute anterior cruciate ligament injury, in Griffin PP (ed): American Academy Orthopaedic Surgeons *Instructional Course Lectures, XXXVI.* Park Ridge, American Academy Orthopaedic Surgeons, 1987, pp 201–203.

39. DeHaven KE: Meniscus repair—open vs. arthroscopic. *Arthroscopy* 1985;1:173–174.

40. DeHaven KE: Diagnosis of acute knee injuries with hemarthrosis. *Am J Sports Med* 1980;8:9–14.

41. Gillquist J, Hagberg G, Oretorp N: Arthroscopy in acute injuries of the knee joint. *Acta Orthop Scand* 1977;48:190–196.

42. Kennedy JC, Weinberg HW, Wilson AS: The anatomy and function of the anterior cruciate ligament: As determined by clinical and morphological studies. *J Bone Joint Surg* 1974;56A:223–235.

43. Lynch MA, Henning CE, Glick KR Jr: Knee joint surface changes: Long-term follow-up meniscus tear treatment in stable anterior cruciate ligament reconstructions. *Clin Orthop* 1983;172:148–153.

44. Noyes FR, Bassett RW, Grood ES, et al: Arthroscopy in acute traumatic hemarthrosis of the knee: Incidence of anterior cruciate tears and other injuries. *J Bone Joint Surg* 1980;62A:687–695.

45. Noyes FR, McGinniss GH: Controversy about treatment of the knee with anterior cruciate laxity. *Clin Orthop* 1985;198:61–76.

46. Paterson FW, Trickey EL: Meniscectomy for tears of the meniscus combined with rupture of the anterior cruciate ligament. *J Bone Joint Surg* 1983;65B:388–390.

47. Warren RF, Levy IM: Meniscal lesions associated with anterior cruciate ligament injury. *Clin Orthop* 1983;172:32–37.

48. Hanley ST, Warren RF: Arthroscopic meniscectomy in the anterior cruciate ligament-deficient knee. *Arthroscopy* 1987;3:59–65.

49. Higgins RW, Steadman JR: Anterior cruciate ligament repairs in world class skiers. *Am J Sports Med* 1987;15:439–447.

50. Allen PR, Denham RA, Swan AV: Late degenerative changes after meniscectomy: Factors affecting the knee after operation. *J Bone Joint Surg* 1984;66B:666–671.

51. Bourne RB, Finlay JB, Papadopoulos P, et al: The effect of medial meniscectomy on strain distribution in the proximal part of the tibia. *J Bone Joint Surg* 1984;66A:1431–1437.

52. Seedhom BB, Hargreaves DJ: On the "bucket handle" tear; Partial or total meniscectomy? A quantitative study. *J Bone Joint Surg* 1979;61B:381–389.

53. Seedhom BB, Hargreaves DJ: Transmission of the load in the knee joint with special reference to the role of the menisci: Part II. Experimental results, discussions and conclusions. *Eng Med* 1979;8:220–228.

54. Smillie IS: *Injuries of the Knee Joint,* ed 5. Edinburgh, Churchill Livingstone, 1978.

55. Arnoczky SP, Warren RF: The microvasculature of the meniscus and its response to injury: An experimental study in the dog. *Am J Sports Med* 1983;11:131–141.

56. Arnoczky SP, Warren RF: Microvasculature of the human meniscus. *Am J Sports Med* 1982;10:90–95.

57. Cabaud HE, Rodkey WG, Fitzwater JE: Medial meniscus repairs: An experimental and morphologic study. *Am J Sports Med* 1981;9:129–134.

58. Cassidy RE, Shaffer AJ: Repair of peripheral meniscus tears: A preliminary report. *Am J Sports Med* 1981;9:209–214.

59. DeHaven KE, Black KP, Griffiths HJ: Open meniscus repair: Technique and two to nine year results. *Am J Sports Med* 1989;17:788–795.

60. Giove TP, Miller SJ III, Kent BE, et al: Non-operative treatment of the torn anterior cruciate ligament. *J Bone Joint Surg* 1983;65A:184–192.

61. Hamberg P, Gillquist J, Lysholm J: Suture of new and old peripheral meniscus tears. *J Bone Joint Surg* 1983;65A:193–197.

62. Lipscomb AB, Anderson AF: Tears of the anterior cruciate ligament in adolescents. *J Bone Joint Surg* 1986;68A:19–28.

63. Aglietti P, Buzzi R, Bassi PB: Arthroscopic partial meniscectomy in the anterior cruciate deficient knee. *Am J Sports Med* 1988;16:597–602.

64. Shields CL Jr, Silva I, Yee L, et al: Evaluation of residual instability after arthroscopic meniscectomy in anterior cruciate deficient knee. *Am J Sports Med* 1987;15:129–131.

65. Sommerlath K: The importance of the meniscus in unstable knees: A comparative study. *Am J Sports Med* 1989;17:773–777.

66. Losse G, Daniel D, Malcom L, et al: The effect of meniscus surgery on anterior laxity of the knee. *Orthop Trans* 1983;7:280–281.

67. Markolf KL, Kochan A, Amstutz HC: Measurement of knee stiffness and laxity in patients with documented absence of the anterior cruciate ligament. *J Bone Joint Surg* 1984;66A:242–252.

68. Gollehon DL, Warren RF, Wickiewicz TL: Acute repairs of the anterior cruciate ligament: Past and present. *Orthop Clin North Am* 1985;16:111–125.

69. Hawkins RJ, Misamore GW, Merritt TR: Followup of the acute nonoperated isolated anterior cruciate ligament tear. *Am J Sports Med* 1986;14:205–210.

70. Noyes FR, McGinniss GH, Grood ES: The variable functional disability of the anterior cruciate ligament-deficient knee. *Orthop Clin North Am* 1985;16:47–67.

71. Fetto JF, Marshall JL: The natural history and diagnosis of anterior cruciate ligament insufficiency. *Clin Orthop* 1980;147:29–38.

72. Feagin JA Jr: The syndrome of the torn anterior cruciate ligament. *Orthop Clin North Am* 1979;10:81–90.

73. McDaniel WJ Jr, Dameron TB Jr: The untreated anterior cruciate ligament rupture. *Clin Orthop* 1983;172:158–163.

74. McDaniel WJ Jr, Dameron TB Jr: Untreated ruptures of the anterior cruciate ligament: A follow-up study. *J Bone Joint Surg* 1980;62A:696–705.

75. Noyes FR, Mooar PA, Matthews DS, et al: The symptomatic anterior cruciate-deficient knee: Part I. The long-term functional disability in athletically active individuals. *J Bone Joint Surg* 1983;65A:154–162.

76. Fairbanks TJ: Knee joint changes after meniscectomy. *J Bone Joint Surg* 1948;30B:664–670.

77. Jacobsen K: Osteoarthrosis following insufficiency of the cruciate ligaments in man: A clinical study. *Acta Orthop Scand* 1977;48:520–526.

78. Sherman MF, Warren RF, Marshall JL, et al: A clinical and radiographical analysis of 127 anterior cruciate insufficient knees. *Clin Orthop* 1988;227:229–237.

79. Balkfors B: The course of knee-ligament injuries. *Acta Orthop Scand* 1982;198(suppl):1–99.

80. Chick RR, Jackson DW: Tears of the anterior cruciate ligament in young athletes. *J Bone Joint Surg* 1978;60A:970–973.

81. Hughston JC, Andrews JR, Cross MJ, et al: Classification of knee ligament instabilities: Part I. The medial compartment and cruciate ligaments. *J Bone Joint Surg* 1976;58A:159–172.

82. Jokl P, Kaplan N, Stovell P, et al: Nonoperative treatment of severe injuries to the medial and anterior cruciate ligaments of the knee. *J Bone Joint Surg* 1984;66A:741–744.

83. Pattee GA, Fox JM, Del Pizzo W, et al: Four to ten year followup of unreconstructed anterior cruciate ligament tears. *Am J Sports Med* 1989;17:430–435.

84. Odensten M, Hamberg P, Nordin M, et al: Surgical or conservative treatment of the acutely torn anterior cruciate ligament: A randomized study with short-term follow-up observations. *Clin Orthop* 1985;198:87–93.

85. Kannus P, Järvinen M: Conservatively treated tears of the anterior cruciate ligament: Long-term results. *J Bone Joint Surg* 1987;69A:1007–1012.

86. Indelicato PA, Bittar ES: A perspective of lesions associated with ACL insufficiency of the knee: A review of 100 cases. *Clin Orthop* 1985;198:77–80.

87. Noyes FR, Matthews DS, Mooar PA, et al: The symptomatic anterior cruciate-deficient knee: Part II. The results of rehabilitation, activity modification, and counseling on functional disability. *J Bone Joint Surg* 1983;65A:163–174.

88. Buss DD, Min R, Skyhar MJ, et al: Conservatively treated anterior cruciate ligament injuries. Presented at the Annual Meeting of the American Orthopaedic Society for Sports Medicine, New Orleans, Feb 11, 1990.

89. Liljedahl S-O, Lindvall N, Wetterfors J: Early diagnosis and treatment of acute ruptures of the anterior cruciate ligament: A clinical and arthrographic study of forty-eight cases. *J Bone Joint Surg* 1965;47A:1503–1513.

90. Darrach W: Internal derangements of the knee. *Ann Surg* 1935;102:129–137.

91. Farquharson-Roberts MA, Osborne AH: Partial rupture of the anterior cruciate ligament of the knee. *J Bone Joint Surg* 1983;65B:32–34.

92. Monaco BR, Noble HB, Bachman DC: Incomplete tears of the anterior cruciate ligament and knee locking. *JAMA* 1982;247:1582–1584.

93. McDaniel WJ: Isolated partial tear of the anterior cruciate ligament. *Clin Orthop* 1976;115:209–212.

94. Sandberg R, Balkfors B: Partial rupture of the anterior cruciate ligament: Natural course. *Clin Orthop* 1987;220:176–178.

95. Noyes FR, Mooar LA, Moorman CT III, et al: Partial tears of the anterior cruciate ligament: Progression to complete ligament deficiency. *J Bone Joint Surg* 1989;71B:825–833.

96. Cabaud HE, Rodkey WG, Feagin JA: Experimental studies of acute anterior cruciate ligament injury and repair. *Am J Sports Med* 1979;7:18–22.

97. Buckley SL, Barrack RL, Alexander AH: The natural history of conservatively treated partial anterior cruciate ligament tears. *Am J Sports Med* 1989;17:221–225.

98. Kennedy JC, Hawkins RJ, Willis RB, et al: Tension studies of human knee ligaments: Yield point, ultimate failure, and disruption of the cruciate and tibial collateral ligaments. *J Bone Joint Surg* 1976;58A:350–355.

99. Noyes FR, DeLucase JL, Torvik PJ: Biomechanics of anterior cruciate ligament failure: An analysis of strain-rate sensitivity and mechanisms of failure in primates. *J Bone Joint Surg* 1974;56A:236–253.

100. Jackson DW: The future of anterior cruciate surgery, in Jackson DW, Drez D Jr (eds): *The Anterior Cruciate Deficient Knee: New Concepts in Ligament Repair*. St. Louis, CV Mosby, 1987, pp 315–318.

101. Sgaglione NA, Warren RF, Wickiewicz TL, et al: Primary repair with semitendinosus tendon augmentation of acute anterior cruciate ligament injuries. *Am J Sports Med* 1990;18:64–73.

102. Gollehon DL, Torzilli PA, Warren RF: The role of the posterolateral and cruciate ligaments in the stability of the human knee: A biomechanical study. *J Bone Joint Surg* 1987;69A:233–242.

103. Sullivan D, Levy IM, Sheskier S, et al: Medial restraints to anterior-posterior motion of the knee. *J Bone Joint Surg* 1984;66A:930–936.

104. Warren RF, Marshall JL: Injuries of the anterior cruciate and medial collateral ligaments of the knee: A retrospective analysis of clinical records—part I. *Clin Orthop* 1978;136:191–197.

105. Warren RF, Marshall JL: Injuries of the anterior cruciate and medial collateral ligament of the knee: A long-term follow-up of 86 cases—part II. *Clin Orthop* 1978;136:198–211.

106. Clancy WG Jr, Ray JM, Zoltan DJ: Acute tears of the anterior

cruciate ligament: Surgical versus conservative treatment. *J Bone Joint Surg* 1988;70A:1483–1488.

107. Dandy DJ, Flanagan JP, Steenmeyer V: Arthroscopy and the management of the ruptured anterior cruciate ligament. *Clin Orthop* 1982;167:43–49.

108. DeHaven KE: Arthroscopy in the diagnosis and management of the anterior cruciate ligament deficient knee. *Clin Orthop* 1983;172:52–56.

109. Bach BR Jr, Warren RF: "Empty wall" and "vertical strut" signs of ACL insufficiency. *J Arthroscopy* 1989;5:137–140.

110. Robson AWM: Ruptured crucial ligaments and their repair by operation. *Ann Surg* 1903;37:716–718.

111. Battle WH: A case after open section of the knee joint for irreducible traumatic dislocation. *Clin Soc London Trans* 1900;33:232–233.

112. Pringle JH: Avulsion of the spine of the tibia. *Ann Surg* 1907;46:169–178.

113. Jones R, Smith SA: On rupture of the crucial ligaments of the knee, and on fractures of the spine of the tibia. *Br J Surg* 1913–14;1:70–89.

114. Cabaud HE, Feagin JA, Rodkey WG: Acute anterior cruciate ligament injury and augmented repair: Experimental studies. *Am J Sports Med* 1980;8:395–401.

115. Järvinen M, Kannus P: Clinical and radiological long-term results after primary knee ligament surgery. *Arch Orthop Trauma Surg* 1985;104:1–6.

116. Solonen KA, Rokkanen P: Operative treatment of torn ligaments in injuries of the knee joint. *Acta Orthop Scand* 1967;38:67–80.

117. Weaver JK, Derkash RS, Freeman JR, et al: Primary knee ligament repair: Revisited. *Clin Orthop* 1985;199:185–191.

118. Youmans WT: The so-called "isolated" anterior cruciate ligament tear or anterior cruciate ligament syndrome: A report of 32 cases with some observation on treatment and its effect on results. *Am J Sports Med* 1978;6:26–30.

119. Kaplan N, Wickiewicz TL, Warren RF: Primary surgical treatment of anterior cruciate ligament ruptures: A long-term follow-up study. *Am J Sports Med* 1990;18:354–358.

120. Cross MJ, Paterson RS, Capito CP: Acute repair of the anterior cruciate ligament with lateral capsular augmentation. *Am J Sports Med* 1989;17:63–67.

121. Eriksson E: Sports injuries of the knee ligaments. Their diagnosis, treatment, rehabilitation, and prevention. *Med Sci Sports* 1976;8:133.

122. Lysholm J, Gillquist J, Liljedahl SO: Long-term results after early treatment of knee injuries. *Acta Orthop Scand* 1982;53:109–118.

123. Renström P, Arms SW, Stanwyck TS, et al: Strain within the anterior cruciate ligament during hamstring and quadriceps activity. *Am J Sports Med* 1986;14:83–87.

124. Straub T, Hunter RE: Acute anterior cruciate ligament repair. *Clin Orthop* 1988;227:238–250.

125. Lindemann K: Über den plastischen Ersatz der Kreuzbander durch gestielte Sehnenverpflanzung. *Z Orthop* 1949–50;79:316–334.

126. Lange M: *Orthopadische-chirurgische Operationslehre. Neueste Operations ver Fahren.* Munchen, JF Bergmann, 1968, pp 203–205.

127. Slocum DB, Larson RL: Pes anserinus transplantation: A surgical procedure for control of rotatory instability of the knee. *J Bone Joint Surg* 1968;50A:226–242.

128. Cho KO: Reconstruction of the anterior cruciate ligament by semitendinosus tenodesis. *J Bone Joint Surg* 1975;57A:608–612.

129. Ellison AE: Distal iliotibial-band transfer for anterolateral rotatory instability of the knee. *J Bone Joint Surg* 1979;61A:330–337.

130. Losee RE, Johnson TR, Southwick WO: Anterior subluxation of the lateral tibial plateau: A diagnostic test and operative repair. *J Bone Joint Surg* 1978;60A:1015–1030.

131. Noyes FR, Butler DL, Paulos E, et al: Intra-articular cruciate reconstruction: I. Perspectives on graft strength, vascularization, and immediate motion after replacement. *Clin Orthop* 1983;172:71–77.

132. Clancy WG Jr, Narechania RG, Rosenberg TD, et al: Anterior and posterior cruciate ligament reconstruction in rhesus monkeys. *J Bone Joint Surg* 1981;63A:1270–1284.

133. Clancy WG Jr, Nelson DA, Reider B, et al: Anterior cruciate ligament reconstruction using one-third of the patellar ligament, augmented by extra-articular tendon transfers. *J Bone Joint Surg* 1982;64A:352–359.

134. Noyes FR, Torvik PJ, Hyde WB, et al: Biomechanics of ligament failure: II. An analysis of immobilization, exercise, and reconditioning effects in primates. *J Bone Joint Surg* 1974;56A:1406–1418.

135. Butler DL, Grood ES, Noyes FR, et al: On the interpretation of our anterior cruciate ligament data. *Clin Orthop* 1985;196:26–34.

136. Bonamo JJ, Krinick RM, Sporn AA: Rupture of the patellar ligament after use of its central third for anterior cruciate reconstruction: A report of two cases. *J Bone Joint Surg* 1984;66A:1294–1297.

137. Hughston JC: Complications of anterior cruciate ligament surgery. *Orthop Clin North Am* 1985;16:237–240.

138. Langan P, Fontanetta AP: Rupture of the patellar tendon after use of its central third. *Orthop Rev* 1987;16(5):61–65.

139. Sachs RA, Daniel DM, Stone ML, et al: Patellofemoral problems after anterior cruciate ligament reconstruction. *Am J Sports Med* 1989;17:760–765.

140. Lipscomb AB, Johnston RK, Snyder RB, et al: Evaluation of hamstring strength following use of semitendinosus and gracilis tendons to reconstruct the anterior cruciate ligament. *Am J Sports Med* 1982;10:340–342.

141. Donaldson WF III, Warren RF, Wickiewicz T: A comparison of acute anterior cruciate ligament examinations: Initial versus examination under anesthesia. *Am J Sports Med* 1985;13:5–10.

142. Souryal TO, Moore HA, Evans JP: Bilaterality in anterior cruciate ligament injuries: Associated intercondylar notch stenosis. *Am J Sports Med* 1988;16:449–454.

143. Gollnick PD, Ericksson E, Harmark T, et al: Rehabilitation of the knee following surgery. *Med Sci Sports* 1976;8:133–134.

144. Noyes FR: Functional properties of knee ligaments and alterations induced by immobilization: A correlative biomechanical and histological study in primates. *Clin Orthop* 1977;123:210–242.

145. Noyes FR, Grood ES: The strength of the anterior cruciate ligament in humans and rhesus monkeys: Age-related and species-related changes. *J Bone Joint Surg* 1976;58A:1074–1082.

146. Paulos L, Noyes FR, Grood E, et al: Knee rehabilitation after anterior cruciate ligament reconstruction and repair. *Am J Sports Med* 1981;9:140–149.

147. Noyes FR, Mangine RE, Barber S: Early knee motion after open and arthroscopic anterior cruciate ligament reconstruction. *Am J Sports Med* 1987;15:149–160.

148. Alm A, Liljedahl SO, Strömberg B: Clinical and experimental experience in reconstruction of the anterior cruciate ligament. *Orthop Clin North Am* 1976;7:181–189.

149. Butler DL: Anterior cruciate ligament: Its normal response and replacement. *J Orthop Res* 1989;7:910–921.

150. Lindahl O, Movin A: The mechanics of extension of the knee-joint. *Acta Orthop Scand* 1967;38:226–234.

151. Jurist KA, Otis JC: Anteroposterior tibiofemoral displacements during isometric extension efforts: The roles of external load and knee flexion angle. *Am J Sports Med* 1985;13:254–258.

152. Kain CC, McCarthy JA, Arms S, et al: An in vivo analysis of the effect of transcutaneous electrical stimulation of the quadriceps and hamstrings on anterior cruciate ligament deformation. *Am J Sports Med* 1988;16:147–152.

153. Henning CE, Lynch MA, Glick KR Jr: An in vivo strain gage study of elongation of the anterior cruciate ligament. *Am J Sports Med* 1985;13:22–26.

154. Smidt GL: Biomechanical analysis of knee flexion and extension. *J Biomech* 1973;6:79–92.

155. Andersson C, Odensten M, Good L, et al: Surgical or non-surgical treatment of acute rupture of the anterior cruciate ligament: A randomized study with long-term follow-up. *J Bone Joint Surg* 1989;71A:965–974.

156. Odensten M, Lysholm J, Gillquist J: The course of partial anterior cruciate ligament ruptures. *Am J Sports Med* 1985;13:183–186.

The Early Recognition, Diagnosis, and Treatment of the Patella Infera Syndrome

Frank R. Noyes, MD

Edward M. Wojtys, MD

Introduction

The patellar infera syndrome, a complication that may follow major knee ligament surgery, fractures about the knee joint, high tibial osteotomy, and other injuries and surgical procedures, occurs more often than has been recognized previously. This potentially disabling syndrome must be recognized early in its course so that prompt treatment can be initiated. Our experience has shown that early treatment of the syndrome is beneficial in that it may limit the progression of the patella infera and return lower-extremity function to normal. However, if the syndrome is not recognized and treatment is delayed, the prognosis is much poorer.

In 1986, Wojtys and associates[1] described a group of patients in whom patella infera developed after trauma or surgery about the knee joint and in whom the condition was untreated and progressed to a chronic patella infera state accompanied by disabling patellofemoral arthrosis and significant functional limitation. The patients were typically young athletic individuals who experienced an initial traumatic episode involving the knee, such as anterior cruciate ligament injury, patellofemoral subluxation, meniscus tear, or tibial fracture. Patella infera developed soon after the injury or early in the postoperative course. The developmental patella infera resulted from early joint arthrofibrosis with limited knee motion and quadriceps weakness. Most of the patients in this groups were referred many months after the onset of the condition, by which time disabling patellofemoral arthrosis and permanent patella infera already existed.

This study represented the first report of the patella infera syndrome in the English literature, although the condition was originally described by Caton and associates[2] in the French literature in 1982. In that initial report, the abnormally low patellar position was in itself a complication of a disease, injury, or surgery and produced secondary symptoms of patellofemoral arthrosis that resulted in a disabling condition in 50% of the population studied. Paulos and associates[3] reported on patients with postoperative arthrofibrosis, labeling the condition "infrapatellar contracture syndrome." It is our belief that this clinical condition was identical to the patella infera syndrome we described in 1986. We also believe the term infrapatellar contracture syndrome is incorrect; the true patella infera syndrome typically involves contractures of all the tissues about the knee joint, including suprapatellar, peripatellar, infrapatellar, and fat pad tissues that limit mediolateral patellar mobility and knee flexion and other extra-articular connective tissues.[4–8]

Windsor and associates[9] reported on 45 total knee arthroplasties performed after proximal high tibial osteotomy and noted that 80% of the knees had patella infera before the surgery. They postulated that postoperative plaster immobilization of the knee in extension after the osteotomy allowed the quadriceps muscle and patellar ligament to relax and shorten. These authors also considered the development of adhesions and scarring around the patellar ligament after the osteotomy to be another important factor in the development of the patella infera. After total knee replacement, the patella infera was believed to be a contributing deleterious factor in the knees that did not fare well. Interestingly, patella infera had previously been recognized as a frequent sequela of poliomyelitis.[10]

On the basis of our previous studies and clinical experience, we interpret the patella infera syndrome to be a series of events that can occur after any knee trauma or surgery. Typically, an early developmental patella infera is associated with soft-tissue contractures and concomitant quadriceps weakness; joint stiffness and limited knee motion are usually present because of the associated arthrofibrotic state. Permanent shortening of the patellar ligament occurs when the initial condition is not recognized and promptly treated; this is followed months to years later by disabling patellofemoral arthrosis. This arthrosis is caused by many factors, including disuse effects, patellofemoral incongruence, and altered patellofemoral contact stresses resulting from the patella's low-lying position. It is therefore, the purpose of this report to (1) define the pathomechanics of the patella infera syndrome, which form the basis of the treatment program; (2) describe the clinical symptoms and radiographic criteria that accompany the syndrome so that developmental patella infera can be diagnosed early; and (3) provide treatment recommendations for patients in the acute stage of the syndrome and for those in the chronic state after significant functional limitations have developed.

Patients and Methods

We have treated two groups of patients for the patella infera syndrome. Group 1 consisted of five patients in whom an early developmental patella infera evolved after anterior cruciate ligament surgery. The syndrome was recognized soon after its onset; all underwent prompt treatment designed specifically for this complication (Table 1). There were two men and three women, with a mean age of 20 years (range, 14 to 26 years).

Group 2 consisted of 15 patients with the chronic form of the syndrome in whom an early developmental patella infera was not recognized or successfully treated early in its course. A permanent patella infera ensued in these knees, accompanied by disabling patellofemoral arthrosis (Tables 2 to 4). There were five men and 10 women, with a mean age of 23 years (range, 14 to 34 years). Eleven patients were referred to us 61 to 942 weeks after the initial knee injury. Four patients were treated elsewhere by orthopaedists who diagnosed the patella infera syndrome after reading our initial report.[1] Most of these patients were young athletic individuals; one was a collegiate cross-country runner, one was a competitive gymnast, and all had routinely participated in athletics before being injured.

In group 2 (chronic state), the initial injury was diagnosed as an anterior cruciate ligament tear in four patients, an anterior cruciate ligament tear and concomitant medial collateral ligament tear in two patients, a tibial plateau and/or femur fracture in three patients, a partial quadriceps rupture in two patients, a torn meniscus in two patients, and a patellar dislocation and osteochondral fracture, a patellar subluxation, an iliotibial band syndrome, and anterior knee pain in one patient each. Table 3 lists the treatment of the initial injury. Nine patients underwent a surgical procedure as part of the initial treatment.

The postoperative rehabilitation that the patients in group 2 participated in before referral to us was categorized into three types: (1) no program; (2) a minimal, nonsupervised, nonprogressive program; and (3) a maximal, supervised, comprehensive, progressive program designed to restore muscle function and joint motion (Table 3). Overall, we determined that the rehabilitation program was none to minimal in 73% (11 of 15 patients). After the initial injury or surgery, 12 patients reported severe pain and 13 reported severe swelling. Of the three patients who sustained ligamentous injury and underwent surgery, all noted severe swelling in and around the knee joint and all had difficulty in regaining knee motion. We diagnosed the patella infera condition in this group from 25 to 942 weeks (mean, 191 weeks) after the initial injury.

Our treatment was designed to correct the severe quadriceps weakness that was present in all patients. The comprehensive rehabilitation program required two to three sessions every week (daily sessions in the most severe cases), and consisted of carefully supervised exercises involving the entire lower extremity. We restricted the quadriceps exercises to isometrics, leg lifts, and active quadriceps contraction with electrical muscle stimulation, and avoided progressive resistance exercises and isokinetic exercises to protect the damaged patellofemoral joint.[11] Additionally, we provided a comprehensive phased program to overcome any limitations in range of knee motion.[12]

Electromyographic and nerve conduction studies were obtained for four patient to rule out an underlying neurologic abnormality. Patellar ligament biopsy procedures were performed in three patients at the time of subsequent surgical procedures. A 4 × 10-mm biopsy specimen of the patellar ligament was removed and fixed for electron microscopic evaluation. Needle muscle biopsy specimens were obtained from the right and left vastus lateralis muscle in five patients by means of a technique previously described.[13] Subjective, objective, and functional data from our knee rating system[14] were collected on 11 of 15 patients during their first visit and during their most recent follow-up visit.

Radiographic Techniques for Measuring the Vertical Position of the Patella

We recently published a study[15] on the normal vertical height ratio of the patella measured on lateral radiographs in 102 right and left knees of 51 patients. In addition, the original measurements for 50 right and left knees reported by Jacobsen and Bertheussen[16] using the Insall-Salvati[13] patellar height index were obtained. The ratio for the right knee was compared to the ratio for the left knee to establish the variability in this second population of knees because Jacobsen and Bertheussen did not report this comparison in their original publication.

The vertical height of the patella was determined by the method described by Caton and associates[2] and by Linclau[17] (Fig. 1). This method relies on readily identifiable and reproducible anatomic landmarks.[13,16,18,19] The distance between the most ventral (anterior-superior) rim of the tibial plateau and the lowest end of the patellar articular surface is measured (Fig. 1, numerator, point A) and divided by the maximum length of the patellar articular surface (Fig. 1, denominator, point B). An alternative method was used to determine the numerator. Described previously by Blackburne and Peel,[18] this method locates the tibial reference point at an anterior central location on the tibial plateau (Fig. 1, point C).

To ensure that the radiographic technique used was acceptable in terms of positioning and magnification, a reproducibility study was performed on three patients who had lateral radiographs of the knee taken on three different days. A 60-degree knee-flexion po·tion was selected to ensure that a nominal tension was present in the extensor mechanism and patellar ligament. This

Table 1
Summary of data for group 1

Case	Sex	Age (yr)	Phased Rehabilitation Program			Decrease in Patellar Height Ratio (%)		
			Extension Case	Manipulation	Surgical Release* (wk)	Before Release	After Release	At Latest Follow-up
1	M	14	Yes	Yes	15	56	35	45
2	F	26	No	Yes	9	16	47	37
3	M	24	Yes	No	36	29	13	13
4	F	19	Yes	No	10	37	30	31
5	F	14	No	Yes	20	22	22	22

*Time between anterior cruciate ligament surgery and release.

Table 2
Group 2: Initial data

Case	Sex	Age (yr)	Mechanism of Injury	Sport or Activity	Time Between Injury and Initial Visit (wk)	Diagnosis at Initial Visit*
6	F	16	Twisted knee	Cheerleading	0	Medial meniscus tear
7	F	18	Hyperextension	Work	0	ACL and medial meniscus tears
8	F	21	Blunt trauma	Motor vehicle accident	0	Tibial plateau fracture
9	M	28	Knee "popped" during squat	Weightlifting	0	Partial quadriceps rupture
10	F	28	Patellar contusion	Grocery shopping	0	Patellar dislocation; osteochondral fracture of patella
11	F	21	Overuse	Work	20	Anterior knee pain
12	F	14	Twisted knee	Volleyball	0	Acute patellofemoral subluxation
13	F	34	Patellar contusion	Walking, hit by dog	1.5	Partial quadriceps rupture; chondromalacia patellae
14	M	21	Twisted knee	Work	0	Medial meniscus tear; arthritis
15	M	20	Twisted knee	Parachute landing	0	Torn ACL
16	M	17	Blunt trauma	Motorcycle accident	0	Fractures of tibia, fibula, and femur; extensive lacerations
17	F	27	Twisted knee	Softball	0	ACL, MCL, and medial and lateral meniscus tears
18	F	32	Twisted knee	Racketball	0	ACL, MCL, and medial and lateral meniscus tears
19	M	18	Blunt trauma	Motorcycle accident	0	Femur fracture
20	F	31	Overuse	Running	0	Iliotibial band syndrome

*ACL, anterior cruciate ligament; MCL, medial collateral ligament.

Table 3
Group 2: Treatment of injury*

Case	Immobilization		Surgery	Rehabilitation	Pain	Swelling
	Method	Time				
6	Cast (2)	8 wk	Open meniscectomy (1)	None	Severe	Severe
7	Cast-brace (2)	4 wk	Reconstruction, meniscectomy (1)	Maximal (3)	Severe	Severe
8	Cast (2)	6 wk	Open reduction and internal fixation (1)	Maximal (3)	Severe	Severe
	Traction (2)	6 wk				
9	Not done	—	Not done	Minimal (1)	Severe	Severe
10	Cast (1)	6 wk	Not done	Minimal (2)	Severe	Severe
11	Not done	—	Open meniscectomy (1)	None	Moderate	Minimal
12	Immobilizer (2)	6 wk	Arthrotomy; patelloplasty (1)	Minimal (3)	Moderate	Severe
13	Immobilizer (1)	—	Not done	Minimal (2)	Severe	Severe
14	Long leg cast (3)	5 wk	Open meniscectomy (2)	Minimal (1)	Severe	Severe
	Cylinder cast (3)	6 wk				
15	Cast (1)	6 wk	Not done	Minimal (2)	Severe	Severe
16	Cast-brace (2)	—	External fixation, femoral pins, traction (1)	Minimal (3)	Severe	Severe
17	Immediate motion (2)	—	Acute augmented repair (1)	Maximal (3)	Severe	Severe
18	Cast-brace (2)	9 wk	Reconstruction (1)	Minimal (3)	Severe	Severe
19	Traction (1)	10 days	Not done	Minimal (2)	Severe	Severe
	Cast (1)	4 wk				
20	Injection (1)	—	Not done	Unknown	Moderate	Minimal

*Numbers in parentheses indicate order of treatment.

Table 4
Group 2: Data from our institution

Case	Time Since Injury (wk)	Diagnosis	Patellar Height Ratio (%)*	Time Between Injury and Diagnosis of Patella Infera (wk)
6	400	Chronic tear of ACL, posterior cruciate ligament, and posterolateral ligament complex†	24	400
7	83	Patella infera, patellofemoral arthrosis, reflex sympathetic dystrophy	32	25
8	127	Patella infera, patellofemoral arthrosis	30	127
9	68	Patella infera, partial quadriceps rupture	36	68
10	67	Patellofemoral arthrosis, patella infera, quadriceps atrophy	62	52
11	61	Patellofemoral arthrosis, patella infera	54	61
12	103	Patellofemoral arthrosis, patella infera, quadriceps atrophy	33	103
13	—	—	75	52
14	942	Patella infera, reflex sympathetic dystrophy, chronic tear of posterior cruciate ligament	45	942
15	384	Chronic tears of ACL, posterior cruciate ligament, and fibular collateral ligament, patella infera†	28	384
16	88	Quadriceps contracture, patella infera	26	88
17	—	—	41	53
18	—	—	72	32
19	411	Patella infera, patellofemoral arthrosis	36	411
20	—	—	89	66

*See Figure 1. For patients not examined at our institution but described to us by other physicians, the first abnormal ratio detected is shown.
†ACL, anterior cruciate ligament.

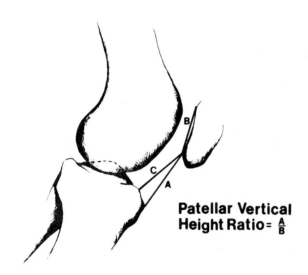

Patellar Vertical Height Ratio $= \frac{A}{B}$

Fig. 1   Method used to determine patellar vertical height. (Reproduced with permission from Noyes FR, Wojtys EM, Marshall MT: The early diagnosis and treatment of the developmental patella infera syndrome. *Clin Orthop* 1991:263:108–119.)

produced a proximal glide of the patella and allowed measurement of patellar height. The lateral radiographs of the right and left knee pairs were taken in a position so as to superimpose both femoral condyles and to have neutral tibial rotation. When these conditions were not met, it was difficult to identify the same anatomic points on the radiographs. Because the tibial reference point was usually the most difficult one to identify, the measurements were made at two different tibial points (Fig. 1, points A and C). The change in the vertical height ratio of the patella ranged from 0% to 9%, with an average difference of 3%.

Phased Rehabilitation Program for Loss of Knee Motion

A phased rehabilitation treatment program was used for patients with lost knee motion[12] (all five patients in group 1 and five patients in group 2). This program included treatment methods used in addition to our normal motion program, which consists of lower-extremity stretching, active and passive range-of-motion exercises, electrical muscle stimulation, and the use of a continuous passive motion device.[20]

Mild limitations of extension were caused by joint pain, hemarthrosis, or hamstring musculature spasm. Knees with less than 15 degrees of extension had developed rigid soft-tissue contractures with proliferation and ingrowth of fibrous tissue in the suprapatellar, peripatellar, infrapatellar, and femoral notch regions. The treatment programs varied for these limitations, depending on the amount of restriction and the length of time the restriction had been present.

Mild limitation of extension (less than 15 degrees and present either in the early postoperative period or at the patient's first visit) was initially treated with a hanging weight program. With the patient sitting on a table with the knee extended and a small support under the foot, 5 to 9 kg of weight was placed over the anterior aspect of the patella for ten to 15 minutes, six to eight times every day. The amount of weight was gradually increased each week to stretch the posterior capsular tissues more aggressively. If the knee did not respond to this treatment, a series of serial extension casts was initiated. The cast, which extended from midthigh to the ankles, was used for a total of 36 to 48 hours. Every 12 hours a wedge was inserted into the cast to extend the tissues gradually. The cast was eventually converted to a night splint that was worn for an additional seven to ten days. Some patients required more than one cast treatment to regain full extension.

Knees with more severe limitations of extension underwent a different treatment program. Because of the existence of rigid soft-tissue contractures, the use of extension casts before any arthroscopic debridement was avoided because of the potentially deleterious effects of high tibiofemoral compressive forces from the casts on the articular cartilage. Our experience shows that these knees usually fail to improve with an extension-cast treatment program. Therefore, we first performed an arthroscopic debridement that involved removal of suprapatellar, peripatellar, and infrapatellar scar tissues and tissues within the notch that block knee extension. After the debridement, these knees began the hanging weight program previously described. If extension was not gained after two weeks, extension casts were implemented for 36- to 48-hour periods.

Knees with limitations in flexion were also treated according to the amount of motion lost. Mild losses of flexion, seen in the early postoperative period after ligamentous surgery, resulted from intra-articular adhesions and contracture of peripatellar tissues. These were treated as soon as possible by gentle manipulation and patellar mobilization with the patient under anesthesia. Any postoperative effusion was aspirated and anti-inflammatory agents were used to control joint inflammation and pain. Failure to initiate early treatment for mild flexion limitations ultimately led to more severe restrictions accompanied by fibrotic scar tissue. These knees, which demonstrated a "hard" resistant block to attempted gentle manipulation, underwent arthroscopic debridement. Using the technique described by Sprague and associates,[21,22] we performed a comprehensive lysis of intra-articular adhesions, medial and lateral retinacular release, and resection of fat-pad scar tissues. After manipulation or arthroscopic debridement, the joint effusion and pain were allowed to recede for a few days. Patients who after one week had not recovered the motion gained were again hospitalized, and a continuous epidural anesthetic was used for three to five days along with intensive physical therapy to regain motion.

Case Studies

Group 1

Case 1 A 14-year-old male gymnast sustained an acute anterior cruciate ligament rupture and underwent an arthroscopically assisted anterior cruciate ligament allograft reconstruction and repair of a lateral peripheral tear of the meniscus.[15] Although a knee motion program was initiated immediately, a limitation developed early in the postoperative course and, at the seventh week, the range of motion was 20 to 90 degrees. A contracture of the peripatellar soft tissues was noted, accompanied by limited patellar mobility. Ten weeks after surgery, lateral radiographs showed a 33% decrease in patellar height. The patient underwent gentle manipulation and patellar mobilization under anesthesia and regained a range of motion from 5 to 135 degrees. The motion again became limited, however, and by the 14th postoperative week was only 10 to 50 degrees. Repeat radiographs showed progression of the patellar infera to 56% of normal (Fig. 2). An arthroscopically assisted open release of contracted peripatellar and infrapatellar tissues was performed. The patellar ligament was not under tension and had a buckled, wavy appearance because of the contracted tissues. Fat-pad scar tissue, originating between the inferior pole of the patella and the intermeniscal ventral area of the tibia, allowed no tension in the patellar ligaments. After the soft-tissue release, the patella returned to a more proximal position but a permanent shortening of the patellar ligament had occurred; postoperative radiographs showed a 35% decrease in the vertical height ratio. The microscopic appearance of the fibrotic fat-pad tissues is shown in Figure 3. The patient achieved a full range of knee motion by the 20th postoperative week. The vertical height ratio at the three-year follow-up examination was decreased by 45% compared with that of the opposite side (Fig. 2, *right*) and moderate patellofemoral crepitus was noted. The patient returned to competitive sports without symptoms or limitations on function.

Case 2 A 26-year-old woman underwent arthroscopically assisted allograft anterior cruciate ligament reconstruction and open repair of the medial collateral ligament and the medial capsular ligament after sustaining a twisting injury while snow skiing.[15] Nine weeks after surgery, a contracture of peripatellar tissues developed; lateral radiographs showed a 16% decrease in patellar height. The range of knee motion was 5 to 90 degrees with limited patellar mobility. The patient underwent an extensive arthroscopic release of contracted peripatellar and fat-pad tissues; this was followed by use of passive range-of-motion device and four days of treatment with a continuous epidural anesthetic. One week later drainage developed from an arthroscopic portal from which *Staphylococcus aureus*

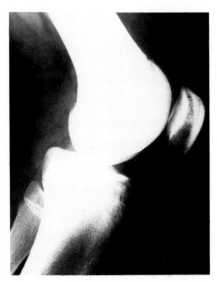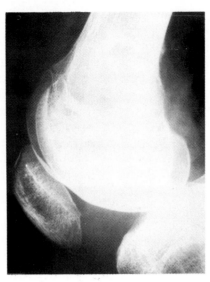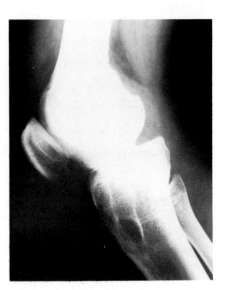

Fig. 2 Group 1, Case 1. **Left,** Radiograph of normal knee. **Center,** Radiograph 14 weeks after anterior cruciate ligament reconstruction shows a 56% decrease in the patellar height ratio. **Right,** Radiograph 36 months after anterior cruciate ligament reconstruction shows a 45% decrease in the patellar height ratio. (Reproduced with permission from Noyes FR, Wojtys EM, Marshall MT: The early diagnosis and treatment of the development patella infera syndrome. *Clin Orthop* 1991;263:108–119.)

was cultured. The patient was returned to the operating room and underwent a limited open drainage of the joint. There was no evidence of abscess formation and the infection resolved with antibiotic treatment. The range of motion was 0 to 95 degrees with normal patellar mobility. After leaving the hospital, the patient failed to perform the prescribed motion program and a third manipulation was required three weeks later to regain a range of 0 to 95 degrees. She remained noncompliant with all aspects of our rehabilitation program and, 13 weeks postoperatively, the vertical height ratio showed a 47% decrease. Twenty months after surgery, the patient had 0 to 115 degrees of motion, a 37% decrease in patellar height, and moderate patellofemoral crepitus. The patient played softball and volleyball with no symptoms and reported pain only with flexion past 115 degrees.

Case 3 A 24-year-old man ruptured his anterior cruciate ligament while snow skiing and underwent an open medial one-third patellar tendon autograft reconstruction elsewhere.[15] The patient was treated with a limited knee motion program (35 to 60 degrees) for the first eight weeks. Fourteen weeks after surgery, his range of motion was 25 to 95 degrees. The patient failed to gain further motion and was referred to us during the 26th postoperative week.

Lateral radiographs showed a 29% decrease in patellar height and a range of motion of 25 to 97 degrees. The patient underwent an arthroscopic release of peripatellar soft tissues and debridement of extensive fat-pad and intra-articular adhesions. Marked fibrillation and gross articular cartilage damage were present on

the undersurface of the patella and femoral sulcus. Postoperatively, the patella showed only a 13% decrease in the vertical height ratio. The postoperative range of motion was 10 to 115 degrees. Serial extension casts (applied for only one to three days) were required to gain full knee extension.

At a follow-up examination 30 months postoperatively, the range of motion was 5 to 125 degrees. There was moderate patellofemoral crepitus, but no symptoms with light recreational activities; the patient was able to water-ski and bicycle with no problems.

Case 4 A 19-year-old woman underwent an arthroscopically assisted anterior cruciate ligament reconstruction that used a patellar tendon autograft for an acute anterior cruciate ligament rupture.[15] Because of an abnormally high Q-angle, a lateral-third graft of the patellar tendon was used. Four weeks after surgery, the range of knee motion was limited to 30 to 85 degrees. A lateral radiograph showed a 37% decrease in patellar height. Early arthrofibrosis was diagnosed and a closely supervised motion program was used in an attempt to gain knee motion. After ten weeks, an arthroscopic release of peripatellar and fat-pad tissues was performed. After the procedure, the range of motion improved to 5 to 130 degrees. By 24 weeks postoperatively, the vertical height ratio was decreased to 30%. After two years, the patient was able to play several sports with no pain. There was moderate patellofemoral crepitus, 0 to 130 degrees of knee motion, and a 31% decrease in patellar height.

Case 5 A 14-year-old female gymnast underwent an

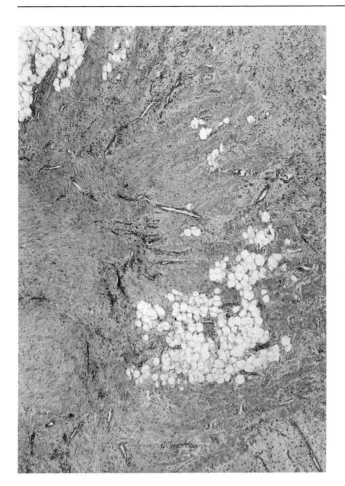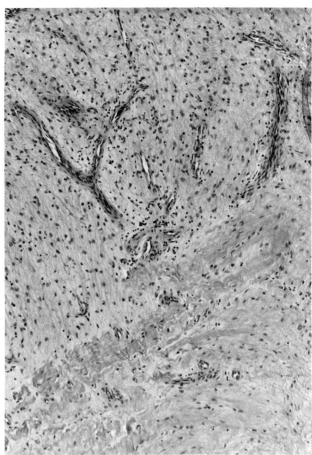

Fig. 3 Same patient shown in Figure 2 (Group 1, Case 1). **Left,** Extensive replacement of the fat pad with immature and mature fibro-connective tissue (× 40). **Right,** High-power photomicrograph shows fibroblastic and endothelial proliferation with dense collagen fiber formation (× 100). (Reproduced with permission from Noyes FR, Wojtys EM, Marshall MT: The early diagnosis and treatment of the development patella infera syndrome. *Clin Orthop* 1991;263:108–119.)

arthroscopically assisted anterior cruciate ligament autograft that used the central third of the patellar ligament and repair of a medial meniscus tear.[15] The patient started immediate range of motion but experienced pain when performing the exercises. During the next several weeks, a limitation in patellar mobility occurred, with significant atrophy of the quadriceps muscle and difficulty with attempted active quadriceps contraction. There was no evidence of neurologic abnormality, tourniquet-induced quadriceps weakness, or reflex sympathetic dystrophy. Four weeks after surgery, a lateral radiograph showed a 22% decrease in patellar height. The patient was treated with daily physical therapy that included range-of-motion exercises, bicycling, and use of an electrical muscle stimulator. Patellar mobility continued to be limited and the need for medial and lateral release of the patella and fat-pad tissues became apparent but was delayed until the 19th week because of the patient's loss of voluntary quadriceps function.

After an arthroscopic fat-pad resection and release of contracted peripatellar tissues, the range of motion was 0 to 135 degrees. Lateral radiographs showed a 22% decrease in patellar height, indicating no further progression in the interval before arthroscopic release. Nine months after surgery, the patient had a full range of motion, no pain, had returned to running, and was expected to return to gymnastics. There was no further progression in the patella infera.

Group 2

Case 11 A 21-year-old woman complained of anterior left knee pain after standing at work for eight to ten hours a day. A medial meniscectomy was eventually performed elsewhere. After surgery, the patient performed occasional straight leg raises for a period of three weeks. Because of continued anterior knee pain, swelling, and giving way, she was examined at our institution nine months later. At that time she had mod-

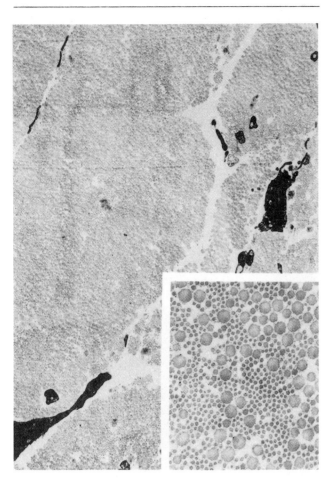

Fig. 4 Group 2, Case 11. Transverse section of collagen fibrils from patellar tendon. A low-power photomicrograph ($\times$ 12,000), shows the presence of small immature collagen fibrils. This is better demonstrated at a greater magnification (inset, $\times$ 79,920.)

erate to severe limitations on the activities of daily living.

Our examination showed severe quadriceps atrophy, moderate patellar compression pain, and moderate peripatellar soft-tissue tenderness. Radiographs demonstrated a 54% decrease in patellar height. After three months of an intensive, supervised quadriceps rehabilitation program and anti-inflammatory medications, she continued to have severe patellofemoral pain. An arthroscopic examination showed diffuse fibrillation on and fragmentation of the undersurface of the patella. Electron microscopy of a biopsy specimen from the patellar tendon showed a reorganization of the collagen fibers and newly formed small-diameter collagen fibrils throughout the cross section (Fig. 4). Nine months of intensive quadriceps rehabilitation followed. Because of continued severe anterior knee pain and an 83% decrease in patellar height, the patient then underwent a Maquet osteotomy and patellar tendon lengthening. Wire internal-fixation struts between the patella and tibial tubercle were used to allow immediate motion and early functional use of the extremity. Despite intensive postoperative therapy, significant quadriceps weakness developed and the patella again showed a distal migration to a 66% decrease three months after surgery. This patient continues to walk with one crutch and is in a long-term rehabilitation program.

Case 8 A 21-year-old woman sustained a fracture of the tibial plateau in an automobile accident. The fracture was treated by open reduction and internal fixation, and the patient was placed in traction for four weeks and then in a hinged cast brace for six weeks. Significant anterior knee pain and swelling were experienced postoperatively. She underwent in-patient therapy and was then placed on a home program of isometrics and leg raises. One year after the injury, the patient noted muscle weakness and anterior knee pain; four years after the injury she was referred here with increasing pain and severe patellofemoral crepitus.

Radiographs showed a 44% decrease in patellar height. The patient began a rehabilitation program that included isometrics, leg raises, electrical muscle stimulation, and light swimming. One month later, the patient underwent arthroscopic debridement of the knee. The undersurface of the patella showed diffuse articular cartilage fibrillation and fragmentation. The medial femoral condyle demonstrated mild softening over the entire weightbearing surface, and the lateral tibial plateau showed moderate fibrillation changes over the surface. The patient continued the rehabilitation program but still experienced patellofemoral symptoms. She continues to have moderate limitations on the activities of daily living, including pain and swelling on walking less than three blocks.

Case 7 An 18-year-old female collegiate cross-country runner complained of activity-related anterior knee pain; radiographs revealed normal patellar height. She was treated with leg raises and continued to run 40 to 50 miles per week. Nine months later, she sustained a hyperextension injury after stumbling into a hole while running across a field. An anterior cruciate ligament rupture and medial meniscus tear were diagnosed. The patient was placed in a long leg cast for ten days and then underwent repair of the anterior cruciate ligament elsewhere. Postoperatively, she was immobilized for four weeks in a long leg cast. For four additional weeks, she was in a cast-brace motion program. Weightbearing was forbidden for six months and only partial weightbearing was allowed for an additional six months. Fifty-four weeks postoperatively, the pain and limitation of knee motion were severe enough that another surgical procedure was performed to remove adhesions and free the quadriceps mechanism. A similar, repeat open arthrotomy procedure was performed one week later. The patient was placed postoperatively in a cylinder cast for eight weeks. A subsequent bone scan revealed a reflex sympathetic dystrophy pattern. She was then referred to us. Our examination showed a range of motion from 30 to 60 degrees and a decrease in patellar height of 32% (Fig. 5, *left* and *center*). Intensive rehabilitation was required to regain quadriceps function. Two arthroscopies and release of contracted scar tissues were required to restore a normal range of motion. A recent physical examination showed severe patellofemoral crepitus and pain with activities of daily living, and repeat radiographs showed a 37% decrease in patellar height (Fig. 5, *right*).

Results

Group 1

Subjective Symptoms and Functional Rating The subjective symptoms and functional ratings obtained at follow-up for group 1 are shown in Table 5. All the patients had returned to sports activities and all had completely resolved their giving-way symptoms. No problems were reported with activities of daily living, and, although all patients had moderate patellofemoral crepitus, all could participate in moderate sports activities[14] with no pain or swelling.

Results of Early Phased Rehabilitation Program All the patients required early arthroscopic debridement and release of contracted suprapatellar, peripatellar, infrapatellar, and fat-pad tissues (Table 1). The average decrease in patellar height before the arthroscopic debridement was 32% (range, 16% to 56%). The arthroscopic release failed to restore the patella to its normal height; the average decrease after release was 29% (range, 13% to 47%). However, the rehabilitation program was effective in restoring lower-limb function, as indicated by the symptoms and functional results previously discussed. A full range of motion was reestablished in three patients; two still lacked complete flexion at follow-up. Patient 2 was noncompliant with her rehabilitation program and, although she returned to sports activities, still lacks 20 degrees of flexion. Patient 3 lacked 10 degrees of flexion and 5 degrees of extension; the delay in initiating this patient's treatment program and the significant patellofemoral articular cartilage deterioration were believed to be the major contributory factors.

Group 2

Subjective Symptoms and Functional Rating The subjective symptoms and functional rating scores for group 2 are shown in Table 6. Final ratings were obtained at a mean of 36 months (range, eight to 94 months) for the 11 patients we treated. Ten of these 15 patients also required arthroscopic debridement and release of contracted joint tissues to restore joint motion and patellar mobility.

The average pain score at the first visit was 1.8, indicating constant pain with activities of daily living. Typically, the anterior knee pain was related to the established patellofemoral arthrosis. The average score at follow-up was 1.6; none of the patients had any lessening of their pain symptoms. Little improvement was noted at follow-up for swelling; however, giving-way symptoms were lessened in five patients.

None of the patients could perform any sports activities when first examined. At follow-up, one patient was able to play volleyball with moderate problems, and another was able to run (against medical advice) with severe problems. The remaining patients refrained from sports activities because of their symptoms. The follow-up mean scores showed no improvement in the

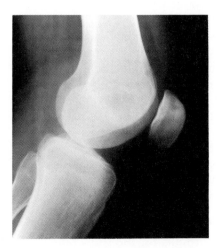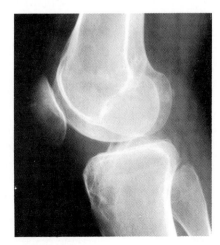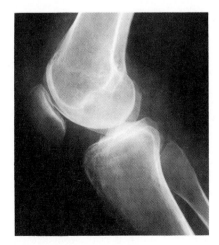

Fig. 5 Group 2, Case 7. **Left,** Radiograph of noninvolved knee. **Center,** Radiograph 83 weeks after injury shows a 32% decrease in patellar height. **Right,** Radiograph 99 weeks after injury shows a 37% decrease in patellar height.

Table 5
Results in group 1

Data	Case 1	Case 2	Case 3	Case 4	Case 5
Months since surgery	36	20	30	24	9
Pain*	10	8	8	10	10
Swelling*	10	8	10	10	10
Giving-way*	10	10	10	10	10
Walking†	40	40	40	40	40
Stairclimbing†	40	30	30	40	40
Kneeling†	40	30	30	40	40
Running‡	100	80	80	100	80
Patellofemoral crepitus	Moderate	Moderate	Moderate	Moderate	Moderate
Range of knee motion (degrees)	Full	0 to 115	5 to 125	Full	Full

*Based on a scale of 0 to 10, with 10 indicating a normal knee and ability to perform strenuous work and sports activities and 8 indicating ability to perform moderate work and sports activities but symptoms with strenuous activities.[14]
†Based on a scale of 0 to 40, with 40 indicating normal, unlimited ability and 30 indicating some limitations.[14]
‡Based on a scale of 0 to 100, with 100 indicating that the patient is fully competitive and 80 indicating some limitations and guarding.[14]

activities of daily living, including walking, kneeling, and stair climbing.

Surgical Procedures Table 7 contains a list of surgical procedures performed in the 15 patients. Twenty-nine operations were performed before the establishment of the patella infera diagnosis and before the patient was referred here for treatment. Twenty-one surgical procedures were performed after the diagnosis of patella infera. The average number of operations was three per patient (range, zero to eight). Five patients underwent a subsequent Maquet osteotomy because of significant patellofemoral arthrosis and symptoms that worsened after the patella infera was diagnosed.

Results of Diagnostic Studies Four patients from group 2 underwent electromyography; results were normal in two cases and abnormal in the other two, showing evidence of a chronic mild muscle denervation that was attributable to possible tourniquet ischemia (Patients 10 and 11). In one case (Patient 14), in which the symptoms included diffuse aching pain of the entire lower limb, pain to light touch, and cold intolerance about the knee joint, reflex sympathetic dystrophy was diagnosed. The patient was treated with a continuous spinal epidural; this relieved the symptoms.

Biopsy specimens of the vastus lateralis muscle in the involved and noninvolved limbs showed a significant decrease in the percentage of type I (slow-twitch) fibers in the involved limb. Type II (fast-twitch) fibers showed a corresponding increase in three of the five patients. Only Patients 6 and 11 showed no differences between limbs in the percentages of the two fiber types.

Patellar ligament biopsy specimens showed different results. The specimen from Patient 6 showed a homogeneous population of mature collagen fibrils. The pattern, which is consistent with a normal fibril-diameter profile (Fig. 6), indicated that the shortened patellar ligament had completed the remodeling process. In contrast, a transverse section from Patient 11 showed both mature fibrils and a large population of smaller fibrils. This pattern was interpreted to indicate that a structural reorganization of the collagen fibrils had occurred in the shortened patellar ligament (Fig. 4). The specimen from Patient 16 was poorly sectioned and the results were inconclusive as to fibril diameters.

Arthroscopic Findings Ten of the 15 patients underwent arthroscopic debridement of the knee joint, at which time the articular cartilage surfaces were graded.[20] For the patellofemoral surface, six patients had major loss of articular cartilage with bone exposed and four patients had major fissuring and fragmentation. Seven patients showed cartilage fibrillation and fragmentation to the medial tibiofemoral joint and six patients showed cartilage fragmentation and fibrillation to the lateral tibiofemoral joint.

Physical Findings Ten of the 15 patients demonstrated moderate to severe patellofemoral compression pain and 13 had moderate to severe patellofemoral crepitus. Four patients had contractures of the peripatellar tissues with limited medial-lateral patellar mobility. Five patients had range-of-motion limitations at their first visit. All had losses of extension; the mean limitation was 14 degrees (range, 5 to 22 degrees). Flexion limitations were present in four patients; one patient had 45 degrees of flexion, one had 50 degrees, and two had 100 degrees. At follow-up, improvements in the motion range were seen in three patients. Reflex sympathetic dystrophy developed in one patient (Case 14), and the motion limitations remained unchanged. Another patient (Case 9) who had not yet undergone a quadriceps reconstruction, actually lost 10 degrees of extension.

Radiographic Measurements: Patellar Vertical Height Ratios

Table 8 shows the results for the study populations obtained by three methods used for calculating patellar vertical height ratios. The data show essentially no difference in the ratios between right and left knees; however, a large variation in the ratios existed from one individual to another in the study populations.

The right-left difference in patellar height ratios for 95% of the population (2 SD) ranged from 11% to 15%, depending on the methods used for calculation. These data show that a greater decrease in the ratio would be diagnostic for developmental patellar infera.

Discussion

Pathomechanics of the Patella Infera Syndrome

In our experience and in reported studies, anterior cruciate ligament surgery remains the most frequent factor initiating the patella infera syndrome.[23,24] Typically, the postoperative course is complicated by limited knee motion, joint stiffness, and significant quadriceps muscle weakness. Contracture of peripatellar soft tissues and quadriceps weakness were the two

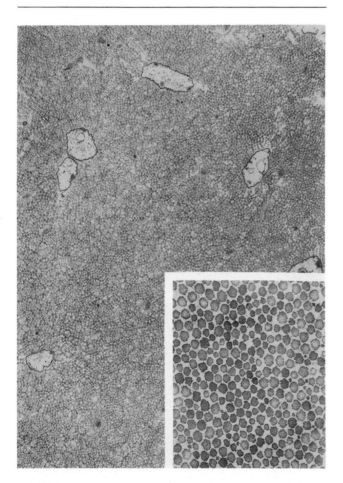

Fig. 6 Group 2, Case 6. Transverse section of collagen fibrils from patellar tendon. A low-power photomicrograph (× 10,350) shows the relative homegeneity of the collagen fibril diameter. This is better demonstrated at a higher magnification (inset, × 67,800). This normal appearance indicates that the shortened patellar tendon has already completed the remodeling process with maturation of the collagen fibrils.

Table 6
Group 2: Symptoms and functional rating

Data	Mean Rating (No. = 11)*	
	First Visit	Latest Visit
Pain	1.8 ± 1.1	1.6 ± 1.2
Swelling	2.4 ± 1.5	2.5 ± 1.8
Giving-way	2.9 ± 2.6	4.2 ± 2.3
Walking	18.5 ± 11.4	16.4 ± 11.2
Stairs	15.5 ± 10.4	13.6 ± 11.2
Kneeling	10.9 ± 10.5	5.5 ± 9.3

*Based on a scale of 0 to 10 for pain, swelling, and giving-way and a scale of 0 to 40 for walking, stairclimbing, and kneeling.[14] Data for the other four patients are not available.

Table 7
Group 2: Surgical procedures

Procedure	No. Before Patella Infera Diagnosis	No. After Patella Infera Diagnosis
Arthroscope, patelloplasty, debridement*	8	10
ACL reconstruction†	4	2
Other ligament reconstruction	3	—
Meniscectomy	4	—
Extensor mechanism realignment	4	2
Patellar ligament repair	2	—
Open reduction and internal fixation	3	—
Patellar ligament lengthening	—	1
Maquet osteotomy	—	5
Total knee replacement	1	—
Skin expander	—	1
Total	29	21

*Includes lateral releases alone or combined with medial reefing and vastus medialis oblique alignment.
†ACL, anterior cruciate ligament.

Table 8
Three methods of computing patellar vertical height ratios*

Data	Methods		
	Linclau[17]	Blackburne and Peel[18]	Insall and Salvati[15]†
No. of subjects	51	51	50
Right knee			
Mean	1.04 ± 0.13	0.84 ± 0.14	1.05 ± 0.11
Range	0.75 to 1.36	0.61 to 1.33	0.86 to 1.28
Left knee			
Mean	1.06 ± 0.15	0.84 ± 0.14	1.04 ± 0.10
Range	0.80 to 1.46	0.64 to 1.30	0.85 to 1.26
Difference			
Mean	−0.02 ± 0.07	0.0003 ± 0.06	0.014 ± 0.05
Range	−0.21 to 0.135	−0.193 to 0.19	0.123 to 0.107
Within 2 SD	15%	14%	11%

*Adapted with permission from Noyes FR, Wojtys EM, Marshall MT: The early diagnosis and treatment of the developmental patella infera syndrome. *Clin Orthop* 1991;263:108–119.
†Calculated from the original data of Jacobsen and Bertheussen.[16] Includes 95% of population.

most significant contributing factors in our series, which underscores the importance of early knee motion and quadriceps rehabilitation after knee surgery.[23,25] The cases reported in this study show that permanent shortening of the patellar ligament may occur within a relatively short period if the developmental patellar infera syndrome is not recognized and treated immediately.

The proposed pathomechanics of the patella infera syndrome are summarized in Figure 7. Numerous physical signs alert the examiner to the onset of developmental patellar infera, including (1) an inability to perform a strong voluntary quadriceps contraction in the first one to three weeks after knee surgery or trauma; (2) decreased passive medial-lateral and cephalad-caudad patellar mobility indicating peripatellar and infrapatellar soft-tissue contractures; (3) decreased palpable tension in the patellar ligament with failure of the patella to displace proximally on quadriceps contraction; and (4) a distal malposition of the involved patella compared with the opposite side. In addition, the fat-pad

and peripatellar tissues may demonstrate warmth and tenderness on palpation. Any patient with postoperative limitations in knee joint motion caused by periarticular and extra-articular contractures is also likely to have developmental patella infera. Reflex sympathetic dystrophy should be suspected in patients who also complain of cold intolerance, burning pain, rest pain, increased pain with weightbearing or quadriceps contraction, and pain with light skin pressure about the knee, such as that induced by the weight of a bed sheet or clothing.[26-28] There may not be obvious atrophic changes of the skin and extremity to suggest the diagnosis of reflex sympathetic dystrophy.[3]

In the initial stages of developmental patellar infera, lateral radiographs may reveal a decrease in the patellar vertical height ratio of only a few millimeters. A repeat radiograph should be obtained one to two weeks later to ascertain any further descent of the patella to establish the diagnosis. Our results indicate that there is normally little or no difference between the right and left patellar height ratios in the same individual; a dif-

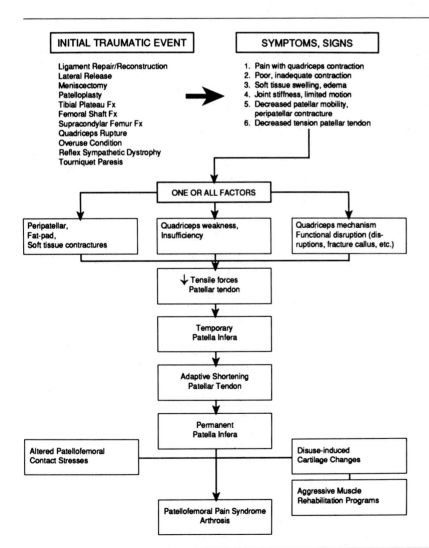

Fig. 7 Pathomechanics for developmental patella infera, patellar ligament shortening, and arthrosis. (Reproduced with permission from Noyes FR, Wojtys EM, Marshall MT: The early diagnosis and treatment of the developmental patella infera syndrome. *Clin Orthop* 1991;263:108–119.)

ference of more than 15% can be considered abnormal.[15] Because there is a wide normal variation in patellar vertical height from one person to another, the ratio must be compared with that of the opposite, uninvolved knee or a preoperative radiograph of the involved knee.

Many authors have discussed the deleterious effects of postoperative soft-tissue contractures of the knee joint.[1,5,6,8,29-31] However, the progression to a permanent patellar infera state and the additional morbidity have not been sufficiently recognized. Treatment of acute cases of arthrofibrosis must include attention to all the tissues that limit patellar mobility and knee motion.[4-8] Additionally, if knee flexion is not restored in the first few months after surgery, a permanent quadriceps contracture may also occur.[23,32-35]

Treatment of Patella Infera in the Initial Stages

Patients with a developing knee arthrofibrosis, in our experience, can often avoid a surgical release of soft tissues by undertaking a closely supervised therapy program.[15] The program (Fig. 8) includes aspirations of joint effusions that inhibit quadriceps contraction, patellar mobilization, and exercises to restore quadriceps muscle function. As a preventive measure, patients should be taught the technique of patellar mobilization as a routine part of the postoperative rehabilitation program. Medial-lateral and proximal-distal patellar mobilization should be performed four to six times daily for eight weeks after surgery. Patellar mobility should be determined on a weekly basis by the therapist and physician. We have found the use of electrical stimulation to the quadriceps muscle intermittently throughout a 24-hour period to be helpful in the re-

habilitation program, particularly for those patients who find it difficult to initiate a good voluntary quadriceps contraction. If early arthrofibrosis is developing, the seriousness of the condition, the need for close monitoring of the daily rehabilitation program, and potential inpatient treatment should be explained to the patient. If loss of joint motion persists, the use of a continuous epidural anesthetic for four to five days should be considered.[23]

If progressive distal descent of the patella is demonstrated on repeat radiographs, or if a significant patellar infera position remains in concert with generalized arthrofibrosis, then early release of contracted soft tissues is necessary to restore patellar height before permanent shortening of the patellar ligament occurs. The arthroscopic procedure must include release of suprapatellar adhesions, medial and lateral peripatellar tissues, and infrapatellar and fat-pad tissues. Postoperatively, a continuous epidural anesthetic is frequently used. Systemic corticosteroids may be required in more resistant cases to prevent recurrence. Although knee motion can usually be restored, future problems can be expected (all of our patients had varying degrees of crepitation and articular cartilage deterioration to the patellofemoral joint).

We believe that developmental patella infera is largely preventable; in an ongoing study of 207 consecutive knees after anterior cruciate ligament reconstruction treated with an immediate motion program postoperatively,[23] only one patient developed patella infera. There is a distinct group of knees that shows an exaggerated inflammatory soft-tissue response postoperatively. This response is characterized by excessive pain, tissue edema, warmth about the knee, and a lim-

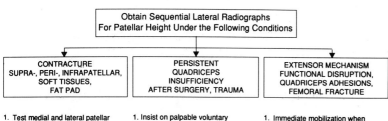

Fig. 8 Treatment recommendations for avoiding developmental patella infera syndrome. (Reproduced with permission from Noyes FR, Wojtys EM, Marshall MT: The early diagnosis and treatment of the developmental patella infera syndrome. *Clin Orthop* 1991;263:108–119.)

itation of knee motion. Treatment of this exaggerated inflammatory reaction is required early in its course and includes control of pain and therapeutic measures to lessen soft-tissue edema. This is the type of case that appears destined for a serious motion complication. The primary mistake is not to recognize the potential seriousness of any early joint contracture after knee surgery. Recognition of the arthrofibrotic condition many weeks to months after surgery means that treatment is much more difficult and often unsuccessful.

It is not possible for us to determine how rapidly the permanent shortening of the patellar ligament occurs, or the reasons why one patient develops patellar ligament shortening whereas another patient in similar circumstances does not. We performed the surgical procedure on ten of the 15 patients in group 2 many months after the patella infera was established. At surgery, the shortened patellar ligament had a normal gross appearance and was under visible tension. Many authors have alluded to Wolff's law of soft tissue.[24-26] Significant biochemical alterations in the chemical composition of soft tissues and increased turnover of collagen have been reported in disuse states.[32,33,36] Akeson and associates[33] postulated that abnormal cross-links between collagen fibers develop at abnormal locations, affecting the geometric alignment and microarchitecture of collagen fibers, decreasing their extensibility. Our transmission electron micrographic studies showed an abnormal cross-sectional distribution of fiber sizes, which we interpreted as indicating that newly formed small-diameter fibers had replaced mature fibers as a part of the overall remodeling process.

The early and rather prolonged effects of immobilization and disuse on skeletal muscle, which we found in our patients, have been reported by other investigators.[35,37,38] However, the pathomechanics involved are still unclear. Fitts and Brimmer,[34] Booth,[37] Eriksson and Häggmark,[38] Edström,[39] and Sargeant and associates[40] all showed a larger loss in type I fibers than in type II fibers, a finding that agreed with the results of the vastus lateralis muscle biopsies we performed. It is important to recognize that biochemical abnormalities in muscle enzymes, and concomitant muscular weakness, occur early in the postinjury or postoperative period.[38]

It is now recognized that a patellar infera position after a Hauser-type procedure may be itself a factor in the subsequent development of a patellofemoral arthrosis. Although one study[41] reported good or excellent results with Hauser procedures, other studies[42,43] suggested that, with time, there is a deterioration in the results. In a ten- to 25-year follow-up study, Hampson and Hill[43] found patella crepitus in 37 of 44 patients who had undergone Hauser procedures and osteoarthritis in 30 of 42 patients. The loss of vertical height of the patella may be a factor in altering patellofemoral contact stresses, producing areas of increased stress (proximal portion) and areas of decreased stress (distal portion). We speculate that disuse-induced articular cartilage changes are an additional factor in the subsequent development of the patellofemoral arthrosis.

Treatment of Patella Infera in the Chronic State

All our chronic cases included established patellofemoral arthrosis and patella infera, which necessitated initial nonsurgical treatment and activity modification. We recommend salvage-type surgical procedures only as a last resort. Initially, we treated patients with a rehabilitation program to overcome the serious muscle deficits that had developed. Local anesthetic injections in peripatellar soft tissues were frequently used to determine the contribution of pain related to the soft tissues apart from the pain originating from the patellofemoral joint. Arthroscopic release of painful contracted tissues was frequently performed. The question as to the efficacy of lengthening the patellar ligament to restore the vertical height of the patella cannot be answered in this series of patients. Patellar ligament lengthening was used in a few select cases in which there were no superimposed patellofemoral articular cartilage alterations. However, it is first necessary to reestablish muscle function and joint motion to lessen the possibility of postoperative shortening of the patellar ligament that occurred in one of our cases. We performed a tibial tubercle elevation procedure on select patients in this series in an attempt to avoid patellectomy. In other patients, particularly those who had undergone many previous operations, a patellectomy or patellar osteochondral allograft procedure, with simultaneous restoration of the patellar height, is planned when symptoms warrant consideration of these salvage-type procedures.

Acknowledgments

Randall Gall, MD, Bernard Morrey, MD, Mark Siegel, MD, Terry Habig, MD, and Jesse DeLee, MD, provided case histories, Klaus Jacobsen, MD, provided original radiographic data; and Paul Gikas, MD, provided electron microscopic analysis.

References

1. Wojtys EM, Noyes FR, Gikas P: Patella baja syndrome. Presented at the 53rd Annual Meeting of the American Academy of Orthopaedic Surgeons, New Orleans, Feb 20–25, 1986.
2. Caton J, Deschamps G, Chambat P, et al: Les rotules basses: A propos de 128 observations. *Rev Chir Orthop* 1982;68:317–325.
3. Paulos LE, Rosenberg TD, Drawbert J, et al: Infrapatellar contracture syndrome: An unrecognized cause of knee stiffness with patella entrapment and patella infera. *Am J Sports Med* 1987;15:331–341.
4. Enneking WF, Horowitz M: The intra-articular effects of im-

mobilization of the human knee. *J Bone Joint Surg* 1972;54A: 973–985.

5. Light KE, Nuzik S, Personius W, et al: Low-load prolonged stretch vs. high-load brief stretch in treating knee contractures. *Phys Ther* 1984;64:330–333.

6. Nicoll EA: Quadricepsplasty. *J Bone Joint Surg* 1963;45B:483–490.

7. Payne R: Neuropathic pain syndromes with special reference to causalgia and reflex sympathetic dystrophy. *Clin J Pain* 1986;2:59–73.

8. Rorabeck CH, Kennedy JC: Tourniquet-induced nerve ischemia complicating knee ligament surgery. *Am J Sports Med* 1980;8:98–102.

9. Windsor RE, Insall JN, Vince KG: Technical considerations of total knee arthroplasty after proximal tibial osteotomy. *J Bone Joint Surg* 1988;70A:547–555.

10. Conner AN: The treatment of flexion contractures of the knee in poliomyelitis. *J Bone Joint Surg* 1970;52B:138–144.

11. Grood ES, Suntay WJ, Noyes FR, et al: Biomechanics of the knee-extension exercises: Effect of cutting the anterior cruciate ligament. *J Bone Joint Surg* 1984;66A:725–734.

12. Noyes FR, Barber SD, Mangine RE: Bone-patellar ligament-bone and fascia lata allografts for anterior cruciate ligament reconstruction. *J Bone Joint Surg* 1990:72A:1125–1136.

13. Insall J, Salvati E: Patella position in the normal knee joint. *Radiology* 1971;101:101–104.

14. Noyes FR, Barber SD, Mooar LA: A rationale for assessing sports activity levels and limitations in knee disorders. *Clin Orthop* 1989;246:238–249.

15. Noyes FR, Wojtys EM, Marshall MT: The early diagnosis and treatment of the developmental patellar infera syndrome. *Clin Orthop* 1991;263:108–119.

16. Jacobsen K, Bertheussen K: The vertical location of the patella: Fundamental views on the concept patella alta, using a normal sample. *Acta Orthop Scand* 1974;45:436–445.

17. Linclau L: Measuring patellar height. *Acta Orthop Belg* 1984;50:70–74.

18. Blackburne JS, Peel TE: A new method of measuring patellar height. *J Bone Joint Surg* 1977;59B:241–242.

19. Lancourt JE, Cristini JA: Patella alta and patella infera: Their etiological role in patellar dislocation, chondromalacia, and apophysitis of the tibial tubercle. *J Bone Joint Surg* 1975;57A:1112–1115.

20. Noyes FR, Stabler CL: A system for grading articular cartilage lesions at arthroscopy. *Am J Sports Med* 1989;17:505–513.

21. Sprague NF III, O'Connor RL, Fox JM: Arthroscopic treatment of postoperative knee fibroarthrosis. *Clin Orthop* 1982;166:165–173.

22. Sprague NF III: Motion-limiting arthrofibrosis of the knee: The role of arthroscopic management. *Clin Sports Med* 1987;6:537–549.

23. Noyes FR, Mangine RE, Barber S: Early knee motion after open and arthroscopic anterior cruciate ligament reconstruction. *Am J Sports Med* 1987;15:149–160.

24. Noyes FR, Torvik PJ, Hyde WB, et al: Biomechanics of ligament failure: II. An analysis of immobilization, exercise, and reconditioning effects in primates. *J Bone Joint Surg* 1974;56A:1406–1418.

25. Noyes FR, Butler DL, Paulos LE, et al: Intra-articular cruciate reconstruction: I. Perspectives on graft strength, vascularization,

and immediate motion after replacement. *Clin Orthop* 1983;172:71–77.

26. Noyes FR: Functional properties of knee ligaments and alterations induced by immobilization: A correlative biomechanical and histological study in primates. *Clin Orthop* 1977;123:210–242.

27. Kozin F, Genant HK, Bekerman C, et al: The reflex sympathetic dystrophy syndrome: II. Roentgenographic and scintigraphic evidence of bilaterality and periarticular accentuation. *Am J Med* 1976;60:332–338.

28. Kozin F, Ryan LM, Carerra GF, et al: Reflex sympathetic dystrophy syndrome (RSDS): III. Scintigraphic studies, further evidence for the therapeutic efficacy of systemic corticosteroids, and proposed diagnostic criteria. *Am J Med* 1981;70:23–30.

29. Bennett GE: Lengthening of the quadriceps tendon. *J Bone Joint Surg* 1922;4:279–316.

30. Benum P: Operative mobilization of stiff knees after surgical treatment of knee injuries and posttraumatic conditions. *Acta Orthop Scand* 1982;53:625–631.

31. deAndrade JR, Grant C, Dixon AStJ: Joint distension and reflex muscle inhibition in the knee. *J Bone Joint Surg* 1965;47A:313–322.

32. Akeson WH, Amiel D, LaViolette D: The connective-tissue response to immobility: A study of the chondroitin-4 and 6-sulfate and dermatan sulfate changes in periarticular connective tissue of control and immobilized knees of dogs. *Clin Orthop* 1967;51:183–197.

33. Akeson WH, Woo SL-Y, Amiel D, et al: The connective tissue response to immobility: Biochemical changes in perarticular connective tissue of the immobilized rabbit knee. *Clin Orthop* 1973;93:356–362.

34. Fitts RH, Brimmer CJ: Recovery in skeletal muscle contractile function after prolonged hindlimb immobilization. *J Appl Physiol* 1985;59:916–923.

35. Jokl P, Konstadt S: The effect of limb immobilization on muscle function and protein composition. *Clin Orthop* 1983;174:222–229.

36. Woo SL-Y, Matthews JV, Akeson WH, et al: Connective tissue response to immobility: Correlative study of biomechanical and biochemical measurements of normal and immobilized rabbit knees. *Arthritis Rheum* 1975;18:257–264.

37. Booth FW: Effect of limb immobilization on skeletal muscle. *J Appl Physiol* 1982;52:1113–1118.

38. Eriksson E, Häggmark T: Comparison of isometric muscle training and electrical stimulation supplementing isometric muscle training in the recovery after major knee ligament surgery: A preliminary report. *Am J Sports Med* 1979;7:169–171.

39. Edström L: Selective atrophy of red muscle fibres in the quadriceps in long-standing knee-joint dysfunction: Injuries to the anterior cruciate ligament. *J Neurol Sci* 1970;11:551–558.

40. Sargeant AJ, Davies CT, Edward RH, et al: Functional and structural changes after disuse of human muscle. *Clin Sci Molec Med* 1977;52:337–342.

41. Fielding JW, Liebler WA, Krishne Urs ND, et al: Tibial tubercle transfer: A long-range follow-up study. *Clin Orthop* 1979;144:43–44.

42. Crosby EB, Insall J: Late results of Hauser procedure, abstract. *J Bone Joint Surg* 1975;57A:1027–1028.

43. Hampson WGJ, Hill P: Late results of transfer of the tibial tubercle for recurrent dislocation of the patella. *J Bone Joint Surg* 1975;57B:209–213.

The Posterior Cruciate Ligament and Posterolateral Structures of the Knee: Anatomy, Function, and Patterns of Injury

Daniel E. Cooper, MD

Russell F. Warren, MD

Jon J.P. Warner, MD

Introduction

Compared with the numerous studies of anterior cruciate ligament anatomy, function, and injury, the orthopaedic literature has paid relatively little attention to the posterior cruciate ligament (PCL) and posterolateral structures of the knee. However, the PCL has been considered by some to be the prime stabilizer of the knee.[1-3] Injuries to the PCL and posterolateral structures of the knee can cause disability ranging from almost no functional limitation to severe limitation of the activities of daily living.[4-9] In general, the isolated lesion tends to allow more function, whereas the combined PCL injury more often leads to functional disability.

Both the anatomy and function of the PCL and posterolateral structures can be somewhat confusing. This discussion reviews the anatomy of the region and attempts to clarify the currently accepted anatomic terminology. A detailed overview of the biomechanical function of each structure and the resultant instability produced by selective sectioning is presented. This information is used in a review of mechanism of injury, clinical examination, and symptoms. A clear understanding of the anatomy of the structures and their functional interrelationship enables the clinician to diagnose accurately injuries to the posterior and posterolateral structures of the knee and to treat these injuries successfully.

Anatomy

Posterior Cruciate Ligament

The PCL derives its name from its posterior insertion on the tibia. The PCL lies within the synovial tissue, which is reflected from the posterior capsule and covers the ligament on its medial, lateral, and anterior aspects. Distally, the posterior portion of the PCL blends with the posterior capsule and periosteum. Although it is within the knee, it is, in fact, completely surrounded by a synovial sleeve and is, therefore, entirely extra-articular in an anatomic sense.[5,10-12]

The PCL is located near the longitudinal axis of rotation, just medial to the center of the knee (Fig. 1). It is directed vertically in the frontal plane and angles forward 30 to 56 degrees in the sagittal plane, de-

pending on the degree of knee flexion.[10] The PCL is more vertical in extension and more horizontal in flexion (Figs. 1 and 2). Its prime function is as a restraint to posterior displacement of the tibia, and it plays a role as a secondary restraint to valgus and varus as well as external rotation.[11-13]

The average length of the PCL is 38 mm and its average width is 13 mm.[10] It is narrowest in its middle portion and fans out superiorly and to a lesser extent inferiorly. It is described as being formed from an anterolateral band and a posteromedial band, although these bundles are not completely separable. These

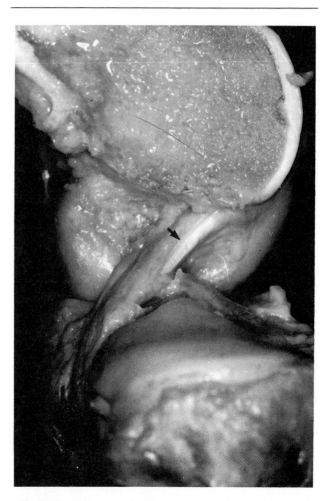

Fig. 1 Sagittal section though the intercondylar notch of the femur, leaving the intact PCL (arrow).

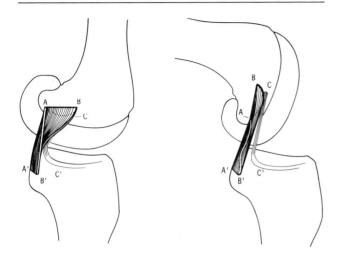

Fig. 2 Illustration demonstrating the changing fiber tension as the knee is flexed to 90 degrees from full extension. (A-A': smaller posteromedial band, B-B': larger anterolateral band, C-C': Ligament of Humphry) (Reproduced with permission from Girgis FG, Marshall JL, Al Monajem ARS, et al: The cruciate ligaments of the knee joints: Anatomical, functional and experimental analysis. *Clin Orthop* 1975; 106:216–231.)

bands are named for their attachment locations on both the femur (anterior or posterior) and on the tibia (medial or lateral) (Fig. 3). In extension, the robust anteromedial bulk of the ligament is lax, whereas the smaller posterolateral band is taut. When the knee is flexed, the posterior band becomes lax and the anterior bulk of the ligament tightens.[3,14] This is somewhat of an oversimplification, because there is actually a gradually changing pattern of fiber tension from anterior to posterior as the knee is extended (Fig. 2).

The PCL originates on the lateral surface of the medial femoral condyle, where its attachment is in the form of a segment of a circle. The general orientation of the attachment is in the horizontal plane with the lower boundary convex and parallel to the lower articular margin of the condyle (Fig. 4). The dimensions of the PCL attachment to the medial femoral condyle average 32 mm in the anteroposterior diameter with most distal fibers at an average of 3 mm proximal to the articular cartilage of the condyle.[10,12]

The tibial attachment of the PCL is into a depression on the posterior tibia between the two tibial plateaus approximately 1 cm below the tibial surface (Fig. 3). The attachment extends distally onto the posterior surface of the tibia. The width of this tibial attachment depends on the width of the intercondylar notch but averages 13 mm (Fig. 5).[10,12]

The anterior meniscofemoral ligament (ligament of Humphry) is less than one third of the diameter of the PCL.[15] Running anterior to the PCL, this ligament arises from the posterior horn of the lateral meniscus and inserts on the femur at the distal edge of the PCL

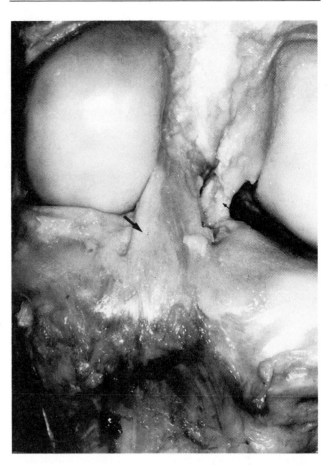

Fig. 3 Posterior view of the PCL demonstrating the tibial insertion site and fiber insertion pattern (arrow).

(Fig. 4). The posterior meniscofemoral ligament (ligament of Wrisberg) may be as large as one-half the diameter of the PCL.[15] It crosses the posterior aspect of the PCL obliquely from the posterior horn of the lateral meniscus to the medial femoral condyle (Fig. 6). Its attachment to the lateral meniscus has been reported to vary, because it can also attach to the tibia or the posterior capsule. In this setting, it only attaches indirectly to the lateral meniscus via the posterior capsular and popliteus attachments to the lateral meniscus.[12,15,16]

Although they are always present in lower mammals, which have no lateral tibiomeniscal attachment, the presence of the meniscofemoral ligaments in humans is somewhat variable and has been reported to be between 70% and 100%.[14,15] The variable insertion of the ligament of Wrisberg into the lateral meniscus has also created some confusion in anatomic reports. It is likely that many observers have considered it a part of the PCL when it inserts directly into the tibia. The absence of the ligaments of Humphry and/or Wrisberg may suggest their limited functional importance in humans. In a study by Girgis and associates,[10] these ligaments

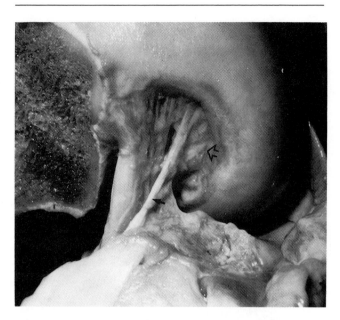

Fig. 4 Sagittal section demonstrating the PCL origin from the femur with its convex inferior border (open arrow). Note the ligament of Humphry and its distinct origin (closed arrow).

were never observed together. In 30% of the specimens, both ligaments were absent. In the remaining 70%, Wrisberg's ligament was found more commonly than Humphry's. This is in contrast with Kaplan,[16] who found one or the other in all knees dissected. Each of these ligaments has a femoral attachment, which is readily distinguishable from that of the PCL (Figs. 4 and 6). When present, the meniscofemoral ligaments may play a minor role as secondary restraints to posterior translation after the PCL is cut (J. Bergfeld, personal communication).

Welch[17] described the PCL as being "perfectly located to remain isometrically under tension throughout the whole range of knee movement." However, it has been demonstrated that no part of the PCL is totally

isometric during a normal range of motion.[18] The femoral location is the primary determinant of a fiber's isometry during flexion and extension. The proximal-distal location of a fiber's femoral attachment has a much stronger effect on its tension than does the anterior-posterior location. The tibial location has a small, but statistically significant, effect. Grood and associates[18] defined a bullet-shaped region whose base lies on the roof of the intercondylar notch and whose nose points posteriorly and slightly distally. The axis of the bullet is near the proximal edge of the femoral insertion of the PCL. Along this axis, anterior-superior attachments (located near the roof of the intercondylar notch) are more isometric than are posterior-inferior attachments located near the cartilage. This information demonstrates that a reconstructed ligament is not totally isometric. Placing the center of the graft as close to the isometric point as possible (at the base of the bullet-shaped region near the roof of the notch) minimizes the strains in that graft and optimizes the likelihood of long-term functional stability.

Posterolateral Structures

Many previous anatomic descriptions have used inconsistent terminology to describe the posterolateral structures of the knee. The terms short lateral ligament and fabellofibular ligament have at times been used interchangeably. We prefer to use the latter term, which is more anatomically correct. Kaplan[19] comprehensively reviewed the anatomy and history of the terminology relating to these structures.

There has also been confusion between the arcuate ligament and the arcuate ligament complex.[1,20] The arcuate ligament is a Y-shaped structure that courses from the fibular head over the popliteus muscle and is continuous with the oblique popliteal ligament of Winslow. Although thin, it is a distinct ligamentous reinforcing structure, and is not the same as the arcuate ligament complex. The arcuate ligament complex, as

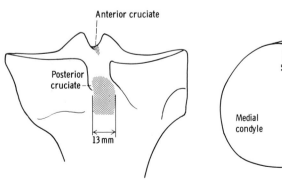

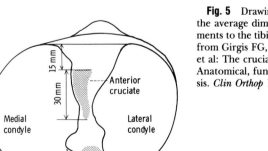

Fig. 5 Drawing of the tibial plateau showing the average dimensions for the cruciate attachments to the tibia. (Reproduced with permission from Girgis FG, Marshall JL, Al Monajem ARS, et al: The cruciate ligaments of the knee joints: Anatomical, functional and experimental analysis. *Clin Orthop* 1975;106:216–231.)

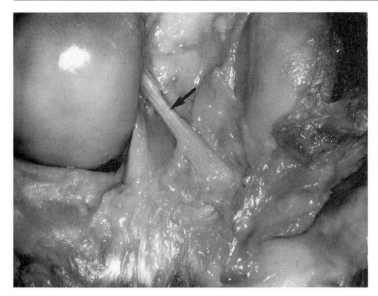
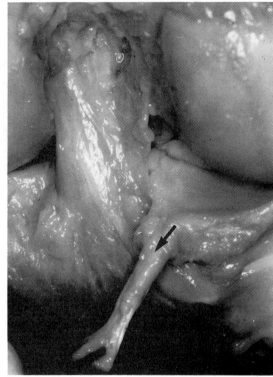

Fig. 6 Left, Posterior view of a right knee demonstrating the ligament of Wrisberg (arrow) and its attachments to the medial femoral condyle and lateral meniscus. **Right,** Same view after the ligament of Wrisberg (arrow) has been sectioned and reflected.

defined by Hughston and associates,[1] refers to the lateral collateral ligament, the arcuate ligament, the tendinous and aponeurotic portions of the popliteus muscle, and the lateral head of the gastrocnemius.[20]

Adding to this confusion is the fact that the anatomy in this region is somewhat variable. When dissecting through the traumatized tissues of an acutely injured knee, the surgeon may find it difficult to identify accurately all components of the posterolateral structures of the knee. The anatomy of the posterolateral aspect of the knee can be organized into three layers (Fig. 7). This concept, reported by Seebacher and associates,[21] was based on 35 dissections.

The most superficial layer (layer 1) has two parts: (1) the iliotibial tract and its expansion anteriorly, and (2) the superficial portion of the biceps and its expansion posteriorly (Fig. 7).[21,22] The biceps insertion divides into a superficial layer and a deep layer with the lateral collateral ligament between the two.[23] Layer 1 is thicker where most of the fibers of the iliotibial tract and biceps are longitudinally oriented. At the level of the distal femur, the peroneal nerve lies deep to layer l, just posterior to the biceps tendon.

Layer 2 is formed anteriorly by the quadriceps retinaculum. Posteriorly, layer 2 is incomplete and is represented by the two patellofemoral ligaments. The proximal ligament joins the terminal fibers of the lateral intermuscular septum, and the distal ligament ends posteriorly at the fabella or at the femoral insertion site of the posterolateral capsular reinforcements and lateral head of the gastrocnemius (Fig. 8).

Layer 3, the deepest layer, is the lateral part of the joint capsule. The capsular attachment to the outer edge of the lateral meniscus is termed the coronary ligament. The popliteus tendon passes through a hiatus in the coronary ligament to attach to the femur just anterior to the femoral attachment site of the lateral collateral ligament. The bare area of the lateral meniscus occurs at this hiatus. Just posterior to the overlying iliotibial tract, the capsule divides into two laminae, the more superficial of which is the original capsule embryologically. This lamina encompasses the lateral collateral ligament and ends posteriorly at the fabellofibular ligament (Fig. 7). The deeper lamina of the posterolateral part of the capsule, which is newer phylogenetically, passes along the edge of the lateral meniscus, forming both the coronary ligament and the hiatus for passage of the popliteus tendon. This inner lamina terminates posteriorly at the Y-shaped arcuate ligament, which spans the junction between the popliteus muscle and its tendon from the fibula to the femur. These two capsular laminae always are separated from each other by the inferior lateral genicular vessels that pass forward in the anteriorly truncated space between them.

Three anatomic variations were found by Seebacher and associates[21]: (1) the arcuate ligament alone reinforcing the capsule in 13% of the knees; (2) the fabel-

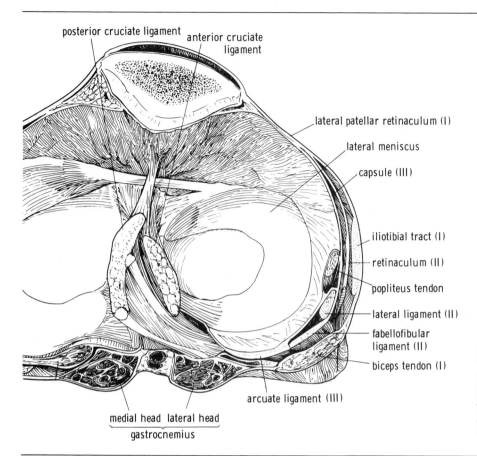

posterior cruciate ligament   anterior cruciate ligament

lateral patellar retinaculum (I)

lateral meniscus

capsule (III)

iliotibial tract (I)

retinaculum (II)

popliteus tendon

lateral ligament (II)

fabellofibular ligament (II)

biceps tendon (I)

arcuate ligament (III)

medial head lateral head
gastrocnemius

Fig. 7 Cross-section demonstrating the layered approach to anatomy of the lateral aspect of the knee. Numerals I, II, and III designate layers 1, 2, and 3. (Reproduced with permission from Seebacher JR, Inglis AE, Marshall JL, et al: The structure of the posterolateral aspect of the knee. *J Bone Joint Surg* 1982;64A: 536–541.)

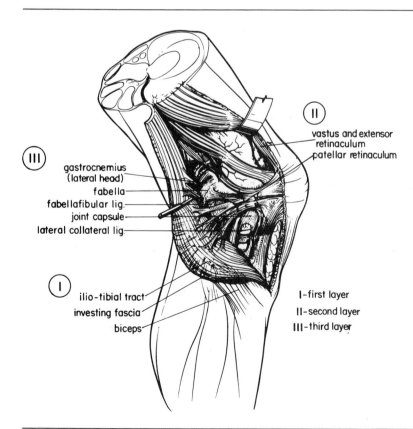

Fig. 8 Drawing of the layer approach to anatomy of the lateral aspect of the knee. (Reproduced with permission from Seebacher JR, Inglis AE, Marshall JL, et al: The structure of the posterolateral aspect of the knee. *J Bone Joint Surg* 1982;64A:536–541.)

II

vastus and extensor retinaculum
patellar retinaculum

III

gastrocnemius (lateral head)
fabella
fabellafibular lig.
joint capsule
lateral collateral lig

I

ilio-tibial tract
investing fascia
biceps

I–first layer
II–second layer
III–third layer

lofibular ligament alone reinforcing the capsule in 20%; and (3) both ligaments reinforcing the posterolateral aspect of the capsule in 67%. When the fabella was large, there was no arcuate ligament and the fabellofibular ligament was robust. Conversely, when the fabella or its cartilaginous remnant was absent, the fabellofibular ligament was also absent and only the arcuate ligament was present. Both the arcuate and fabellofibular ligaments insert on the apex of the fibular styloid process (Figs. 7 and 8).[21]

The popliteus is a dynamic internal rotator of the tibia. In its static role, it restricts posterior tibial translation and varus rotation, as well as external rotation of the tibia on the femur.[16,24] There are variations of the popliteus muscle attachment to the posterior horn of the meniscus.[16,25–27] Last's[25,26] concept was that the popliteus sent firm attachment fibers to the lateral meniscus in the vast majority of knees, thereby functioning to retract the lateral meniscus during knee flexion. However, a more recent study was not in agreement, demonstrating these connections in less than 20%.[27]

The tibial attachment of the popliteus is quite broad and is oriented obliquely so that tension along the tendon is probably transmitted throughout the tibia. Because it is the only major structure that is positioned in an oblique fashion, the popliteus is well suited to prevent external rotation of the tibia (Fig. 9). The popliteus tendon functions as both a static and an active restraint to external rotation, rather than merely as an active muscle for rotation of the tibia.[14,16,26]

Functional Biomechanics

Recent work in biomechanical analysis of the function of the PCL and posterolateral structures has added a great deal to the understanding of their role in the stability of the knee.[13,28–31] However, the great detail in these studies may be somewhat confusing. It is essential for the reader to understand the methods of the different studies and the relative advantages and shortcomings of each method. The two methods most commonly employed for biomechanical analysis of knee ligaments are (1) the assessment of the restraining force that develops in individual ligaments during predetermined displacements of the knee, and (2) the selective cutting approach. Both methods provide important information, but there are significant differences between the two experimental approaches.[32]

By determining the restraining force that develops in individual ligaments during displacements of the knee, the relative importance and function of a single ligament can be assessed in terms of the percentage of the total restraining force that it provides.[13,32] By determining the force necessary to produce a predetermined amount of displacement, the relative importance of a certain structure may be determined by sectioning

that structure and calculating the difference in force required to produce the same distance. The decline in required force correlates directly with the percentage of restraining force that structure contributes to the stability of the knee in the direction tested. Using this method, Butler and associates[13] determined the primary and secondary restraints to various displacements in the knee joint.

In contrast, a selective cutting study attempted to determine the increase in knee joint laxity after transection of a specific ligament. This provided a reliable indication of the resultant stability of the joint after injury to that specific ligament. However, because joint laxity is a result of a complex interaction among all the knee ligaments—an interaction altered when a specific ligament is cut or injured—the change in joint laxity reflected not only the loss of the ligament, but also changes in the interaction of the remaining ligaments.[32]

Selective cutting offers one major advantage over methods that describe the restraining function of individual ligaments as a percentage of overall restraint. It directly measures the changes in motion of the knee that occur when individual or combined ligament sectioning is performed. In addition, the determination of ligament function by measuring changes in motion of the knee within the 90-degree arc of flexion allows us to evaluate abnormalities of motion in a manner similar to that used in clinical testing. This helps to determine the angle of flexion at which clinical laxity testing is most accurate for each ligament being assessed.[28]

Detailed biomechanical analysis of the role of the posterolateral structures and PCL in the stability of the knee have recently been reported by Gollehon and associates[28] and Grood and associates.[30] Both studies measured increases in rotational, angular, and translational displacement after selective sectioning of the PCL and posterolateral structures in randomized orders. These studies contain important information regarding the relative stabilizing roles of these ligamentous structures in the function of the knee and the resultant instability patterns after injury to these structures. The close correlation of data between the two studies is a testimony to the accuracy and reproducibility of the methods.

The following is a discussion of the work performed at our institution and reported by Gollehon and associates.[28] This information is summarized from three viewpoints: (1) For each degree of freedom in the knee, normal parameters and the effects of isolated and combined section of the PCL and posterolateral structures are reviewed. (2) The effect on the 6 degrees of freedom of the knee of each isolated and combined sectioning pattern is given. (3) This information is applied to the clinical setting to determine the most accurate examination techniques for evaluating the PCL and posterolateral structures.

Before the biomechanical data are reviewed, a clar-

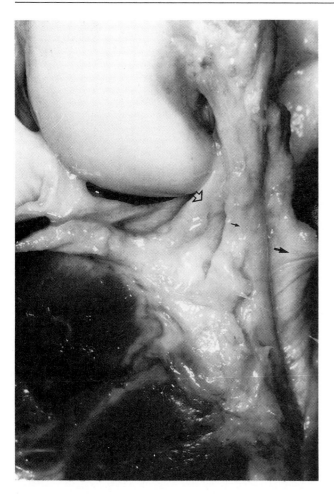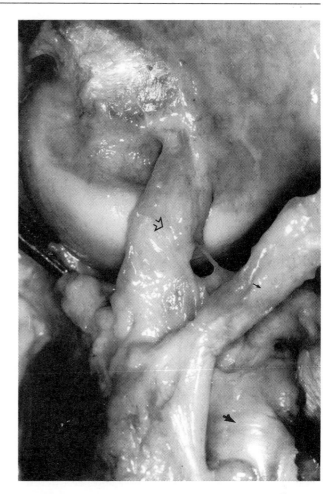

Fig. 9 Anatomy of the posterolateral structures of the knee: Lateral collateral ligament (large arrow), popliteus (open arrow), and biceps insertion (small arrow), which surrounds the lateral collateral ligament. Before (**left**) and after (**right**) sectioning of the lateral collateral ligament.

ification of the anatomic terminology used by Gollehon and associates[28] is needed. To simplify reporting, the authors grouped the structures of the posterolateral aspect of the knee into what they term the "deep ligament complex," which includes the arcuate ligament, the popliteus tendon, the fabellofibular ligament, and the posterolateral capsule, but not the lateral collateral ligament.

Anterior-Posterior Translation With Anterior-Posterior Force

Isolated sectioning of the PCL significantly increases posterior translation at all angles of flexion.[13] The absolute amount of translation increases progressively from 0 to 90 degrees of flexion (Fig. 10). Isolated sectioning of the lateral collateral or deep ligament complex (arcuate ligament, fabellofibular ligament, popliteal tendon, posterolateral capsule) produces no increase in posterior translation at any angle of flexion.[28]

Combined sectioning of the lateral collateral liga-

ment and deep ligament complex results in small (approximately 3 mm) but significant increases in posterior translation at all angles of flexion. At 0 and 30 degrees of flexion, the increase in posterior translation produced by combined sectioning of the lateral collateral ligament and deep ligament complex is similar in magnitude to that produced by isolated sectioning of the PCL (Fig. 10). Combined sectioning of the PCL, deep ligament complex, and lateral collateral ligament results in a significant increase (20 to 25 mm) in posterior translation at all positions of flexion compared with intact knees or knees in which isolated section is performed (Fig. 10).[28] Neither isolated nor combined sectioning of the PCL and posterolateral structures increases anterior tibial translation.

Varus-Valgus Rotation With Varus-Valgus Torque

In the intact knee, the least amount of varus and valgus rotation occurs at full extension.[14,28,30] Varus and valgus rotation increases continually with increasing

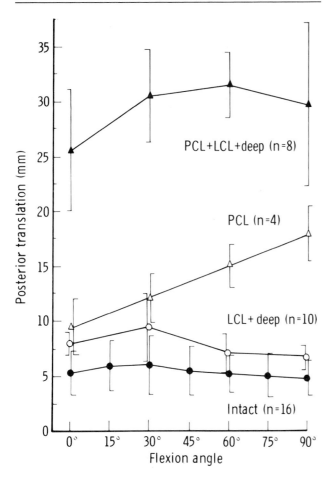

Fig. 10 Posterior translation with posterior force of 100 N. Results of intact knees as well as selected cuttings. (Reproduced with permission from Gollehon DL, Torzilli PA, Warren RF: The role of the posterolateral and cruciate ligaments in the stability of the human knee: A biomechanical study. *J Bone Joint Surg* 1987;69A:233–242.)

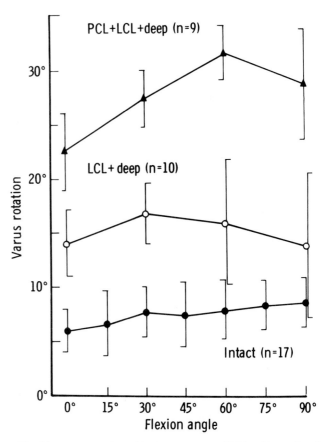

Fig. 11 Varus rotation with varus torque at 10 Nm. (Reproduced with permission from Gollehon DL, Torzilli PA, Warren RF: The role of the posterolateral and cruciate ligaments in the stability of the human knee: A biomechanical study. *J Bone Joint Surg* 1987;69A: 233–242.)

flexion of the knee to 90 degrees. Isolated sectioning of the anterior cruciate ligament or the PCL produces no significant increase in valgus or varus rotation at any angle of knee flexion.[28,29,33] An increase in valgus rotation cannot be produced by isolated or combined sectioning of the lateral collateral ligament, deep posterolateral structures, or PCL.[28]

Compared with the intact knee, a small but significant increase (1 to 4 degrees) in varus rotation occurs at all angles of flexion when only the lateral collateral ligament is sectioned. A similar magnitude of increased varus rotation is produced at 90 degrees of flexion when only the deep ligament complex is sectioned. A larger increase (5 to 9 degrees) occurs with combined sectioning of the lateral collateral ligament and deep ligament complex. An even larger increase in varus rotation (14 to 19 degrees) occurs at all angles of flexion when the PCL is sectioned (Fig. 11). This combined sectioning of the PCL and all posterolateral structures produced varus angulation of more than 30 degrees at 60 degrees of knee flexion (Fig. 11).[28]

Internal-External Rotation of the Tibia With Internal-External Tibial Torque

Total (internal plus external) tibial rotation in intact knees is least at 0 degrees of flexion (approximately 29 degrees of rotation) and greatest at 45 degrees of flexion (approximately 44 degrees of rotation). Internal rotation is greatest at 45 degrees and external rotation is greatest at 90 degrees (Fig. 12).[28]

No increase in internal rotation of the tibia is seen after isolated or combined sectioning of the lateral collateral ligament, deep posterolateral structures, or PCL. No significant increase in internal rotation of the tibia is found after isolated sectioning of the anterior cruciate ligament. Large increases in internal rotation of the tibia (7 to 20 degrees) result when the anterior cruciate ligament, lateral collateral ligament, and deep ligament complex are all sectioned, but these increases are significant only at 30 and 60 degrees of knee flexion.[28]

Isolated sectioning of the deep ligament complex produces a significant increase (6 ± 3 degrees) in external rotation at 90 degrees of flexion. Isolated sec-

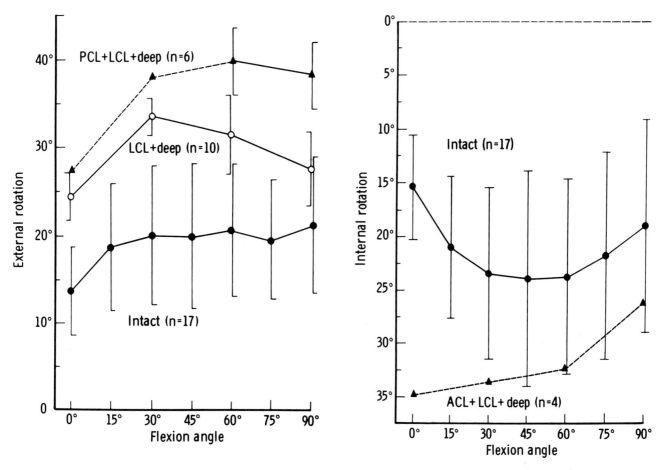

Fig. 12 **Left,** External tibial rotation with external tibial torque at 4.5 Nm. (Reproduced with permission from Gollehon DL, Torzilli PA, Warren RF: The role of the posterolateral and cruciate ligaments in the stability of the human knee: A biomechanical study. *J Bone Joint Surg* 1987;69A:233–242.) **Right,** Internal tibial rotation with internal tibial torque at 4.5 Nm. (Reproduced with permission from Gollehon DL, Torzilli PA, Warren RF: The role of the posterolateral and cruciate ligaments in the stability of the human knee: A biomechanical study. *J Bone Joint Surg* 1987;69A:233–242.)

tioning of the lateral collateral ligament produces significant but smaller increases of 2 to 3 degrees at 0, 30, and 90 degrees of flexion. Sectioning both the lateral collateral ligament and the deep ligament complex significantly increases external rotation at all angles of flexion compared with the intact knee (Fig. 12). Isolated sectioning of the PCL results in no change in external rotation. When the PCL is sectioned after the lateral collateral ligament and deep ligament complex have been cut, a significant increase in external rotation is produced at 60 and 90 degrees of flexion, but no significant increase occurs at 0 or 30 degrees of flexion (Fig. 12).[28]

Coupled Rotations and Translations

When anterior force is applied to the tibia of an intact knee, the tibia rotates internally. Similarly, when posterior force is applied, external rotation of the tibia occurs. These predictable resultant tibial rotations are termed coupled rotations. Anterior and posterior force

produces a maximum total tibial rotation of approximately 16 degrees at 60 to 75 degrees of flexion. As the knee is extended, the coupled total rotation of the tibia decreases to approximately 5 degrees.[28]

An increase in internal rotation with anterior force does not occur after isolated or combined sectioning of the lateral collateral ligament, deep ligament complex, or PCL. When the anterior cruciate ligament is sectioned in addition to the lateral collateral ligament and deep posterolateral structures, there is a significant increase in coupled internal rotation, but only at 30 degrees of flexion (Fig. 13).[28]

Isolated sectioning of the PCL eliminates the coupled external rotation that occurs with posterior force but does not affect the coupled internal rotation that occurs with anterior force. If the posterolateral structures are sectioned with the PCL, then coupled external rotation with posterior force returns and is increased over the intact situation.[28]

Combined sectioning of the lateral collateral liga-

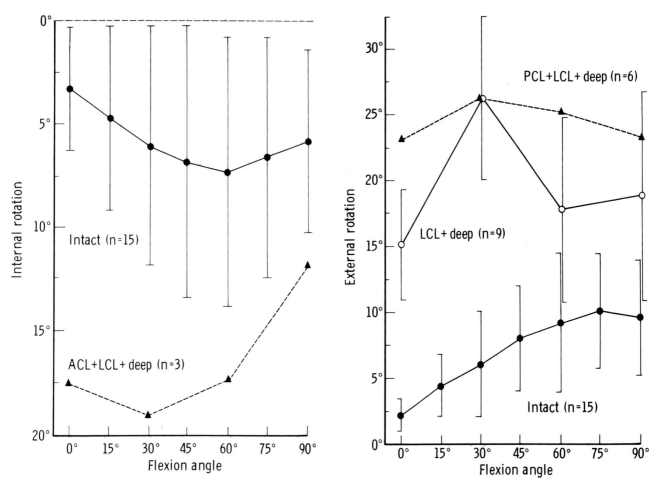

Fig. 13 Left, Coupled tibial rotation with anterior force at 100 N. (Reproduced with permission from Gollehon DL, Torzilli PA, Warren RF: The role of the posterolateral and cruciate ligaments in the stability of the human knee: A biomechanical study. *J Bone Joint Surg* 1987; 69A:233–242.) **Right,** Coupled tibial rotation with posterior force at 100 Nm. (Reproduced with permission from Gollehon DL, Torzilli PA, Warren RF: The role of the posterolateral and cruciate ligaments in the stability of the human knee: A biomechanical study. *J Bone Joint Surg* 1987;69A:233–242.)

ment and deep ligament complex significantly increases the external rotation that occurs with the posterior force at all angles of flexion, with an increase of approximately 20 degrees occurring at 30 degrees of knee flexion. If the PCL is also sectioned, there is a slight but insignificant increase in external rotation.[28]

Just as there are coupled rotations with anterior-posterior force, there are coupled translations with internal-external rotation. When internal tibial torque is applied to the intact knee, coupled anterior translation results. The application of external tibial torque results in coupled posterior translation. This coupled total anterior and posterior translation that results from internal and external tibial torque is least at 0 degrees and greatest at 90 degrees of flexion.[28]

When the lateral collateral ligament and deep ligament complex are sectioned in combination, a significant increase in posterior translation occurs with external torque at all angles of flexion. Combined

sectioning of the lateral collateral ligament, deep ligament complex, and PCL produces an additional increase in this posterior translation (Fig. 14).[28]

Isolated Sectioning

PCL The strength of the PCL is approximately 2,000 N.[34] The PCL is the primary restraint to posterior translation at all degrees between full extension and 90 degrees of flexion.[13] According to Hughston and associates,[1,35] its central location makes it the center of rotation for rotatory instability patterns of the knee.

The results of Gollehon and associates[28] indicate that the PCL is the only isolated ligament that provides initial restraint to primary posterior translation at all angles of flexion. This finding is also supported by data from other studies.[13,30] Sectioning of the PCL produces posterior translation of the tibia at all degrees of flexion of the knee, with the greatest increases occurring between 75 and 90 degrees (Fig. 10). Isolated sectioning

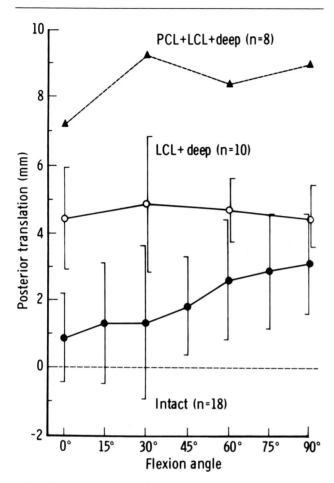

Fig. 14 Coupled posterior translation with external tibial torque at 4.5 Nm. (Reproduced with permission from Gollehon DL, Torzilli PA, Warren RF: The role of the posterolateral and cruciate ligaments in the stability of the human knee: A biomechanical study. *J Bone Joint Surg* 1987;69A:233–242.)

of the PCL produces a smaller amount of posterior translation at 0 and 30 degrees of flexion. This is, in fact, similar in magnitude to the increased posterior translation seen at 0 and 30 degrees after sectioning of the lateral collateral ligament and deep ligament complex (Fig. 10). In addition, sectioning of the PCL has no effect on varus or valgus or external rotation of the tibia as long as the lateral collateral ligament and deep structures are intact.

Lateral Collateral Ligament The lateral collateral ligament is the major restraint to primary varus rotation at all positions of flexion. No change occurs in primary internal rotation of the tibia or in coupled anterior or posterior translation after isolated sectioning of the lateral collateral ligament. However, primary external rotation increases at all angles of flexion except at 60 degrees.[28]

Deep Ligament Complex Sectioning of the deep ligament complex (arcuate ligament, popliteus tendon, fabello-

fibular ligament, and posterolateral capsule) alone does not significantly affect primary or coupled varus and valgus rotation or primary or coupled anterior or posterior translation. Sectioning of the deep ligament complex produces a significant increase in primary external rotation of the tibia at 90 degrees of flexion.[28]

Combined Sectioning

Lateral Collateral Ligament and Deep Ligament Complex When the lateral collateral ligament and deep ligament complex are sectioned in combination, significant primary varus angular rotation of the tibia occurs compared with that seen with isolated sectioning of either the lateral collateral ligament or the deep structures (Fig. 11). The clinical implication of these data on varus rotation is that the small increase in varus rotation that occurs when there is an isolated injury of the lateral collateral ligament or deep posterolateral structures may be difficult to detect. Conversely, a combined injury of the lateral collateral ligament and deep posterolateral structures should not be difficult to recognize because of the increased varus rotation that is present, particularly when the knee is in 30 degrees of flexion. In addition, sectioning of the posterolateral structures (including the lateral collateral ligament) produces a significant increase in primary posterior translation at 0 and 30 degrees of flexion of the knee and a significant increase in primary external rotation at all angles of flexion. The average increase in external rotation depends on the angle of flexion and is greatest at 30 degrees of flexion and decreases with additional flexion. At 90 degrees of flexion, the intact PCL limits the increase in external rotation to less than one half of the increase that occurs at 30 degrees. After combined sectioning of the lateral collateral ligament and deep ligament complex, the increase in posterior translation at 0 and 30 degrees of flexion is similar in magnitude to that seen when only the PCL has been sectioned.[28]

Lateral Collateral Ligament, Deep Structures, and PCL Combined sectioning of the lateral collateral ligament, deep structures, and PCL significantly increases primary posterior translation, varus rotation, and external rotation of the tibia at all angles of flexion when compared with either the intact knee or with the knee with an isolated or lesser combination of ligament sectioning (Figs. 10 to 12).[28]

Clinical Application

These results suggest that, in the clinical setting, posterior translation, varus rotation, and external rotation are the most useful motions for detecting injury to the posterolateral ligament structures, the PCL or both. Thus, complete posterolateral disruption along with an intact PCL would be expected to demonstrate maximum varus rotation, posterior translation, and external rotation at 30 degrees of knee flexion. The abnormal motion after removal of the entire posterolateral complex when the PCL is intact results primarily from abnormalities in the limits of both external rotation and varus angulation. Because the increase in external rotation is greatest at 30 degrees of flexion, the external rotation test should be more sensitive when it is performed with the knee at 30 degrees of flexion. A large increase in external rotation at 90 degrees should alert the examiner to the possibility of a complete tear of the PCL.

Isolated injury to the PCL should cause maximum posterior translation at 75 to 90 degrees of flexion and less posterior translation at 0 to 30 degrees. No change would be expected in primary rotation or varus-valgus angulation. Because the increase in the limit to posterior translation is twice as large at 90 degrees as it is at 30 degrees, the posterior drawer test should be more sensitive for PCL injury when it is performed with the knee at 90 degrees of flexion.

When both the posterolateral structures and the PCL are ruptured, there is a substantial increase in primary posterior translation, external rotation, and varus rotation at all angles of flexion of the knee compared with an intact knee or a knee in which either structure has been injured in isolation.

These findings do not support those in other studies regarding the absence of all so-called rotatory instabilities of the knee once the PCL has been ruptured.[1,2,28,30,35] The PCL provides substantial restraint to primary varus rotation and primary external rotation of the tibia after sectioning of the posterolateral structures. Isolated sectioning of the PCL results in no significant change in any of the measured rotations except for a loss in the coupled external rotation of the tibia. However, when the PCL is sectioned in combination with posterolateral structures, there are substantial increases in coupled external rotation of the tibia, primary varus rotation, primary external rotation, and posterior translation.[28]

Articular Pressure and Chondral Degeneration

Several reports of long-term follow-up of PCL-deficient knees have recently been published.[5,6,8,9,36–38] It appears that with an isolated PCL injury, the functional result may be quite good.[4–8] However, degenerative changes have been found even after these isolated injuries.[5,36] Clancy and associates[36] found a high incidence of patellofemoral and medial compartment articular degenerative changes on arthroscopic inspection after PCL injury. Of the patients with arthroscopic evidence of cartilage degeneration, only 31% had radiographic evidence of arthritis.

There are conflicting data on the association of degenerative changes with degree of laxity. It has been suggested that greater degrees of laxity are more likely to lead to degenerative changes over time. However, this hypothesis has been difficult to confirm in long-term follow-up studies.

There is also controversy as to the relative incidence of degenerative changes after PCL injury and the degree of involvement of each compartment of the knee.[1,36,39] Clancy and associates[36] arthroscopically observed the frequent occurrence of medial compartment degenerative changes. However, a recent long-term follow-up report by Torg and associates[40] indicated that radiographic degenerative changes are much more common in PCL-deficient knees with combined ligament instability patterns, and that the lateral compartment may be involved nearly as often as the medial compartment. It was their finding that the degenerative changes associated with isolated PCL deficiency were mild, did not significantly affect function, and did not necessarily grow worse with time.[40]

Skyhar and associates[41] recently studied the effect of sectioning the PCL and posterolateral structures on the articular contact pressures of the medial, lateral, and patellofemoral compartments of the knee. They found that lateral compartment pressure was not significantly increased by isolated PCL sectioning, but was increased by combined PCL and posterolateral structure sectioning. In contrast, medial compartment pressure was significantly increased by both isolated PCL sectioning and combined PCL and posterolateral structure sectioning. The peak pressure occurred at 60 degrees of knee flexion.

Patellofemoral compartment pressure increased with both isolated PCL sectioning and combined PCL and posterolateral sectioning, with the peak pressure noted at 90 degrees. Quadriceps load required to extend the knee increased with both isolated PCL and combined PCL and posterolateral sectioning. The increase in the patellofemoral pressure is a result of the dropback of the tibia after PCL rupture. This "reverse Maquet" effect results in an alteration in the force vectors that occur during active knee extension. This is reflected by increased quadriceps load during active knee extension and increased patellofemoral contact pressures.

These changes in the patellofemoral and medial compartment pressures raise concerns as to the appropriate treatment for acute PCL ruptures. In particular, an attempt should be made to save the medial meniscus to avoid progressive degenerative changes. Fortunately, tears of the medial meniscus in association with isolated PCL injury are relatively uncommon.[39]

Incidence of Injury

Injury to the PCL is certainly much less common than injury to the anterior cruciate ligament. Because so many isolated injuries are either unreported or undetected, the true incidence of PCL injuries is not known.

In surgical reviews, reported injury to the PCL ranges from 3.4% reported by O'Donoghue[42] to 20% of all ligament injuries in a series reported by Clendenin and associates.[43] These numbers may be skewed by differences in the patient populations. Our experience indicates that the incidence is in the midrange, at about 8%.[44] However, it is important to distinguish between the truly isolated PCL injury and the combined major knee ligament injury in which PCL disruption is only one component. It has been our experience that most PCL injuries are caused by either athletics or vehicular accidents. Industrial accidents account for the remainder. Isolated posterolateral injury is less common than PCL injury.[20,45,46] DeLee and associates[45] reported an incidence of less than 2%. Both PCL and posterolateral injuries are seen more commonly in association with other knee ligament injuries than as an isolated finding.[46-53]

Mechanism of Injury

Injuries to the PCL occur by several mechanisms. A direct blow to the flexed knee is probably the most common mechanism of isolated PCL injury.[3] This may occur in sports when a fall occurs and the knee strikes the ground in a position of flexion. When the foot is dorsiflexed during the fall, PCL injury may be avoided because the force is transmitted to the patella and along the longitudinal axis of the femur. If the foot is plantarflexed, then the blow tends to be sustained by the region of the tibial tubercle, imparting a forceful posterior drawer to the knee and rupturing the PCL. The same mechanism of injury is common during vehicular accidents when the knee strikes the dashboard in a flexed position. Because the anterolateral bundle of the PCL tightens with flexion, it is believed that forced hyperflexion may also cause PCL rupture.

The other mechanisms of PCL injury are more apt to produce combined ligament injuries than isolated PCL disruption. Forced hyperextension is a common mechanism of combined ligament injuries as well as knee dislocation. Girgis and associates[10] demonstrated that the anterior cruciate ligament is the first ligament to rupture in forced hyperextension. Kennedy and Grainger[3] demonstrated that the PCL ruptures at approximately 30 degrees of hyperextension. Therefore, a PCL disruption caused by a pure hyperextension mechanism would also be associated with anterior cruciate ligament disruption.

Severe varus or valgus stress may cause disruption of the PCL in combination with collateral injury. We have been unable to demonstrate that isolated sectioning of the PCL has any effect on varus-valgus stability. The collateral ligaments are the primary restraints to varus and valgus stress, and the PCL is subject to disruption by a varus or valgus rotation only after disruption of the respective collateral ligament.

Injury to the posterolateral corner of the knee most commonly occurs because of a posteriorly directed blow to the anteromedial knee in extension.[20,45,46] Such a blow produces hyperextension and a varus moment about the knee, disrupting the posterolateral structures. In addition, a less common mechanism is severe external rotation of the tibia as a component of injury. These mechanisms explain why cruciate ligament injury is so commonly associated with posterolateral instability.[20,45,46]

Examination

Injuries to the PCL and posterolateral structures of the knee are commonly missed at the time of initial evaluation. It is, therefore, imperative that a thorough examination be performed and that specific tests for PCL and posterolateral instability be done.

Swelling, ecchymosis, induration, and tenderness in the region of the posterolateral corner of the knee are important signs of acute injury. An abrasion over the anteromedial aspect of the knee may be a clue to the mechanism of injury. In addition, because many of these knee ligament injuries represent a violent mechanism of injury with severe ligament disruption, any laceration about the knee should be suspected of communicating with the joint. An air arthrogram on routine radiographs is diagnostic of such a connection (Fig. 15). Local exploration or injection of saline into the joint may be required to prove that no communication exists. The presence of an open knee joint requires prompt, thorough irrigation of the wound and knee joint to prevent sepsis.

In the acutely injured knee, assessment of the neurovascular status is critical. Injuries to the PCL or posterolateral structures are often seen as combined knee ligament injuries or as a component of the injury in a knee dislocation. Arteriography should be considered for knees suspected of dislocation. It must be remembered that a dislocation may occur and then spontaneously reduce without having been documented by radiograph.

Any knee with a varus component to the mechanism of injury should be closely examined for evidence of peroneal nerve damage. The incidence of this in association with lateral and posterolateral ligament disruption varies from 10% to 30%.[20,45,46]

Anterior-Posterior Translation

When assessing anterior or posterior translation of the tibia along the femur, it is helpful to palpate the tibial plateau and femoral condyles to aid in determining the amount and direction of displacement. On the basis of recent selective cutting biomechanical studies,

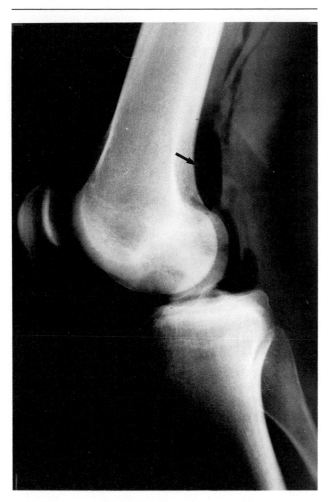

Fig. 15 Lateral radiograph taken after a severe blow to the anteromedial knee. The air arthrogram (arrow) is evidence of an open knee joint. In this case the forces of injury were so violent that the skin was torn and air was drawn into the joint.

it is apparent that the posterior drawer test performed at 80 to 90 degrees of flexion is the best way of assessing the integrity of the PCL.[28,30] Both the degree of displacement and the quality of the endpoint should be assessed.[54] In contrast, the posterior drawer test performed at 30 degrees of flexion is not as specific for the PCL, even though the ligament is a primary restraint.[13] Injury to the posterolateral structures may increase posterior translation slightly at this degree of flexion.

In the study of Gollehon and associates[28] isolated sectioning of either the PCL or the posterolateral structures combined with the lateral collateral ligament produced a similar degree of posterior translation at 30 degrees. It is important to realize that this posterior translation at 30 degrees was only produced by the complete sectioning of the lateral collateral ligament, arcuate ligament, popliteus tendon, fabellofibular ligament, and the posterolateral capsule.

When the Lachman test is performed, it should be recognized that increased translation may occur because of posterolateral or PCL disruption. There should be a sensation of increased anterior translation because of the more posterior resting position of the tibia. However, a solid endpoint to anterior translation indicates that the anterior cruciate ligament is intact.

Butler and associates[13] demonstrated that, for the straight posterior drawer, the PCL provides a mean of 95% of the total restraining force. After loss of the PCL, the secondary restraints to the posterior drawer test are the posterolateral capsule and popliteus complex combined (58%), the medial collateral ligament (16%), and, to a lesser extent, many other structures. The anterior cruciate ligament does not resist the posterior drawer, nor does the PCL resist the anterior drawer.[13] A false-positive response on the anterior drawer test after rupture of the PCL occurs because of a posterior shift in the starting position of the tibia. This is not in agreement with the statement of Hughston and associates[1,2] that an anterior drawer sign in internal rotation is indicative of injury only to the PCL. We do agree that with or without anterior cruciate ligament disruption, internal rotation may diminish the anterior drawer. However, this is more the effect of the collateral and secondary capsular restraints than an effect of the PCL.

Varus-Valgus Rotation

Varus and valgus stress testing should be performed both at full extension and at 30 degrees of flexion. Isolated disruption of the PCL does not affect varus-valgus stability. In contrast, posterolateral disruption significantly affects varus stability, especially at 30 degrees of flexion. Studies have demonstrated that varus instability in full extension can occur because of disruption of the posterolateral structures alone with a completely intact PCL.[28] This contrasts with the concept of Hughston and associates[1,2] that any evidence of varus-valgus instability in full extension is evidence of PCL disruption. It must again be stressed that this laxity is caused by combined injury to the lateral collateral ligament and deep posterolateral structures, and that isolated injury to either does not cause large degrees of varus rotation. Also, although some degree of varus rotation in full extension does not necessarily imply PCL injury, it is probably more common than not that the PCL sustains injury when the lateral collateral ligament and deep posterolateral structures are completely disrupted. Certainly, large degrees of varus rotation in full extension indicate injury to the PCL and, often, the anterior cruciate ligament.

Quadriceps Active Test

The quadriceps active test was described by Daniel and associates[55] as a maneuver that can help clarify the resting position of the tibia in relation to the femur. The test is performed with the patient supine with the knee flexed 90 degrees and the foot resting on the table. In the normal knee or the knee with anterior cruciate ligament disruption, active quadriceps contraction against resistance in this position produces a force vector that is directed slightly posteriorly. Therefore, when the relationship of the tibia to the femur in this position is observed, there should be no anterior translation during the test. In contrast, when the PCL is disrupted, the tibia assumes a resting position that is relatively posterior to its normal position. The force vector of the quadriceps active test is directed slightly anteriorly and produces anterior tibial translation with active quadriceps contraction against resistance. This test can be useful for assessing the knee for PCL injury.

External Rotation Recurvatum Test

The external rotation recurvatum test as described by Hughston and associates[1,56] is performed by placing the patient in the supine position, suspending the lower extremity in extension, and grasping the great toe. A positive result is produced when the knee falls into varus hyperextension and tibial external rotation. Hughston and associates stated that this test is specific for injury to the arcuate ligament complex (lateral collateral ligament, arcuate ligament, popliteus, lateral gastrocnemius). Other authors have criticized this test for not being sensitive enough to injury to the posterolateral corner. This criticism is based on the belief that for this test to give a positive result, there must also be injury to the anterior cruciate ligament and possibly even the PCL (Fig. 16). This is based on the study of Girgis and associates,[10] which showed that the PCL is a check against extreme hyperextension only after the anterior cruciate ligament has been severed.

It has been our experience that this test may give mildly positive results with isolated injury to the posterolateral corner, especially in the knee with physiologic varus alignment. However, when excessive hyperextension and varus are present on the external rotation recurvatum test, we believe that this is evidence of anterior cruciate ligament injury and possibly PCL injury as well.

Posterolateral Drawer Test

The posterolateral drawer test is an attempt to assess the integrity of the posterolateral structures by performing a posterior drawer test with the knee flexed 80 degrees and the foot externally rotated 15 degrees. Hughston and Norwood[56] considered the findings positive when the lateral tibial plateau moves posteriorly on the femoral condyle during the push phase of the test. In contrast, the medial plateau does not move. When asymmetric, this is considered evidence of pathologic external rotation of the tibia. Although posterior tibial translation occurs, Hughston and Norwood[56] believed that the PCL is not injured. In fact, more recent studies have demonstrated that the PCL is a major re-

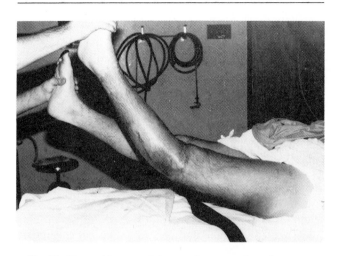

Fig. 16   Knee with severe injury to the posterolateral structures, complete anterior cruciate ligament and PCL disruption. This marked degree of external rotation recurvatum is evidence of anterior cruciate ligament and possibly PCL disruption in addition to the posterolateral disruption.

straint to external rotation at 90 degrees of flexion. When the posterolateral structures are sectioned, external rotation increases approximately 5 degrees at 90 degrees of flexion. When the PCL is subsequently sectioned, external rotation at 90 degrees of flexion increases another 15 degrees. This is good evidence that if the findings are grossly positive, then there is probably damage to the PCL. Because this examination is very difficult to quantitate, it relies on subjective interpretation. With the knee flexed 80 degrees, there is no tension in the lateral collateral ligament, and, thus, there is a degree of physiologic laxity of the lateral compartment. This allows the tibia to rotate externally as a posterior force is applied during this test. The studies of Gollehon and associates[28] and Grood and associates[30] demonstrated this normal coupled external rotation with posterior translation (Fig. 12). In the normal knee, the endpoint to posterior translation is always firm. However, the endpoint to this external rotation is not always firm and is quite variable. Heavy reliance on comparison with the contralateral knee is necessary with this examination.

Tibial External Rotation

When assessing the knee for injury to the posterolateral structures, we assess external rotation of the tibia on the femur at both 30 degrees and 90 degrees of knee flexion. We use the medial border of the foot in its neutral position as a reference point for external rotation. With the knee stabilized at the desired degree of flexion, the foot is externally rotated forcefully. The degree of external rotation of the medial border of the foot relative to the axis of the femur is assessed and compared with the contralateral side. This assessment can be performed with the patient in the supine position, but is somewhat easier with the patient in the prone position.

It is important to point out that the degrees of external rotation of the tibia on the femur, reported in selected cutting studies, are direct measurements of the bony structures and their relationship. However, the clinician is faced with having to assess this external rotation without invasive techniques. Jacobsen[57] found that this measurement of external rotation using the medial border of the foot correlates with knee rotation at a ratio of 3:1. Therefore, in quantitative terms, external rotation measurements using this method are roughly three times the actual amount of tibial rotation at the knee. Mobility of the hindfoot, midfoot, tibiotalar joint, and the bimalleolar axes can all affect this measurement. However, because these factors all affect the clinical assessment, it is important to know the normal parameters of these measurements. Just as in assessing posterior translation, it is important when examining the knee for excessive external rotation to palpate each tibial plateau to determine its relative position to the femoral condyles. Without this assessment it is difficult to distinguish whether the increase in external rotation is caused by posterolateral instability or anteromedial instability.

There is great variability in the degree of maximal external rotation, both at 30 and at 90 degrees of flexion. This lends strong support to the concept of comparison with the normal contralateral side. In examining 100 normal knees with the patients under anesthesia, we found that external rotation using this method averages 29 degrees at 30 degrees of flexion and that the normal range is 10 to 45 degrees.[58] External rotation averages 37 degrees at 90 degrees of flexion with a range of 15 to 70 degrees. There was no significant difference between men and women. External rotation, both at 30 and at 90 degrees, correlated directly with the degree of ligamentous laxity. Therefore, with this examination technique, external rotation at 90 degrees is expected to be slightly greater than that found at 30 degrees.[14,28,30,58] In addition, the normal amount of external rotation varies widely. Patients with ligamentous laxity should be expected to have more external rotation. Knowledge of these findings, as well as comparison with the normal contralateral knee, aids the clinician in accurately assessing the integrity of the posterolateral structures of the knee.

Reversed Pivot Shift

The reversed pivot shift, described by Jakob and associates,[59] is elicited by bringing the knee from a position of 90 degrees of flexion to the fully extended position under a valgus load and with the foot externally rotated. There has been considerable debate regarding the significance of the reversed pivot shift test. Most have considered a positive finding to be indicative of posterolateral injury, and others have even suggested

that PCL injury was necessary to produce a positive reversed pivot shift. However, Jakob and associates[59] reported that this test gave grossly positive results in 3% and mildly positive results in 8% of normal knees in military recruits examined. This report has not received proper attention.

It has been our experience in examining normal knees that as many as 35% have a positive reversed pivot shift phenomenon.[58] This finding directly correlates with ligamentous laxity. This common finding was at first a surprise because the internal rotation of the tibia and concomitant reduction sensation that are found as the knee is extended fully were not consistent with the traditional concept of the screw-home mechanism.[14] It has traditionally been believed that the screw-home mechanism of the knee represents an obligatory tibial external rotation as the knee reaches terminal extension. However, Grood and associates[30] demonstrated that this concept is not completely valid. If the tibia is in either internal or neutral rotation as the knee is extended, then it externally rotates near terminal extension. In contrast, when the tibia is positioned in forced external rotation, there is a coupled internal tibial rotation of nearly 14 degrees as the knee is extended fully.[30] Interestingly, this is the exact position of the tibia in performing the reverse pivot shift test. These findings certainly help to explain the common finding of a positive reversed pivot shift phenomenon in the normal knee when this maneuver is used.

It is important to realize that the reversed pivot shift maneuver may only be a normal variant, rather than a specific test for posterolateral instability. Certainly, any asymmetry is significant. However, finding a reversed pivot shift phenomenon in a knee is not necessarily indicative of posterolateral ligament injury. As stated by the originator of the examination, "the occurrence of a reversed pivot shift is, therefore, only of clinical significance if the sign is observed in one knee only, if the maneuver is painful and reproduces the patient's symptoms, if there are other signs of posterolateral instability and there's appropriate history of trauma."[59]

Voluntary Instability

In addition to ligament stress testing and these examination maneuvers, it may be helpful to ask the patient whether or not he or she is able to reproduce the pattern of instability. At times, patients with posterolateral instability may be able to evoke their instability pattern voluntarily. We have encountered several patients who were able to produce a large reversed pivot shift voluntarily. Shino and associates[60] also observed this and documented the pattern of muscle firing that enables the patient to produce the instability. The biceps appears to be active in the subluxation phase and the popliteus active in the reduction phase.

Limb Alignment

It is important to emphasize that the patient's physiologic limb alignment may affect the degree to which injury to the posterolateral corner of the knee creates disability symptoms. It is normal during the stance phase of gait to have an adduction moment about the knee, even when there is valgus anatomic limb alignment. For patients with varus morphotype knee alignment, this adduction moment may be much greater than in the average person with slight valgus limb alignment. This adduction moment may contribute to the severity of symptoms of posterolateral instability. In addition, varus limb alignment may adversely affect the success of surgical repair or reconstruction of the ligaments of the posterolateral corner of the knee.

Instrumented Testing

Instrumented knee stability testing may be helpful in documenting disruption of the PCL or posterolateral structures. The direction of tibial translation may be determined with an active drawer test at 90 degrees. Anteroposterior translation may also be assessed in full extension and at 30 degrees. In general, the results of instrumented laxity systems are reproducible. However, the exact numerical data are not interchangeable between different systems.

The Genucom system initially offered the promise of accurate noninvasive quantification of external rotation of the tibia, which would be useful in evaluating the knee with posterolateral instability. However, it has been our observation that this system has not given reproducible assessments of external rotation that correlate well with the clinical findings. At present, only anterior and posterior displacements can be determined with instrumented testing.

Radiographic Evaluation

In evaluating the acutely injured knee, plain radiographs may demonstrate evidence of PCL or posterolateral disruption. Posterior translation, sag on the lateral radiograph, or an avulsion off the tibia may signal PCL disruption (Fig. 17). Fibular head avulsion or avulsion of Gerdy's tubercle are evidence of severe lateral or posterolateral disruption (Fig. 18).[45,61] These signs should be distinguished from the lateral capsular sign (Segond's fracture), which is associated with anterior cruciate ligament injury.[62]

In the past, the use of anterior or posterior stress views and varus stress views was not uncommon. However, our experience has been that the clinical examination is usually sufficient to detect this translation and that these stress views are not necessary.

In the knee with chronic PCL deficiency, evidence of patellofemoral arthritis or medial compartment arthritis may be seen. Lateral compartment arthritis is

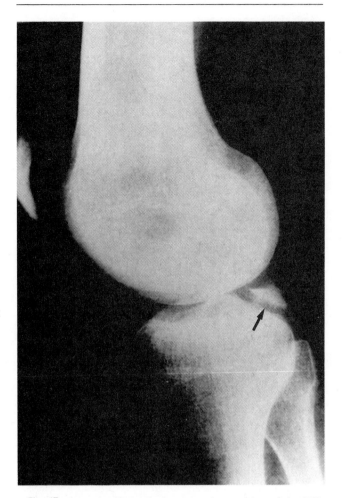

Fig. 17 Lateral radiograph demonstrating avulsion of the PCL from the tibia (arrow).

less common in general, but has a higher incidence when there is marked posterior translation leading to tricompartmental arthritis. Pain may be a predominant symptom in the knee with PCL insufficiency, and a technetium bone scan may be useful in detecting early evidence of osteoarthritis. In addition, a standing anteroposterior or standing 40-degree flexion posteroanterior radiograph can be useful in evaluating early tibiofemoral arthritis.

Magnetic resonance imaging has recently become more widely available as a useful tool in assessing knee ligament injuries. With improved techniques, excellent visualization of intra-articular structures is obtained. The PCL in the normal knee appears as a signal void (black) on magnetic resonance imaging scans. It usually appears somewhat more black than the anterior cruciate ligament, perhaps because of its increased relative thickness and the resultant effect on the appearance of the averaged scan (Fig. 19). In the event of acute injury, the signal increases in the PCL. It commonly appears swollen, and a diffuse or localized increased signal may represent injury. Because the PCL is enclosed within a

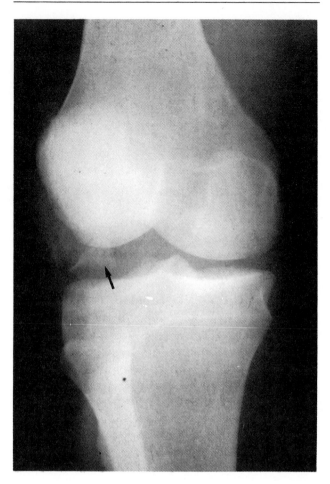

Fig. 18 Anteroposterior radiograph demonstrating avulsion of the fibular head (arrow). This is evidence of severe posterolateral disruption.

synovial sheath, it may have better healing potential than the anterior cruciate ligament.

Chronic Symptoms

Pain is usually the predominant feature of the patient's symptoms.[5,6,9,40,63] Dandy and Pusey[6] reported that 70% of patients complained of pain at a seven-year follow-up examination. Patellofemoral symptoms, also common, were found in 40% to 55%.[5,6,9,40,63]

In addition, patients with chronic PCL insufficiency usually complain of a different type of giving-way than those with anterior cruciate ligament insufficiency. The knee seems to give way because of pain or a sensation of sliding rather than a true buckling sensation such as the pivot shift phenomenon. The patients often complain of a sensation of looseness in the knee and many have difficulty descending stairs.

The symptoms of isolated, acute PCL disruption may require months to resolve completely. Symptoms tend

to be more pronounced if there is a combined injury.[9] There is controversy as to whether or not symptoms are related to the degree of posterior translation.[5,6,38,40] Several long-term reports have demonstrated that there is no statistical correlation of severity of symptoms with degree of posterior translation.[5] It must be remembered that posterior translation exceeding 15 mm represents incompetency of the secondary restraints (posterolateral structures) as well.[28] Most authors report that the ability to return to full function correlates directly with quadriceps strength.[4,7] We believe that severity of symptoms probably reflects a combination of the degree of translation, quadriceps strength, and activity level. Most athletes with isolated PCL injuries are able to return to full participation in sports.[4,5,7,8,40]

Patients with chronic posterolateral instability demonstrate varus and hyperextension in the stance phase of gait.[46] A visible thrust may be present during this phase. Formal gait analysis and standing full-length lower-extremity radiographs may be useful in detecting the abnormal alignment and mechanics. These patients often complain of a sensation of looseness and may also have episodes of giving-way. Many also complain of pain and fatigue caused by ligamentous laxity. Because many patients are unable to lock the knee in full extension, they experience difficulty with ascending and descending stairs or slopes.[46] Twisting or cutting activities may also be difficult.

Treatment

Although it is not our purpose to discuss the historical aspects and current treatment options for PCL and posterolateral knee injuries, we have developed the following guidelines, which are based on the biomechanical, anatomic, and functional data presented.

PCL Instability

In general, we prefer to avoid surgery for isolated acute PCL disruption. It has been our experience and that of others that the majority of these knees return to almost normal function. In addition, the literature indicates that many of the surgical reconstructions for PCL injuries have not proven to be reliable.[35,37,51,58,63-77] Although current reconstruction and rehabilitation techniques are better, it remains to be proven whether or not surgery is indicated solely to prevent the possible occurrence of degenerative changes after PCL injury.

In contrast to this nonsurgical approach for isolated injuries, it is our policy for combined injuries to recommend acute repair, augmentation, or reconstruction as necessary.[78,79] This is because of the well documented poorer outcome for untreated combined injury.[9,40,42]

Because of more successful treatment results, many authors have recommended primary repair with or

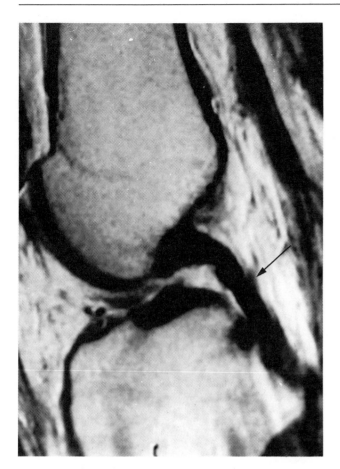 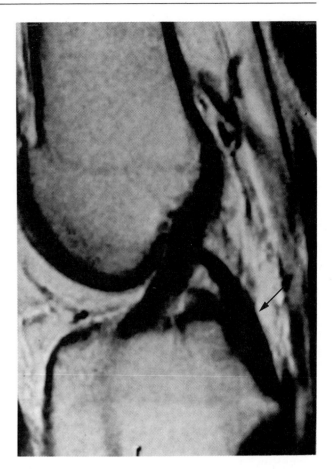

Fig. 19 Magnetic resonance images of the PCL (arrows). The proximal **(left)** and distal **(right)** portions are seen in serial images in this knee.

without augmentation for isolated PCL injuries that involve avulsion with a bony fragment.[53,68,70,74–76,80] However, with the recent reports of good function after nonsurgical treatment of PCL injuries, we have adopted a less aggressive approach to these injuries. If the lesion is truly isolated and posterior translation is less than 10 mm, then we recommend avoiding surgery. Surgery is recommended for these avulsions if there is a combined injury or excessive posterior translation (>15 mm).

For knees with chronic isolated PCL deficiency, quadriceps strengthening and nonsurgical treatment are the general rule. For those who are able to wear high-heeled shoes (boots), the higher heel can make the quadriceps more active during the stance phase of gait and can help to diminish symptoms.

When quadriceps strengthening for PCL deficiency is implemented, distal placement of the resistance pad is ideal because of the anteriorly directed vector of force during quadriceps resistance exercises. Jurist and Otis[81] demonstrated that when the resistance pad is placed at the midleg or distal leg, an anterior force vector causes anterior tibial translation on the femur.

In contrast, proximal pad placement causes a posteriorly directed force during quadriceps resistance exercises and is probably best avoided when rehabilitating the knee with PCL injury. Avoiding proximal pad placement eliminates increases in posterior tibial translation and gives the PCL the optimal situation in which to avoid stressing the PCL and secondary restraints. This pad placement is the opposite of that used for rehabilitation of the anterior cruciate ligament.

Indications for surgery for chronic PCL instability include more than 10 to 15 mm of posterior tibial translation with limiting symptoms that have failed to respond to adequate conservative treatment or evidence of early degenerative changes (cartilage wear, "hot" bone scan) in the symptomatic knee. In general, moderate to severe osteoarthritis is too advanced to gain much benefit from ligament reconstruction. However, if the instability is the major component of the patient's symptoms, ligament reconstruction may relieve these symptoms, although it probably will not affect the arthritic changes. This scenario is more common in knees with anterior cruciate ligament deficiency, and we have encountered relatively few knees with moderate to severe degenerative changes subsequent to isolated PCL injury.

Posterolateral Instability

Our experience supports the findings of others that the treatment of acute posterolateral instability is generally more successful than that of chronic posterolateral instability.[20,45,46] Acute posterolateral instability is not common as a completely isolated finding. More often, it is combined with cruciate ligament injury.[20] We consider a 10- degree difference in external rotation at 30 degrees of flexion to be good evidence of significant posterolateral injury requiring repair. In addition, asymmetry of varus angulation at 30 degrees of knee flexion is a good indicator of posterolateral injury. We believe that it is important to address all components of instability at the time of surgery in order to provide the best opportunity for success. In a review of the results of anterior cruciate ligament reconstruction using the patellar tendon, O'Brien and associates[82] noted that, at the time of follow-up, the only failures demonstrated some element of posterolateral instability.

In dealing with chronic posterolateral instability, we would recommend delayed surgical reconstruction of the ligaments if there is varus alignment and a lateral thrust in the stance phase of gait. A valgus proximal tibial osteotomy is necessary to correct the varus alignment and, therefore, to protect the ligament reconstruction.

Summary

Injuries to the PCL and posterolateral structures of the knee are much less common than anterior cruciate ligament injuries. The physical findings may be subtle and the complex nature of combined instability patterns may confuse the clinical picture. However, the treating physician must have a clear understanding of the mechanism of injury, instability patterns, and resultant disability produced by injury to these structures. It is only through a thorough review of the detailed biomechanical studies that a truly clear understanding of the role of these structures in stability of the knee can be obtained. This knowledge lays the foundation for the physical examination of these injuries. Accurate diagnosis and appropriate treatment can limit the disability that may accompany these instability patterns when they are undetected or untreated.

References

1. Hughston JC, Andrews JR, Cross MJ, et al: Classification of knee ligament instabilities: Part I. The medial compartment and cruciate ligaments. *J Bone Joint Surg* 1976;58A:159–172.
2. Hughston JC, Andrews JR, Cross MJ, et al: Classification of knee ligament instabilities: Part II. The lateral compartment. *J Bone Joint Surg* 1976;58A:173–179.
3. Kennedy JC, Grainger RW: The posterior cruciate ligament. *J Trauma* 1967;7:367–377.
4. Cain TE, Schwab GH: Performance of an athlete with straight posterior knee instability. *Am J Sports Med* 1981;9:203–208.
5. Cross MJ, Powell JF: Long-term followup of posterior cruciate ligament rupture: A study of 116 cases. *Am J Sports Med* 1984;12:292–297.
6. Dandy DJ, Pusey RJ: The long-term results of unrepaired tears of the posterior cruciate ligament. *J Bone Joint Surg* 1982;64B:92–94.
7. Fowler PJ, Messieh SS: Isolated posterior cruciate ligament injuries in athletes. *Am J Sports Med* 1987;15:553–557.
8. Parolie JM, Bergfeld JA: Long-term results of nonoperative treatment of isolated posterior cruciate ligament injuries in the athlete. *Am J Sports Med* 1986;14:35–38.
9. Satku K, Chew CN, Seow H: Posterior cruciate ligament injuries. *Acta Orthop Scand* 1984;55:26–29.
10. Girgis FG, Marshall JL, Al Monajem ARS: The cruciate ligaments of the knee joint: Anatomical, functional and experimental analysis. *Clin Orthop* 1975;106:216–231.
11. Van Dommelen BA, Fowler PJ: Anatomy of the posterior cruciate ligament: A review. *Am J Sports Med* 1989;17:24–29.
12. Warren R, Arnoczky SP, Wickiewicz TL: Anatomy of the knee, in Nicholas JA, Hershman EB (eds): *The Lower Extremity and Spine in Sports Medicine.* St. Louis, CV Mosby, 1986, vol 1, pp 657–694.
13. Butler DL, Noyes FR, Grood ES: Ligamentous restraints to anterior-posterior drawer in the human knee: A biomechanical study. *J Bone Joint Surg* 1980;62A:259–270.
14. Brantigan OC, Voshell AF: The mechanics of the ligaments and menisci of the knee joint. *J Bone Joint Surg* 1941;23:44–66.
15. Heller L, Langman J: The menisco-femoral ligaments of the human knee. *J Bone Joint Surg* 1964;46B:307–313.
16. Kaplan EB: Some aspects of functional anatomy of the human knee joint. *Clin Orthop* 1962;23:18–29.
17. Welsh RP: Knee joint structure and function. *Clin Orthop* 1980;147:7–14.
18. Grood ES, Hefzy MS, Lindenfield TN: Factors affecting the region of most isometric femoral attachments: Part I. The posterior cruciate ligament. *Am J Sport Med* 1989;17:197–207.
19. Kaplan EB: The fabellofibular and short lateral ligaments of the knee joint. *J Bone Joint Surg* 1961;43A:169–179.
20. Baker CL Jr, Norwood LA, Hughston JC: Acute posterolateral rotatory instability of the knee. *J Bone Joint Surg* 1983;65A:614–618.
21. Seebacher JR, Inglis AE, Marshall JL, et al: The structure of the posterolateral aspect of the knee. *J Bone Joint Surg* 1982;64A:536–541.
22. Terry GC, Hughston JC, Norwood LA: The anatomy of the iliopatellar band and iliotibial tract. *Am J Sports Med* 1986;14:39–45.
23. Marshall JL, Girgis FG, Zelko RR: The biceps femoris tendon and its functional significance. *J Bone Joint Surg* 1972;54A:1444–1450.
24. Southmayd W, Quigley TB: The forgotten popliteus muscle: Its usefulness in correction of anteromedial rotatory instability of the knee. A preliminary report. *Clin Orthop* 1978;130:218–222.
25. Last RJ: Some anatomical details of the knee joint. *J Bone Joint Surg* 1948;30B:683–688.
26. Last RJ: The popliteus muscle and the lateral meniscus: With a note on the attachment of the medial meniscus. *J Bone Joint Surg* 1950;32B:93–99.
27. Tria AJ Jr, Johnson CD, Zawadsky JP: The popliteus tendon. *J Bone Joint Surg* 1989;71A:714–716.
28. Gollehon DL, Torzilli PA, Warren RF: The role of the posterolateral and cruciate ligaments in the stability of the human knee: A biomechanical study. *J Bone Joint Surg* 1987;69A:233–242.

29. Grood ES, Noyes FR, Butler DL, et al: Ligamentous and capsular restraints preventing straight medial and lateral laxity in intact human cadaver knees. *J Bone Joint Surg* 1981;63A:1257–1269.

30. Grood ES, Stowers SF, Noyes FR: Limits of movement in the human knee: Effect of sectioning the posterior cruciate ligament and posterolateral structures. *J Bone Joint Surg* 1988;70A:88–97.

31. Markolf KL, Mensch JS, Amstutz HC: Stiffness and laxity of the knee: The contributions of the supporting structures. A quantitative in vitro study. *J Bone Joint Surg* 1976;58A:583–594.

32. Noyes FR, Grood ES, Butler DL, et al: Clinical laxity tests and functional stability of the Knee: Biomechanical concepts. *Clin Orthop* 1980;146:84–89.

33. Sullivan D, Levy IM, Sheskier S, et al: Medial restraints to anterior-posterior motion of the knee. *J Bone Joint Surg* 1984;66A:930–936.

34. Kennedy JC, Hawkins RJ, Willis RB, et al: Tension studies of human knee ligament: Yield point, ultimate failure, and disruption of the cruciate and tibial collateral ligaments. *J Bone Joint Surg* 1976;58A:350–355.

35. Hughston JC, Bowden JA, Andrews JR, et al: Acute tears of the posterior cruciate ligament: Results of operative treatment. *J Bone Joint Surg* 1980;62A:438–450.

36. Clancy WG Jr, Shelbourne KD, Zoellner GB et al: Treatment of knee joint instability secondary to rupture of the posterior cruciate ligament: Report of a new procedure. *J Bone Joint Surg* 1983;65A:310–322.

37. Fleming RE Jr, Blatz DJ, McCarroll JR: Posterior problems in the knee: Posterior cruciate insufficiency and posterolateral rotatory insufficiency. *Am J Sports Med* 1981;9:107–113.

38. Tibone JE, Antich TJ, Perry J, et al: Functional analysis of untreated and reconstructed posterior cruciate ligament injuries. *Am J Sports Med* 1988;16:217–223.

39. Pournaras J, Symeonides PP, Karkavelas G: The significance of the posterior cruciate ligament in the stability of the knee: An experimental study in dogs. *J Bone Joint Surg* 1983;65B:204–209.

40. Torg JS, Barton TM, Pavlov H, et al: Natural history of the posterior cruciate ligament-deficient knee. *Clin Orthop* 1989;246:208–216.

41. Skyhar MJ, Schwartz E, Warren RF, et al: The effects of posterior cruciate ligament and posterolateral complex laxity on articular contact pressures within the knee. Presented at the 56th Annual Meeting of the American Academy of Orthopaedic Surgeons, Las Vegas, Feb 9–14, 1989.

42. O'Donoghue DH: An analysis of end results of surgical treatment of major injuries to the ligaments of the knee. *J Bone Joint Surg* 1955;37A:1–13.

43. Clendenin MB, Delee JC, Heckman JD: Interstitial tears of the posterior cruciate ligament of the knee. *Orthopedics* 1980;3:764–772.

44. Savatsky GJ, Marshall JL, Warren RF, et al: Posterior cruciate ligament injury. Presented at the 47th Annual Meeting of the American Academy of Orthopaedic Surgeons, Atlanta, Feb 7–12, 1980.

45. DeLee JC, Riley MB, Rockwood CA Jr: Acute posterolateral rotatory instability of the knee. *Am J Sports Med* 1983;11:199–207.

46. Hughston JC, Jacobson KE: Chronic posterolateral rotatory instability of the knee. *J Bone Joint Surg* 1985;67A:351–359.

47. DeLee JC, Riley MB, Rockwood CA Jr: Acute straight lateral instability of the knee. *Am J Sports Med* 1983;11:404–411.

48. Grana WA, Janssen T: Lateral ligament injury of the knee. *Orthopedics* 1987;10:1039–1044.

49. Jobe FW: Acute tears of the lateral complex, in American Academy of Orthopaedic Surgeons *Symposium on the Athlete's Knee: Surgical Repair and Reconstruction.* St. Louis, CV Mosby, 1980, pp 164–172.

50. Kannus P: Nonoperative treatment of grade II and III sprains of the lateral ligament compartment of the knee. *Am J Sports Med* 1989;17:83–88.

51. Loos WC, Fox JM, Blazina ME, et al: Acute posterior cruciate ligament injuries. *Am J Sports Med* 1981;9:86–92.

52. Towne LC, Blazina ME, Marmor L, et al: Lateral compartment syndrome of the knee. *Clin Orthop* 1971;76:160–168.

53. Trickey EL: Rupture of the posterior cruciate ligament of the knee. *J Bone Joint Surg* 1968;50B:334–341.

54. Hughston JC: The absent posterior drawer test in some acute posterior cruciate ligament tears of the knee. *Am J Sports Med* 1988;16:39–43.

55. Daniel DM, Stone ML, Barnett P, et al: Use of the quadriceps active test to diagnose posterior cruciate-ligament disruption and measure posterior laxity of the knee. *J Bone Joint Surg* 1988;70A:386–391.

56. Hughston JC, Norwood LA Jr: The posterolateral drawer test and external rotational recurvatum test for posterolateral rotatory instability of the knee. *Clin Orthop* 1980;147:82–87.

57. Jacobsen K: Gonylaxometry: Stress radiographic measurement of passive stability in the knee joints of normal subjects and patients with ligament injuries: Accuracy and range of application. *Acta Orthop Scand* 1981;52(suppl):1–263.

58. Cooper DE: Examination under anesthesia for posterolateral instability. Presented at the 57th Annual Meeting of the American Academy of Orthopaedic Surgeons, New Orleans, Feb 8–13, 1990.

59. Jakob RP, Hassler H, Staeubli HU: Observations on rotatory instability of the lateral compartment of the knee: Experimental studies on the functional anatomy and the pathomechanism of the true and the reversed pivot shift sign. *Acta Orthop Scand* 1981; 52(suppl):1–32.

60. Shino K, Horibe S, Ono K: The voluntarily evoked posterolateral drawer sign in the knee with posterolateral instability. *Clin Orthop* 1987;215:179–186.

61. Jones RW: Styloid process of the fibula in the knee joint with peroneal palsy. *J Bone Joint Surg* 1931;13:258–260.

62. Woods GW, Stanley RF, Tullos HS: Lateral capsular sign: X-ray clue to a significant knee instability. *Am J Sports Med* 1979;7:27–33.

63. Hughston JC, Degenhardt TC: Reconstruction of the posterior cruciate ligament. *Clin Orthop* 1982;164:59–77.

64. Bianchi M: Acute tears of the posterior cruciate ligament: Clinical study and results of operative treatment in 27 cases. *Am J Sports Med* 1983;11:308–314.

65. Eriksson E, Häggmark T, Johnson RJ: Reconstruction of the posterior cruciate ligament. *Orthopedics* 1986;8:217–220.

66. Insall JN, Hood RW: Bone-block transfer of the medial head of the gastrocnemius for posterior cruciate insufficiency. *J Bone Joint Surg* 1982;64A:691–699.

67. Kennedy JC, Galpin RD: The use of the medial head of the gastrocnemius muscle in the posterior cruciate-deficient knee: Indications—technique—results. *Am J Sports Med* 1982;10:63–74.

68. Mayer PJ, Micheli LJ: Avulsion of the femoral attachment of the posterior cruciate ligament in an eleven-year-old boy: Case report. *J Bone Joint Surg* 1979;61A:431–432.

69. McCormick WC, Bagg RJ, Kennedy CW Jr, et al: Reconstruction of the posterior cruciate ligament: Preliminary report of a new procedure. *Clin Orthop* 1976;118:30–31.

70. Meyers MH: Isolated avulsion of the tibial attachment of the posterior cruciate ligament of the knee. *J Bone Joint Surg* 1975; 57A:669–672.

71. Moore HA, Larson RL: Posterior cruciate ligament injuries: Results of early surgical repair. *Am J Sports Med* 1980;8:68–78.

72. Roth JH, Bray RC, Best TM, et al: Posterior cruciate ligament reconstruction by transfer of the medial gastrocnemius tendon. *Am J Sports Med* 1988;16:21–28.

73. Southmayd WW, Rubin BD: Reconstruction of the posterior cruciate ligament using the semimembranosus tendon. *Clin Orthop* 1980;150:196–197

74. Torisu T: Isolated avulsion fracture of the tibial attachment of the posterior cruciate ligament. *J Bone Joint Surg* 1977;59A:68–72.

75. Torisu T: Avulsion fracture of the tibial attachment of the posterior cruciate ligament: Indications and results of delayed repair. *Clin Orthop* 1979;143:107–114.

76. Trickey EL: Injuries to the posterior cruciate ligament: Diagnosis and treatment of early injuries and reconstruction of late instability. *Clin Orthop* 1980;147:76–81.

77. Wirth CJ, Jager M: Dynamic double tendon replacement of the posterior cruciate ligament. *Am J Sports Med* 1984;12:39–43.

78. Levy IM, Riederman R, Warren RF: An anteromedial approach to the posterior cruciate ligament. *Clin Orthop* 1984;190:174–181.

79. Strand T, Mølster AO, Engesaeter LB, et al: Primary repair in posterior cruciate ligament injuries. *Acta Orthop Scand* 1984;55:545–547.

80. Sanders WE, Wilkins KE, Neidre A: Acute insufficiency of the posterior cruciate ligament in children: Two case reports. *J Bone Joint Surg* 1980;62A:129–131.

81. Jurist KA, Otis JC: Anteroposterior tibiofemoral displacements during isometric extension efforts: The roles of external load and knee flexion angle. *Am J Sports Med* 1985;13:254–258.

82. O'Brien SJ, Warren RF, Wickiewicz TL, et al: Reconstruction of the chronically insufficient anterior cruciate ligament using the central third of the patellar ligament. *J Bone Joint Surg* 1990:72A:in press.

Myelomeningocele

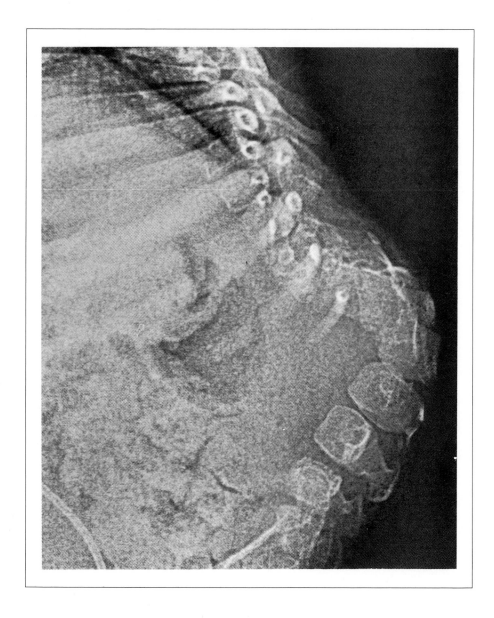

CHAPTER 33

Spine Deformity in Myelomeningocele

Richard E. Lindseth, MD

Introduction

Deformity of the spine occurs so frequently in myelomeningocele that it can be considered part of the disease process.[1-3] The deformity often causes severe disability, thwarting attempts at rehabilitation and negating previous treatment to maintain ambulation.[4] It is rare for a patient with myelomeningocele to reach adulthood without some treatment of the spine. Unfortunately, treatment is very difficult and is associated with frequent complications. In many cases, the surgery performed is not extensive enough or is not done early enough to be effective.

Three main types of spine deformity occur: The first is scoliosis, usually associated with severe lordosis (often the lordosis is more severe than the scoliosis). The second is kyphosis, which usually is congenital in nature and is centered at the upper lumbar spine. The third is congenital malformation of the spine secondary to a lack of segmentation or formation. The sagittal-plane deformities are often of greater significance than the frontal-plane deformities.

Scoliosis and Lordosis

Scoliosis is common, particularly in the higher levels of paraplegia. Almost 100% of patients with thoracic-level paraplegia develop scoliosis, and 85% of the curves are greater than 45 degrees. As the paralysis level drops so does the incidence of scoliosis. At the fourth lumbar level of paraplegia, the incidence of curvature decreases to about 60%, and only about 40% of patients will require surgical intervention.[5]

Several causes have been identified for the scoliosis. A collapsing C-shaped scoliosis is caused by muscle weakness associated with high-level paraplegia. This type of scoliosis can be associated with kyphosis instead of lordosis. This curve pattern occurs at a young age, often in infancy, and is always progressive.

Hydromyelia or hydrosyringomyelia associated with uncompensated hydrocephalus can also cause scoliosis.[6-8] It has been shown that reinserting a shunt improves the scoliosis if it is less than 50 degrees. The scoliosis is usually in the thoracic or thoracolumbar region. It usually is S-shaped and resembles idiopathic scoliosis in appearance. Other symptoms of hydromyelia are back pain, weakness of the upper extremities, and increasing paralysis of the legs.

Another cause of scoliosis is tethered cord syndrome, which can be associated with such intraspinal problems as dermoid tumors, lipoma, or diastematomyelia.[9-11] In my experience, the tethered cord usually causes a dorsal-lumbar or a lumbar scoliosis and a marked increase in lumbar lordosis. Other associated symptoms are increased spasticity in the legs, a higher level of paralysis, and back or leg pain. Results from release of the tethered cord are variable. In most cases, curve progression is stopped; in a few cases, it improves. If the curve is more than 50 degrees, the scoliosis should be corrected and stabilized with spine fusion at the time the tethered cord is released.

In the past, all neuromuscular curves, particularly those of myelomeningocele, were generally classified in a single category, not divided into groups according to level of curve, curve type, and etiology. For this reason, most follow-up studies of the results of spine fusion have been unable to separate the treatment according to the types of curve represented. Overall, scoliosis associated with myelomeningocele can be classified in the same way that curves in idiopathic scoliosis are. There are dorsal, dorsal-lumbar, lumbar, and double primary curves. To use one treatment program for all curves is probably as inappropriate for neuromuscular scoliosis as it is for idiopathic scoliosis. However, it is also an error to use the same guidelines for fusion and instrumentation for neuromuscular disease that are used for idiopathic scoliosis.

Treatment

The treatment of each child is individualized and depends on the level and type of curve, the level of paralysis, the age of the patient, and the patient's ambulatory status. The first step is to determine if there are neurologic causes for the scoliosis. Shunt function should be assessed and the spinal cord evaluated for the presence of hydromyelia and for tethered cord syndrome. Probably the most sophisticated diagnostic method available at present is magnetic resonance imaging of the cervical, dorsal, and lumbar spine. This will identify hydromyelia, syrinx formation, and intraspinal tumors, as well as a tethered cord. If the scoliosis continues to progress after neurologic problems have been corrected, treatment is indicated. If the child is very young, bracing can be tried.[12] However, because the bracing in paralytic scoliosis is passive, not active as it is in idiopathic scoliosis, the brace has a tendency to deform the rib cage and to produce pressure sores

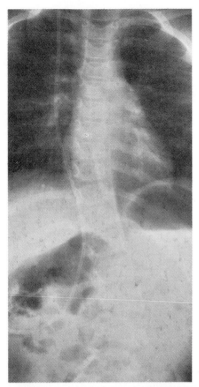
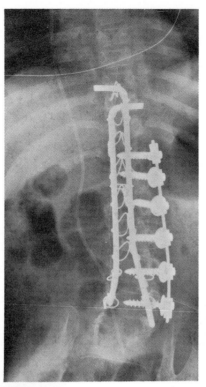
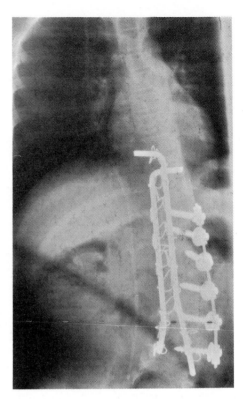

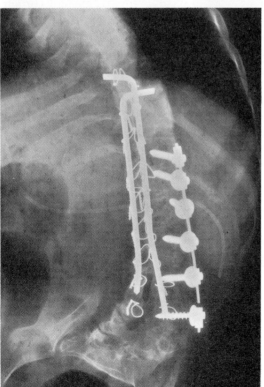

Fig. 1 This child demonstrates most of the problems found in treating scoliosis in a patient with L-4 paraplegia and spasticity caused by an unrecognized tethered cord. **Top left,** Age 5 years. This scoliosis measured 25 degrees. Spastic muscles were released about the hip. **Top center,** The curve progressed to 60 degrees, and an anterior fusion from T-11 to L-4 and a posterior fusion from T-8 to L-4 were performed. Residual pelvic obliquity was 17 degrees. **Top right,** Two years later the lumbosacral curve had increased. **Bottom left,** After a growth spurt at age 16, the curve had increased at both ends of the posterior fusion as a result of the "crankshaft phenomenon." Exploration of the spine at that time showed a solid posterior fusion from T-8 to the sacrum.

in insensate skin. In the infant, bracing produces abdominal compression, which can make it difficult for the child to breath. Although the correction obtained is usually temporary, use of a brace can buy time until about the age of 7 years, when surgery can be carried out more effectively.

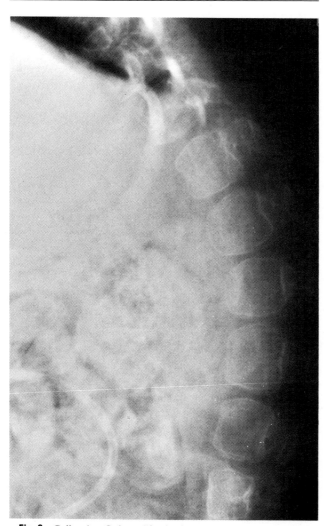

Fig. 2 Collapsing C-shaped kyphosis.

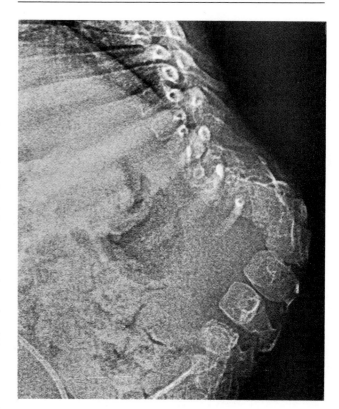

Fig. 3 S-shaped rigid kyphosis.

Most of these children will require surgical correction and spine fusion.[13] Levels of fusion depend on the age of the child, the location of the curve, the level of paralysis, and ambulatory status. It is easy for the surgeon to err in selecting the levels of spinal fusion. It is important not to fuse short. Repeat surgery for curve progression is often the result of spine fusion that ended too short, particularly in the thoracic spine. Usually the thoracic compensatory curve must be fused as well as the primary lumbar curve. Strict attention must be paid to sagittal alignment. The goal is to achieve normal kyphosis and lordosis, in addition to correcting the scoliosis. In general, the fusion should not end in the middle of a sagittal curve, which can greatly affect the sitting balance. This recommendation is similar to that made for instrumentation in idiopathic scoliosis.

Indications for extending the fusion mass to the sacrum are not well established. Lumbosacral arthrodesis is difficult to obtain, and pseudarthrosis and instrument failure are common. Attempts to correct these prob-

lems can require repeated surgical procedures, and improvement is not certain. Patients who were able to walk before surgery may be deprived of that ability by lumbosacral spine fusion.[4] For this reason, the procedure is to be avoided unless it is absolutely necessary. Also, once the lumbosacral spine has been fused, if its residual deformity is 15 degrees or more, the incidence of pressure sores will increase because of the inability of the lumbosacral joint to absorb forces associated with position changes and wheelchair mobility. On the other hand, unless the lumbar scoliosis can be corrected to less than 20 degrees and the overall pelvic obliquity to less than 15 degrees, the lumbosacral joint should be fused or it will continue to show progressive deformity. It is important to treat scoliosis vigorously and early to achieve satisfactory correction.

Most curves require both anterior and posterior fusion, particularly in the area where there is posterior arch insufficiency.[14] This area usually includes most of the lumbar spine. If fusion is carried out in children younger than 10 years of age, it is important to fuse anteriorly all parts of the spine that will be fused posteriorly. If this is not done, the curve will continue to progress as the child grows.[15] Because of the risks of such major surgery in very young children, and because of the resultant extremely short spine, I often try to stabilize the spine without spine fusion by using a Lu-

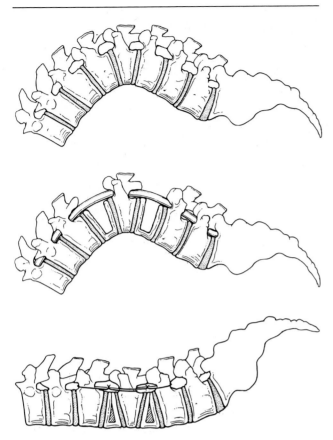

Fig. 4   Top, The C-shaped kyphosis before removal of the ossific nucleus from its vertebrae. **Center,** The spinous process, lamina, pedicle, and ossific nucleus have been removed from the vertebrae above and below the apical vertebrae. The growth plate, disk, and anterior cortex are left intact. **Bottom,** The deformity is reduced by pushing the apical vertebrae forward and tension-band wiring around the pedicles.

que rod followed by postoperative brace treatment. This approach is used when bracing alone fails to control the curve. Complications with this approach include rod breakage, wire breakage, and spontaneous fusion. To provide a definitive solution, reoperation is often necessary. In the interim, however, valuable spine growth often occurs.

The instrumentation used depends on individual preference. I prefer to use the Zielke instrumentation anteriorly, particularly in the lumbar spine, followed by Luque segmental instrumentation posteriorly. This combination gives maximum correction without the need for postoperative immobilization. Many surgeons prefer to do anterior diskectomy and fusion and use instrumentation only on the posterior spine. I find that I get better correction by combining Zielke and Luque instrumentation than I do by using posterior instrumentation alone. The newer posterior instrumentation, which uses pedicle screws, may make it possible to obtain satisfactory correction of the lumbar curve with posterior instrumentation alone, following anterior

diskectomy and bone graft. Although the advantages of newer instrumentations over the typical Harrington rod fusion for idiopathic scoliosis may be limited, I believe that they hold great promise for the child with myelomeningocele. Anterior fusion and instrumentation without posterior fusion is insufficient. An unpublished study that I performed on 50 patients, 25 with anterior fusion only and 25 with anterior and posterior fusion, showed the rates of complication, rod breakage, and pseudarthrosis to be much higher in the group with only anterior fusion.

Postoperative immobilization depends on individual preference and on the instrumentation used. In general, if there is doubt about the stability of the spine or if the lumbosacral joint is being fused, postoperative immobilization by means of a cast or polypropylene brace is indicated.

The following case illustrates most of the problems outlined above. In 1976, a 5-year-old child was discovered to have a 25-degree scoliosis. Because the legs showed increased tone when the child stood, an adductor release was performed (Fig. 1, *top left*). The possibility of a tethered cord was not considered at that time. By 1983, when the child was 12 years of age, the curve had progressed to 60 degrees in the lumbar spine. Anterior fusion with Zielke instrumentation from T-11 to L4 and posterior fusion with Luque instrumentation from T-8 to L4 were done (Fig. 1, *top center*). Despite apparent excellent correction of the curve, the child continued to have a 17-degree pelvic obliquity, which was unrecognized at the time of surgery. Two years later, there was an increase in the lumbosacral curve and an increase in pelvic obliquity (Fig. 1, *top right*). Surgery was performed on the child's spastic foot deformities, still without knowledge of the tethered cord syndrome. By 1989, after a growth spurt, the curve at the upper and lower end of the fusion had increased by means of the "crankshaft phenomenon" caused by a solid posterior fusion, confirmed at surgery, and anterior open growth plates (Fig. 1, *bottom left*).

Congenital Scoliosis

Congenital scoliosis in children with myelomeningocele does not differ significantly from congenital scoliosis in children without myelomeningocele.[16] If the curve is progressive, it should be fused anteriorly and posteriorly, even in infancy. If it is in an area below the level of paralysis, an osteotomy may be indicated to obtain maximum correction. Because developmental scoliosis can occur in addition to the congenital curves in these children, most curves must be treated as outlined in the section on scoliosis and lordosis.

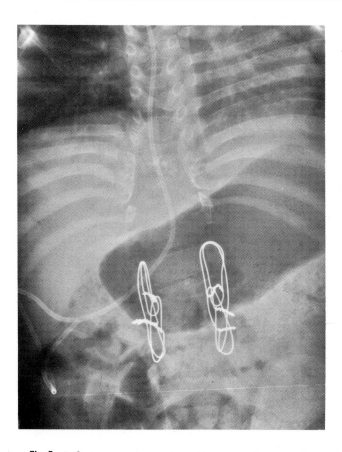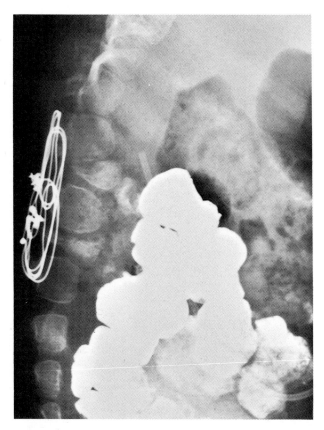

Fig. 5 **Left,** Anteroposterior view of the spine after correction and the position of the pedicle wires. **Right,** Lateral view six months after surgery shows continued correction of the deformity and rapid bone formation in the excised vertebrae.

Kyphosis

Treatment of kyphosis in myelomeningocele patients presents a number of frustrating and demanding problems. These kyphosis problems can be divided into three types. The first type is a collapsing kyphosis, often C-shaped and supple, at least during its initial early stages (Fig. 2). The apex may occur anywhere from the lower dorsal spine to the lumbosacral joint.

The second type of kyphosis is present at birth, is associated with vertebral deformity, and is usually S-shaped, with rigid lordosis at T10 followed by an acutely angled rigid kyphosis at L2 (Fig. 3). This type of kyphosis is always progressive and leads to severe deformity.

The third type of kyphosis is quite rare and is associated with a partial aplasia of the lumbar spine. It can exist in either the proximal or the distal portion of the lumbar spine and is distinguished from sacral agenesis by the presence of the sacrum. Because treatment for this third type is similar to that used for the second type, the two will be discussed together.

Kyphosis is almost always progressive. Attempts at conservative treatment usually fail. However, surgical treatment is also difficult and is often associated with complications. Any attempt to delay surgery until the child is older, to allow use of a particular form of instrumentation, can lead to disaster. The kyphosis steadily progresses, ultimately to a severe deformity, approaching 180 degrees, which is almost impossible to treat. For this reason, it is important to begin treatment early in order to obtain maximum correction.

The goal of treatment is more than just obtaining a satisfactory radiograph. It is also important to increase abdominal height to allow more room for the abdominal contents and to relieve pressure on the diaphragm and the lungs. In addition, the kyphosis must be minimized to lessen the incidence of pressure sores, and the center of gravity must be moved posteriorly to center it over the ischium, which will enable the child to sit without using his or her arms for propping. Conservative treatment, which involves observation to see if the curve gets worse, is usually futile, because the curve generally progresses quite rapidly. It is not unusual to see a 2- or 3-year-old child with a 100-degree kyphosis. Attempts to treat with the brace also tend to

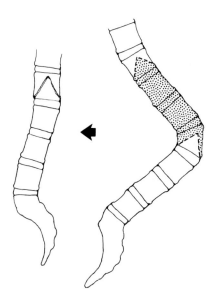

Fig. 6 The rigid S-shaped kyphosis is corrected by excising the vertebrae between the apex of the kyphosis and the lordosis and fusing the apical vertebrae. (Reproduced with permission from Lindseth RE: Myelomeningocele, in Morrissy RT (ed): *Lovell and Winters' Pediatric Orthopaedics*, ed 3. Philadelphia, JB Lippincott, 1990, p 522.)

be futile. If the curve is very small and the skin is in excellent condition, a brace can be used satisfactorily. However, any orthotic device must push over the apical vertebra posteriorly and against the protuberant abdomen anteriorly, leading to pressure sores over the gibbus and increased pressure on the abdominal contents. This pressure decreases the child's appetite and pulmonary reserve, jeopardizing survival. If a brace is tried, it is usually used temporarily as a way of delaying surgery. Kyphosis usually requires surgical correction.

Surgical Treatment of Collapsing Kyphosis

Surgical treatment depends on the type of curve and the age of the patient. Heretofore, the collapsing type of curve has been the most difficult to treat. Posterior spinal fusion without instrumentation usually led to failure because of the tension forces on the fusion mass. Attempts to provide stability by an anterior spinal fusion with a strut graft also failed in the young patient, because although the fusion created an anterior unsegmented bar, growth continued posteriorly, and with growth, the kyphosis increased. If the surgeon waits until the child is older to carry out an anterior-posterior spinal fusion with instrumentation along the dorsal-lumbar spine, the curve often becomes so severe that satisfactory correction is difficult, if not impossible, to achieve. Recently, I developed another approach that may solve the problem. The results of a 2.5-year study indicate that this approach appears to be accomplishing the desired result. It can be performed at any age,

even shortly after birth. If it is performed in an older child, posterior Luque instrumentation is advisable, because it decreases the need for postoperative immobilization.[17]

The procedure is performed posteriorly by removing the ossific nucleus from the vertebra above and the vertebra below the apical vertebra, which is left intact. The posterior elements of the vertebrae to be excised are removed with a rongeur. The surgeon then uses a curette to remove the cancellous bone from these vertebrae, using the pedicle as a conduit (Fig. 4, *top* and *center*). This procedure is similar to the eggshell procedure described by Heinig and Boyd.[18] The epiphysis of the end plate, the cortical bone at the end plate, and the cortical bone anteriorly are left intact. Cortical bone is removed laterally and posteriorly. The apical vertebra is then pushed forward, correcting the kyphosis. Segmental wiring is then used to create a tension band between the pedicle of the apical vertebra and the vertebrae above and below the osteotomy (Fig. 4, *bottom*). A posterior spinal fusion can be done at this time. Because the anterior growth centers are left, further growth of the spine tends to continue the correction, producing a gradual lordosis. Approximately 100 degrees of kyphosis can be corrected in this fashion. After surgery, the immature child is kept in a body jacket for a period of one year. Initially, the child is maintained in a supine, prone, or lateral position. The head can be elevated to a level of 60 degrees as long as the weight of the child is pushing backward to avoid undue stress on the wires. After one month, the child is allowed to sit up in the jacket. Bone forms rapidly in the ossific nucleus in the area of resected vertebrae and can stabilize very quickly (Fig. 5). The surgeon may be tempted to use Luque instrumentation posteriorly in the young child to provide more complete stabilization of the osteotomies. However, if the spine is fused for the length of the instrumentation, the lumbar spine will not grow, and this area will not be long enough to allow adequate room for the abdominal contents. In the older child, however, use of posterior instrumentation is appropriate.

Surgical Treatment of Rigid Kyphosis

Treatment of the rigid form of kyphosis requires a different approach. Because both the kyphosis and the proximal lordosis are rigid, it is necessary to correct both deformities. In this situation, the vertebrae between the kyphosis and lordosis, usually two in number, are excised.[19] The apical vertebra is then fused to the distal end of the thoracic spine at the level of the resection (Fig. 6).[5] In a young child, only this area is fused, and the osteotomy is held in position by tension-band wiring around the pedicle. It is also important that the paraspinous muscles be sutured behind this area of the spine to add a corrective force. In an older child, instrumentation can be used to maximize correction and stability.[8] When this procedure was performed in children under the age of 5 years, the residual kyphosis was rarely progressive. After long-term follow-up, additional surgery was necessary in only two of 25 cases. In both patients who required additional surgery, the initial curve exceeded 120 degrees, and, because of this, the initial correction was insufficient. In children more than 5 years old at the time of surgery, progression of kyphosis is more likely. If the patient is more than 8 years old when the surgery is performed, I recommend that the spine be fused and instrumented from the dorsal to the lumbosacral spine.

Spine deformity in myelomeningocele is frequent, progressive, and disabling. Treatment almost always requires surgery. If possible, the causes of the deformity should be identified and corrected before surgical correction of the spine itself is attempted. In selecting the procedure performed and the instruments used, it is important to consider the location of the deformity, frontal and sagittal alignment, the age of the patient, and the patient's ambulatory status.

References

1. Drummond DS, Moreau M, Cruess RL: The results and complications of surgery for the paralytic hip and spine in myelomeningocele. *J Bone Joint Surg* 1980;62B:49–53.
2. Hull WJ, Moe JH, Winter RB: Spinal deformity in myelomeningocele: Natural history, evaluation and treatment, abstract. *J Bone Joint Surg* 1974;56A:1767.
3. Sriram K, Bobechko WP, Hall JE: Surgical management of spinal deformities in spina bifida. *J Bone Joint Surg* 1972;54B:666–676.
4. Mazur J, Menelaus MB, Dickens DR, et al: Efficacy of surgical management for scoliosis in myelomeningocele: Correction of deformity and alteration of functional status. *J Pediatr Orthop* 1986;6:568–575.
5. Lindseth RE: Myelomeningocele, in Morrissy RT (ed): *Lovell and Winters' Pediatric Orthopaedics*, ed 3. Philadelphia, JB Lippincott, 1990, p 522.
6. Hall PV, Campbell RL, Kalsbeck JE: Meningomyelocele and progressive hydromyelia: Progressive paresis in myelodysplasia. *J Neurosurg* 1975;43:457–463.
7. Hall PV, Lindseth RE, Campbell RL, et al: Myelodysplasia and developmental scoliosis: A manifestation of syringomyelia. *Spine* 1976;1:48–56.
8. Hall PV, Lindseth RE, Campbell RL, et al: Scoliosis and hydrocephalus in myelocele patients: The effects of ventricular shunting. *J Neurosurg* 1979;50:174–178.
9. Bunch WH, Scarff TB, Dvonch V: Progressive loss in myelomeningocele patients. *Orthop Trans* 1983;7:185.
10. Heinz ER, Rosenbaum AE, Scarff TB, et al: Tethered spinal cord following meningomyelocele repair. *Radiology* 1979;131:153–160.
11. McLaughlin TP, Banta JV, Gahm NH, et al: Intraspinal rhizotomy and distal cordectomy in patients with myelomeningocele. *J Bone Joint Surg* 1986;68A:88–94.
12. Bunch WH: The Milwaukee brace in paralytic scoliosis. *Clin Orthop* 1975;110:63–68.
13. Osebold WR, Mayfield JK, Winter RB, et al: Surgical treatment of paralytic scoliosis associated with myelomeningocele. *J Bone Joint Surg* 1982;64A:841–856.
14. McMaster MJ: Anterior and posterior instrumentation and fusion of thoracolumbar scoliosis due to myelomeningocele. *J Bone Joint Surg* 1987;69B:20–25.
15. Dubousset J, Herring JA, Shufflebarger H: The crankshaft phenomenon. *J Pediatr Orthop* 1989;9:541–550.
16. Winter RB, Moe JH, Eilers VE: Congenital scoliosis: A study of 234 patients treated and untreated. Part I: Natural history. Part II: Treatment. *J Bone Joint Surg* 1968;50A:1–47.
17. Heydemann JS, Gillespie R: Management of myelomeningocele kyphosis in the older child by kyphectomy and segmental spinal instrumentation. *Spine* 1987;12:37–41.
18. Heinig CF, Boyd BM Jr: One stage vertebrectomy or eggshell procedure. *Orthop Trans* 1985;9:130–131.
19. Lindseth RE, Stelzer L Jr: Vertebral excision for kyphosis in children with myelomeningocele. *J Bone Joint Surg* 1979;61A:699–704.

Hip Deformities in Myelomeningocele

Luciano S. Dias, MD

Introduction

Nearly one third to one half of children with myelomeningocele will, at some time during their growth, have a hip dislocation or subluxation. Hip contractures, such as abduction, adduction, external rotation, and flexion, that interfere with bracing and ambulation can also be serious problems.

In treating these deformities, the objective is to improve function and mobility. A deformity alone, with no impairment in function, should be left untreated. Treatment must be individualized.[1]

Hip Flexion Contracture

Hip flexion contracture occurs more frequently in children with myelomeningocele at the high lumbar and thoracic levels and is caused by either the unopposed action of the hip flexors (iliopsoas, sartorius, and rectus femoris) or by contractures produced when the child remains seated for prolonged periods of time. Spasticity of the hip flexors, caused by tethering of the spinal cord, is another main cause of flexion contractures and may be more common than is generally acknowledged. Hip flexion contracture and knee flexion contracture are commonly seen in association. When both are present, surgical treatment of both deformities should be done at the same time. Any deformity of more than 20 degrees can impair ambulation because maintaining an upright position produces a severe lumbar lordosis with anterior pelvic tilt, which increases the demand on the upper extremity during standing and walking. In children with high lumbar or thoracic level myelomeningocele, surgical correction is achieved by an anterior hip release with tenotomy of the sartorius, rectus femoris, iliopsoas, and tensor fascia latae and, if necessary, an anterior capsulotomy.[2]

In the child with low lumbar level myelomeningocele, it is important to preserve hip flexor power for independent ambulation. If a significant flexion contracture is present, one of two approaches is used. The first is extension osteotomy at the subtrochanteric level, preserving the hip flexor musculature. This approach is used for children older than 10 to 11 years of age because, if it is done earlier, remodeling will lead to a recurrence of the deformity. The second approach is a hip flexor release with a free tendon graft for the

sartorius (using the fascia lata) and an intramuscular lengthening of the iliopsoas tendon, above the rim.

Hip Flexion-Abduction-External Rotation Contracture

This deformity is quite common in children with myelomeningocele at the thoracic level with total paralysis of the lower-extremity muscles. When the deformity interferes with bracing, a radical hip release, including division of all the hip flexors, abductors, and external rotators, and an extensive capsulotomy, can correct the deformity.

Hip Abduction Contracture

Unilateral hip abduction contracture is a common cause of pelvic obliquity leading to scoliosis. It is generally secondary to a contracture of the iliotibial band and tensor fascia lata. Surgical correction is achieved by dividing the tensor fascia lata proximally and, if necessary, by releasing the iliotibial band distally (the Ober-Yount procedure).[3,4]

Adduction Contracture

Adduction contracture is frequently seen in association with hip subluxation and dislocation. Unilateral adduction contracture can cause pelvic obliquity. Adductor myotomy, through a transverse inguinal incision, should restore abduction to at least 45 to 60 degrees. On occasion, a valgus subtrochanteric osteotomy may be necessary to correct the deformity and allow bracing.

After undergoing any of the soft-tissue release procedures described above, the child should be immobilized in a hip spica cast for a period of two to three weeks. It is important to have the child stand in the cast for prolonged periods to decrease osteopenia and the pathologic fractures that can occur after cast removal. After cast removal, it is also important to institute a physical therapy program to improve the joint's range of motion, bracing to allow ambulation, and night splinting, in a total-body splint, to prevent recurrence of the deformities.

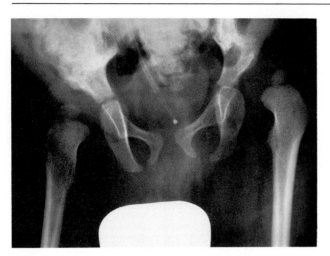 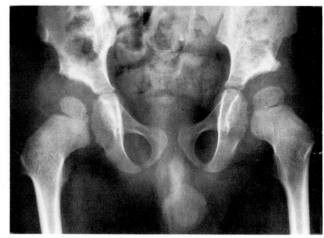

Fig. 1 Left, Radiograph of a 4-year-old child with L4-level myelomeningocele, bilateral hip dislocation, and severe acetabular dysplasia. **Right,** Same child, 18 months after an open reduction, Albee acetabuloplasty, and external oblique transfer.

Hip Dislocation and Subluxation

Hip dislocation or subluxation is common in children with myelomeningocele. About 50% of these patients will have a hip dislocation or subluxation during their growing years.

True congenital dislocations are seen in children with sacral level myelomeningocele, and teratologic dislocations are more common in children with myelomeningocele at the thoracic level. The most common type of hip subluxation and dislocation, however, is the paralytic type associated with low lumbar level myelomeningocele. This problem, which affects 50% to 75% of these children, is the result of an imbalance between strong hip flexors and adductors, innervated at L1 to L4, and weak or completely paralyzed hip abductors and extensors, innervated at L5 to S2.[5-11]

Several authors have questioned the concept of reducing dislocated hips.[12] Feiwell and associates[13,14] showed that reducing the hip did not improve its range of motion or reduce the amount of bracing necessary for ambulation. They believed it was more important to maintain a level pelvis and flexible hips than to reduce the hips.

There is little doubt that a dislocated hip associated with low lumbar level myelomeningocele in a child with normal balance and normal upper-extremity function will not deter this child from walking. Reducing the hips improves the quality of ambulation, decreases the need for external support, improves trunk alignment, and decreases the amount of energy required for walking. These goals are well accepted by Menelaus,[8] Lee and Carroll,[15] Yngve and Lindseth[16] and others. Lindseth reported that, of 47 patients who underwent triple transfer (adductor, external oblique, tensor fascia lata), 22 required less bracing after surgery and 28, com-

pared with eight before the surgery, were able to walk without a walker or crutches.[16]

It is established that bilateral or unilateral hip dislocation or subluxation associated with high level myelomeningocele does not require extensive surgical treatment.[8] Soft-tissue contractures should be corrected to permit bracing and allow some degree of ambulation. At maturity, most of these children will use a wheelchair or have very limited ability to walk.

If a child with low lumbar level myelomeningocele has bilateral hip subluxation and/or dislocation, surgical treatment is indicated. The exception to this rule is when the dislocation is high, associated with severe acetabular dysplasia. In this instance, because the procedure required to achieve stabilization—an extensive soft-tissue release, in association with pelvic and femoral procedures—has a high risk for complications, such as hip stiffness, and a low success rate, the surgery is contraindicated. On the other hand, if bony abnormalities are not severe and the dislocation is not high, an attempt should be made to reduce these hips surgically. A common problem with these children is a progressive hip flexion contracture that can markedly interfere with their mobility later in life.[15]

To achieve a high success rate, the following should be done at the time of surgery: (1) correct the muscle imbalance by muscle transfers—iliopsoas transfer[10] or external oblique transfer[17]; (2) release contractures; (3) correct bony deformities, such as acetabular dysplasia and coxa valga (Fig. 1); and (4) correct capsular laxity by capsular plication. It has been documented by Lee and Carroll[15] that the association of the iliopsoas transfer with adductor release and open reduction with capsulorrhaphy and acetabuloplasty leads to a high success rate (83%).

It is important to emphasize that such extensive pro-

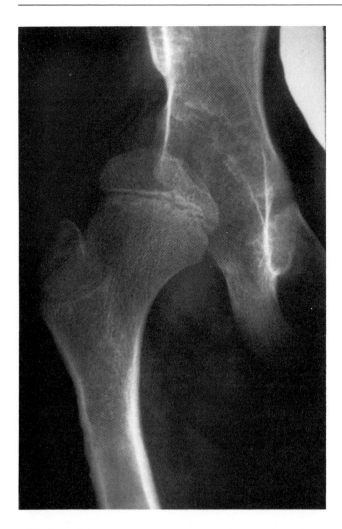 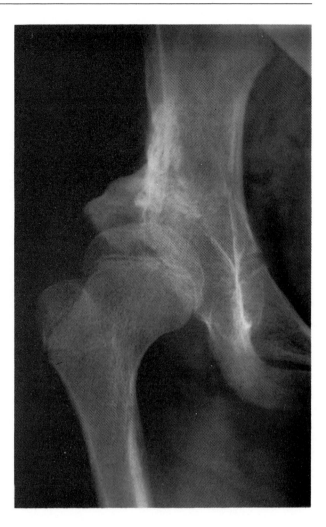

Fig. 2 **Left,** This 11-year-old child with L4-level myelomeningocele had significant hip subluxation and acetabular dysplasia. This patient had previously undergone external oblique transfer. **Right,** Eleven months after open reduction with a shelf procedure.

cedures are reserved for children who have demonstrated the ability to walk with a below-knee orthosis. Because this is rarely achieved by a child with spina bifida who is younger than 2 years of age, most of these operations will be performed on children older than 2 years.

Two types of muscle transfers available to the orthopaedic surgeon are the iliopsoas transfer to the greater trochanter, as described by Sharrard[18,19] and Menelaus,[20] and the external oblique transfer, as described originally by Thomas and associates,[17] and popularized by McKay,[21] Yngve and Lindseth,[16] and Dias and Nordland.[22] Two other muscle transfers, in addition to the above, are the adductor transfer to the ischium and the tensor fascia lata, as described by Yngve and Lindseth.[16]

I favor the external oblique transfer as a good substitute for paralyzed abductors of the hip. Because its nerve supply is not from the spinal segment that innervates the gluteus medius and minimus muscles, the external oblique is less likely to be paralyzed when these

muscles are. Its aponeurosis is long and broad, its surfaces are well adapted for gliding movement, and after transfer its mechanical action on the greater trochanter is direct.

The external oblique transfer has four advantages over the iliopsoas transfer: (1) A weak hip is not further weakened by eliminating the iliopsoas as a hip flexor. (2) Muscle power is added to the hip by taking the muscle from the abdominal wall, where its absence is well tolerated. (3) External oblique transfer functions synergistically; the iliopsoas transfer functions antagonistically. In electromyelographic gait studies in children who underwent this transfer, the external oblique muscle showed good activity during the swing and stance phase of the gait cycle. (4) The external oblique transfer does not violate the ilium, and pelvic osteotomies can be done without any technical difficulty.

In conjunction with the tendon transfer, any degree of adduction deformity present should be corrected by an extensive adductor release (longus, gracilis, and

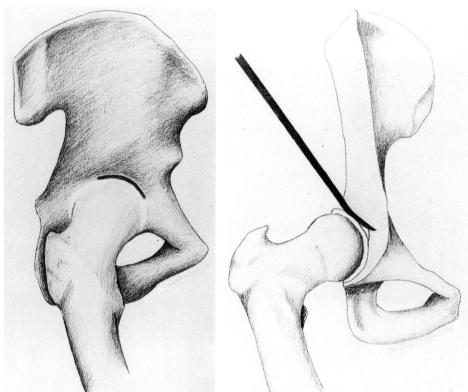

Fig. 3 **Left**, The costochondral junction, where the labrum is to be detached from the ilium. **Right**, The osteotome is inserted to push the labrum down, making space for the bone graft.

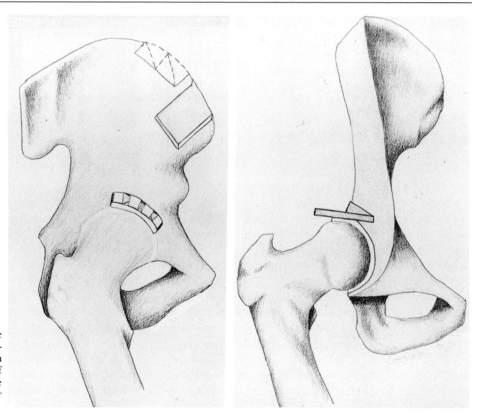

Fig. 4 **Left**, The triangular bone graft and the rectangular graft are inserted snugly, pushing the labrum down. **Right,** Anteroposterior view of Albee shelf with grafts in place. The rectangular graft will provide further lateral coverage.

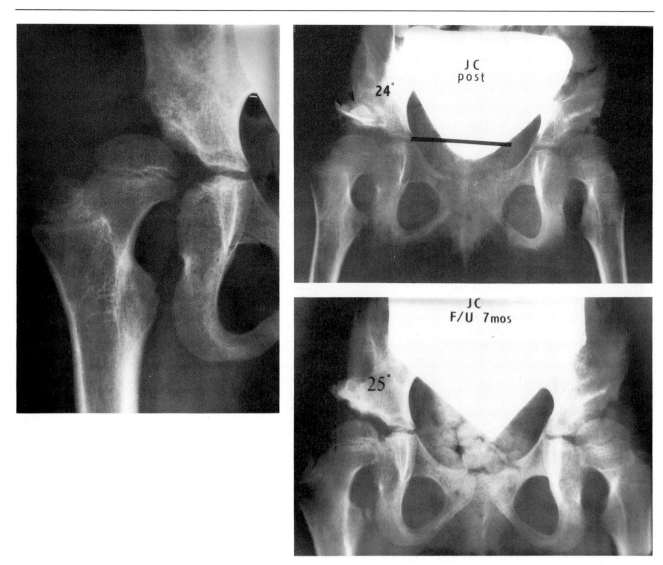

Fig. 5 Left, This 6-year-old child with L4-level myelomeningocele has hip subluxation and acetabular dysplasia. **Top right,** Eight weeks after surgery, the rectangular and triangular grafts can be seen clearly. **Bottom right,** Seven months after surgery the graft is well incorporated. Hip coverage is excellent.

brevis, if necessary). Correction of the acetabular dysplasia is important. The three types of pelvic procedures available are the Chiari pelvic osteotomy,[23] the shelf procedure (Fig. 2), as described by Staheli,[24] and the Albee shelf procedure. The Albee acetabuloplasty was first described in 1915.[25] Lee and Carroll[15] reported their experience in 1985. If exposure of the hip joint shows the acetabulum to be insufficient anteriorly and laterally, the insufficiency can be corrected by the following technique. By means of a freer-elevator or a 0.25-in osteotome at the costochondral junction (Fig. 3, *left*), between the labrum and the bony portion of the acetabulum, the labrum is gradually detached from the acetabulum to a depth of about 2 cm. At this point, the labrum is pushed down, making it fit more snugly over the femoral head (Fig. 3, *right*). Three triangular

pieces of bone graft are then removed from the ilium and placed parallel to each other, so that they push the labrum down laterally and anteriorly.

A modification of this technique was recently developed. A unicortical, rectangular bone graft, measuring approximately 2.5 by 3 cm, is removed from the ilium (Fig. 4, *left*). Before the triangular piece of bone graft is inserted, this rectangular piece is inserted so that it fits snugly into a slot in the ilium, with its cortical surface facing distally. The three triangular pieces are then inserted above it. Then, as in the shelf procedure, spongy bone is applied over the bone graft. After the graft is inserted, a snug, tight capsulorrhaphy is performed (Fig. 4, *right*). In children more than 6 years old, or when more than 20 to 30 degrees of abduction is necessary to maintain a concentric reduction of the hip, a varus derotation osteotomy is also indicated.

In my experience with this procedure over the last four years, a good radiologic result has been achieved in 81% of the cases. As described by Yngve and Lindseth,[16] at least 80% of the patients showed functional improvement (Fig. 5). Further studies will be necessary to determine the degree of functional improvement. The use of gait analysis before and after surgery may provide information that will allow better selection of patients. After surgery, the child is immobilized in a hip spica cast with the hip in abduction of 25 to 30 degrees, extension, and internal rotation. Six weeks later, the spica cast is removed and intensive physical therapy initiated for range of motion and ambulation. A total-body splint is applied to place the hips in 25 degrees of abduction and 15 to 20 degrees of internal rotation.

Hip subluxation and dislocation in spina bifida are difficult to treat. Redislocation is not unusual, no matter what procedure is performed to maintain reduction. Stiffness after a single surgical procedure is rare, but it is common after repeated operations. For this reason, it is important to obtain a concentric, stable reduction and a more balanced musculature with one operation.

Late hip dislocation associated with low lumbar or sacral level myelomeningocele should be viewed as a sign of unstable neurologic function, and the possibility of tethered cord syndrome must be evaluated carefully. If a tethered cord is diagnosed, it is important to release the tethered cord before proceeding with surgical treatment of the dislocated hip.

References

1. Curtis BH: The hip in the myelomeningocele child. *Clin Orthop* 1973;90:11–21.
2. Menelaus MB: The hip in myelomeningocele: Management directed towards a minimum number of operations and a minimum period of immobilisation. *J Bone Joint Surg* 1976;58B:448–452.
3. Ober FR: An operation for the relief of paralysis of the gluteus maximus muscle. *JAMA* 1927;88:1063–1064.
4. Yount CC: The role of the tensor fasciae femoris in certain deformities of the lower extremities. *J Bone Joint Surg* 1926;8:171–193.
5. Carroll NC: Hip instability in children with myelomeningocele. *Orthop Clin North Am* 1978;9:403–408.
6. Dias LS, Hill JA: Evaluation of treatment of hip subluxation in myelomeningocele by intertrochanteric varus derotation femoral osteotomy. *Orthop Clin North Am* 1980;11:31–37.
7. Donaldson WF: Hip problem in the child with myelomeningocele, in *American Academy of Orthopaedic Surgeons Symposium on Myelomeningocele*. St. Louis, CV Mosby, 1972, pp 176–185.
8. Menelaus MB: *Conditions Affecting the Hip: Paralytic Dislocation of the Hip in Orthopaedic Management of Spina Bifida Cystica*. Edinburgh, ES Livingstone, 1971.
9. Rueda J, Carroll NC: Hip instability in patients with myelomeningocele. *J Bone Joint Surg* 1972;54B:422–431.
10. Sharrard WJW: Congenital paralytic dislocation of the hip in children with myelo-meningocele, abstract. *J Bone Joint Surg* 1959;41B:622.
11. Sharrard WJW: *Pediatric Orthopaedics and Fractures*. Oxford, Blackwell Scientific Publications, 1971.
12. Barden GA, Meyer LC, Stelling FH III: Myelodysplastics: Fate of those followed for twenty years or more. *J Bone Joint Surg* 1975;57A:643–647.
13. Feiwell E, Sakai D, Blatt T: The effect of hip reduction on function in patients with myelomeningocele: Potential gains and hazards of surgical treatment. *J Bone Joint Surg* 1978;60A:169–173.
14. Feiwell E: Surgery of the hip in myelomeningocele as related to adult goals. *Clin Orthop* 1980;148:87–93.
15. Lee EH, Carroll NC: Hip stability and ambulatory status in myelomeningocele. *J Pediatr Orthop* 1985;5:522–527.
16. Yngve DA, Lindseth RE: Effectiveness of muscle transfer in myelomeningocele hips measured by radiographic indices. *J Pediatr Orthop* 1982;2:121–125.
17. Thomas LI, Thompson TC, Straub LR: Transplantation of the external oblique muscle for abductor paralysis. *J Bone Joint Surg* 1950;32A:207–217.
18. Sharrard WJW: Posterior iliopsoas transplantation in the treatment of paralytic dislocation of the hip. *J Bone Joint Surg* 1964;46B:426–444.
19. Sharrard WJW: Long-term follow-up of posterior iliopsoas transplant for paralytic dislocation of the hip, abstract. *J Bone Joint Surg* 1970;52B:779.
20. Menelaus MB: Posterior iliopsoas transfer, abstract. *J Bone Joint Surg* 1966;48B:592.
21. McKay DW: McKay hip stabilization in myelomeningocele. *Orthop Trans* 1977;1:87.
22. Dias LS, Nordland T: Triple transfer and varus osteotomy for hip subluxation and dislocation in spina bifida: A preliminary report. *Orthop Trans* 1987;11:50–51.
23. Chiari K: Medial displacement osteotomy of the pelvis. *Clin Orthop* 1974;98:55–71.
24. Staheli LT: Slotted acetabular augmentation. *J Pediatr Orthop* 1981;1:213–217.
25. Albee FH: The bone graft wedge: Its use in the treatment of relapsing, acquired and congenital dislocation of the hip. *NY State Med J* 1915;102:433–435.

Foot Deformities in Myelomeningocele

James C. Drennan, MD

Management of the patient with myelomeningocele has been considerably refined in the past decade.[1] The current emphasis is on improved functional outcomes, and it is now recognized that treating the total child in a multidisciplinary environment offers the best way of optimizing the functional outcome.

Foot deformities are the most common orthopaedic abnormality in patients with myelomeningocele. Approximately 85% of these children develop paralytic malformation secondary to neuromuscular imbalance.[2] The lower lumbar and sacral roots, which innervate the muscles of the foot and ankle, are the most common neurologic levels of paralysis in myelodysplasia. The muscle imbalance creates an uneven distribution of forces across the growth cartilage of the hindfoot bones (Hueter-Volkmann law). This imbalance causes severe

osseocartilaginous deformity and can further complicate the orthopaedic management of these patients. Lack of sensation is associated with undersized feet, and autonomic dysfunction causes vasomotor instability. Thickened capsules, which encompass the narrow joints, are caused by the absence of movement in utero.

The objectives of orthopaedic treatment are obtaining braceable plantigrade feet and muscle balance. Surgical correction and the use of orthotics are intended to allow the myelodysplastic child to approximate the expected motor milestones of the average child,[3] for example, to be able to stand by 12 months of age. Correction of foot deformities must be considered in the perspective of the total child and is of particular importance for patients with ambulatory potential.[4,5] To achieve long-term correction of a foot deformity, the

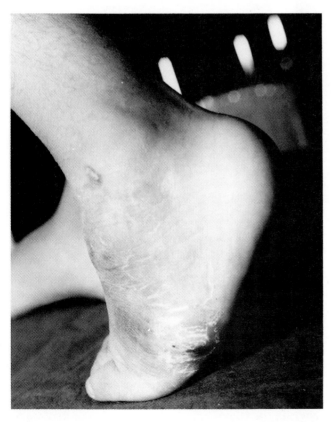 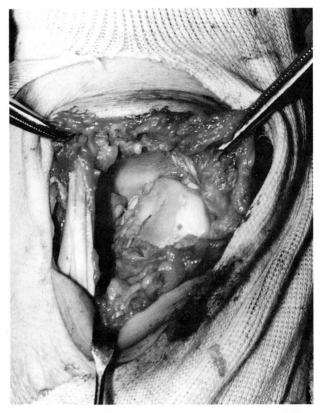

Fig. 1 **Left,** Rigid recurrent equinovarus deformity limits weightbearing to the lateral border of the forefoot with resultant soft-tissue ulceration under the base of the fifth metatarsus. **Right,** Talectomy permits satisfactory alignment of the hindfoot but does not address residual forefoot deformity.

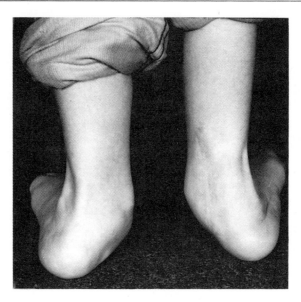

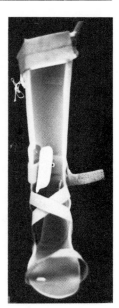

Fig. 2 Left, Severe hindfoot valgus results from overcorrection of talipes equinovarus. **Right,** The T-strap principle, added to a polypropylene ankle-foot orthosis, controls either hindfoot varus (illustrated) or valgus.

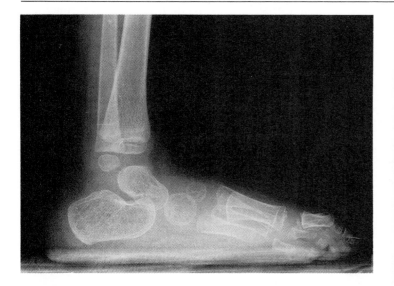

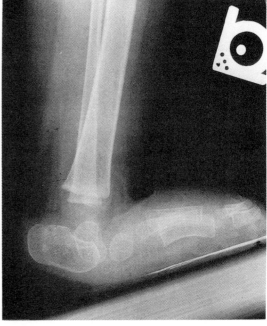

Fig. 3 Lateral views of congenital convex pes valgus demonstrate that the apex of deformity is in line with the anterior border of the tibia.

surgeon must understand the cause of the particular deformity and respect the possible risks of the proposed treatment.

Management, begun soon after birth, involves careful serial manipulations, and well-padded, long leg holding casts. The casts extend beyond the toes to protect the insensate digits from pressure ulceration. This casting gently stretches the contracted skin and neurovascular structures to keep them from limiting the degree of surgical correction. Surgery is generally re-

served until the child is 8 to 9 months of age, at which time the entire deformity is corrected with single procedure. After surgery, a four-month period of immobilization with long leg casts and Kirschner-wire fixation allows accommodation of the newly lengthened soft tissues and permits remodeling of the hindfoot bones by altering the compressive and tensive forces that act on the growth cartilage of the realigned hindfoot (Hueter-Volkmann law).

Familiarity with the general principles of both tendon

transfers and tenotomies will help the surgeon avoid the risk of recurrent deformity or the creation of a secondary iatrogenic muscle imbalance. Tenotomies are most appropriate when the individual muscle cannot be controlled voluntarily. The sole exception to this rule is the tibialis posterior, which should be lengthened to minimize the risk of creating iatrogenic hindfoot valgus. A single active muscle should be transferred to the midline to neutralize its rotational effect. As an example, an isolated tibialis anterior should be transferred to the os calcis both to correct the forefoot muscle imbalance and to assist in orthotic management. Bony procedures, limited to children over the age of 3 years, consist primarily of osteotomies to avoid further shortening of the small foot. Arthrodeses are generally contraindicated because they place additional rotational stress on the neighboring insensate joints. In rare cases, a Symes amputation may be necessary because of significant loss of bony architecture secondary to recurrent osteomyelitis.

Specific Types of Foot Deformity

Equinovarus

This rigid, severe form of clubfoot, most commonly found with an L4 level myelomeningocele, is associated with retained activity or contracture of the tibialis anterior and tibialis posterior muscles. After serial manipulations and castings, surgical correction is accomplished through a Cincinnati transverse incision.[6] The procedure includes extensive capsular and tendon releases, lengthening of the tibialis posterior and the Achilles tendons, and transfer of the active tibialis anterior to the dorsal midfoot. Feet with equinovarus can demonstrate a marked degree of subtalar rotational deformity. The traditional Turco technique[7] is inadequate because it does not allow sufficient subtalar rotation to correct the hindfoot alignment. After four months of K-wire fixation of the talocalcaneal and talonavicular joints, coupled with long leg casting, an ankle-foot orthosis is employed.

Recurrent or residual deformities can require additional surgery. Recurrent problems in a young child can be treated by a tedious repeat posteromedial release. If there is excessive surgical scarification of the medial heel soft tissue, a talectomy (Fig. 1) performed through an anterolateral approach may be more appropriate.[8] Residual hindfoot varus can be corrected by the Dwyer closing calcaneal osteotomy.

Children with myelomeningocele assume a tripod upright stance with a wide standing base. This posture, coupled with the loss of tibialis posterior power through injudicious tenotomy or transfer, can lead to the development of progressive secondary hindfoot valgus and overload the medial malleolar skin (Fig. 2).[9] This unfortunate complication may be improved by a

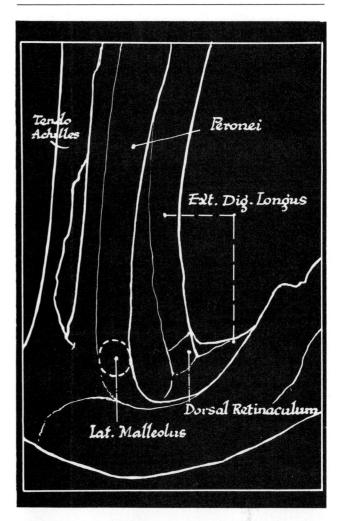

Fig. 4 The subluxed perinei and contracted dorsal retinaculum at the apex of the rigid deformity. (Reproduced with permission from Drennan JC, Sharrard WJW: The pathological anatomy of convex pes valgus. *J Bone Joint Surg* 1971;53B:457.)

medial displacement, horizontal calcaneal osteotomy.[10] In children more than 5 years of age, residual forefoot adduction can be managed by metatarsal osteotomies or by appropriate shortening of the lateral column of the foot through the os calcis or cuboid. Ankle arthrodesis and triple arthrodesis should be avoided because of the considerable risk of neuropathic joints developing, both proximal and distal to the site of the arthrodesis.

Congenital Convex Pes Valgus

Congenital vertical talus is characterized by a rigid hindfoot equinus and forefoot dorsiflexion and eversion.[11] The dislocation of the navicular onto the anterior talar neck occurs at the apex of the medial longitudinal arch. A more severe rocker-bottom deformity develops when the lateral longitudinal arch demonstrates an accompanying dislocation of the calcaneocuboid joint. Paresis of the tibialis posterior muscle is believed to cause this severe foot deformity. The hind-foot is plantar-flexed directly beneath the tibia, and the midfoot dorsal dislocation occurs in a direct line with the anterior border of the tibia. The contracted dorsal retinaculum acts as the fulcrum about which the fore-foot is drawn into dorsiflexion. This fixed deformity is exacerbated by the peroneal tendons, which bowstring across the midfoot and act as perverted dorsiflexors as well as everters (Figs. 3 and 4).

After pulmonary soft-tissue serial casting, surgical correction is undertaken when the child is 9 months of age through a Cincinnati incision that can be extended laterally to include the calcaneocuboid joint. In a one-stage open reduction, all extrinsic muscles to the foot are lengthened, except for the tibialis posterior muscle, which is shortened. To balance the hindfoot and fore-foot musculature, the tibialis anterior is transferred to the talar neck and the peroneus longus is transferred to the navicular. This complex surgery requires exten-sive capsular releases, particularly when the calcaneo-cuboid joint is dislocated. The choice of two- or three-pin K-wire fixation is determined by the presence or absence of calcaneocuboid deformity. After plaster im-mobilization, the patient is fitted with an ankle-foot orthosis, which includes a modified Gillette heel[12] to guard against recurrent hindfoot valgus. If surgery is delayed until the child is more than 5 years of age, the surgeon may have to excise the navicular to shorten the excessively lengthened medial longitudinal arch. Occasionally an older child requires an extra-articular subtalar arthrodesis in concert with staged metatarsal osteotomies to correct residual hindfoot valgus.

Equinus Deformity

Equinus can develop because of failure to protect a flail foot from the plantar-producing effects of gravity or because of retained sacral reflex activity in the un-opposed triceps surae and long-toe flexors. Flail equinus is best treated by use of proper prophylactically weightbearing foot-positioning and ankle-foot orthot-ics, which extend beneath the toes to prevent the de-velopment of forefoot equinus. Mild deformity is man-aged by repeat manipulation and serial casting until the foot can be properly maintained in an ankle-foot or-

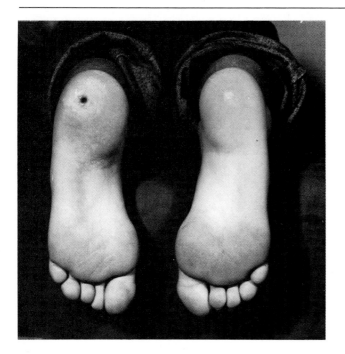

Fig. 5 Active teenagers who lack protective sensation, have in-creasing rigid foot deformity, and develop inadequate distribution of weightbearing over the diminished plantar surfaces are susceptible to clinical problems related to pes cavus.

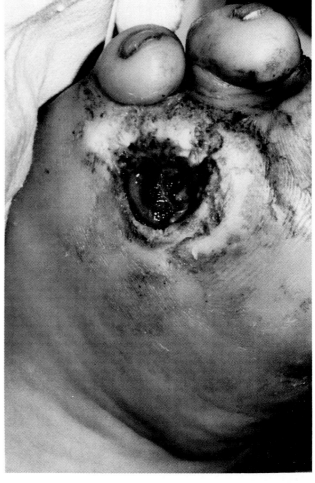

thosis. Paralytic equinus in excess of 20 degrees of fixed plantar flexion requires posterior release to permit proper orthotic fittings. Reflex equinus is less common, is more difficult to manage, and has a tendency to recur. Radical excision of 2 to 4 cm of the offending tendons can be performed early, with repeated efforts directed towards a formal transfer of the tendons into the distal tibia.[13]

Cavus

Calcaneal cavus progresses rapidly because of the unopposed retained activity of the long-toe dorsiflexors and tibialis anterior. The os calcis drifts into dorsiflexion, which shortens the posterior level arm of the os tuber as the calcaneus migrates beneath the tibia. The most appropriate management is early transfer of the conjoined tendon of the tibialis anterior and the hypertrophied peroneus tertius through the interosseous membrane to the os calcis. The other dorsiflexors are selectively lengthened. For older children, a Mitchell posterior displacement calcaneal osteotomy,[14] combined with metatarsal osteotomies, offers an effective option.

Pes cavus describes forefoot equinus, which is generally not a problem until adolescence, when plantar ulceration secondary to excessive localized skin pressure can develop under the os calcis or metatarsal heads (Fig. 5). Shoe fitting can also be difficult. The hindfoot is in neutral alignment, and the forefoot deformity can be managed by appropriate metatarsal osteotomies and use of orthotics.

Cock-up Toe Deformities

Cock-up toe deformity, most common in the great toe, reflects a loss of intrinsic muscle stability of the metatarsophalangeal joint. The problem includes hyperextension of the metatarsophalangeal joint as well as fixed flexion of the interphalangeal joint. Surgical management includes lengthening the extensor hallucis longus, dorsal metatarsophalangeal capsulotomy, and tenodesis of the long-toe flexor to the first phalanx. K-wire fixation is required for four weeks.

Hindfoot valgus

Weightbearing anteroposterior and lateral radiographs are used to determine whether the hindfoot valgus is located at the level of the ankle joint or in the subtalar area. Ankle valgus in excess of 7 degrees requires surgical management to avoid progressive skin embarrassment over the medial malleolus. Tenodesis of the Achilles tendon to the distal fibula is recommended in patients under the age of 8 years.[15] For patients between the ages of 8 and 12 years, multiple, small sta-

plings on the distal medial tibial epiphysis can be effective.[16] In older adolescents, a closing wedge supramalleolar osteotomy corrects ankle valgus. In this age group, this type of supramalleolar osteotomy prevents migration of the correction, which would result in progressive distal tibial diaphyseal deformity. For pure rotational correction, the procedure can be successfully employed in patients as young as 4 years of age.[17] Hindfoot valgus localized to the subtalar joint is best managed by a medial displacement calcaneal osteotomy.

References

1. Drennan JC, Banta JV, Bunch WH, et al: Symposium: Current concepts in the management of myelomeningocele. *Contemp Orthop* 1989;19:63–88.
2. Sharrard WJW, Grosfield I: The management of deformity and paralysis of the foot in myelomeningocele. *J Bone Joint Surg* 1968; 50B:456–465.
3. Drennan JC, Bondurant M: Paralytic disorders, in *American Academy of Orthopaedic Surgeons Atlas of Orthotics*, ed 2. St. Louis, CV Mosby, 1985, pp 322–330.
4. Asher M, Olson J: Factors affecting the ambulatory status of patients with spina bifida cystica. *J Bone Joint Surg* 1983;65A: 350–356.
5. Hoffer MM, Feiwell E, Perry R, et al: Functional ambulation in patients with myelomeningocele. *J Bone Joint Surg* 1973;55A: 137–148.
6. Crawford AH, Marxen JL, Osterfeld DL: The Cincinnati incision: A comprehensive approach for surgical procedures of the foot and ankle in childhood. *J Bone Joint Surg* 1982;64A:1355–1358.
7. Turco VJ: Resistant congenital club foot: One-stage posteromedial release with internal fixation. A follow-up report of a fifteen-year experience. *J Bone Joint Surg* 1979;61A:805–814.
8. Menelaus MB: Talectomy for equinovarus deformity in arthrogryposis and spina bifida. *J Bone Joint Surg* 1971;53B:468–473.
9. Lin RS: Application of the varus T-strap principle to the polypropylene ankle foot orthosis. *Orthot Prosthet* 1982;36:67–70.
10. Koutsogiannis E: Treatment of mobile flat foot by displacement osteotomy of the calcaneus. *J Bone Joint Surg* 1971;53B:96–100.
11. Drennan JC, Sharrard WJW: The pathological anatomy of convex pes valgus. *J Bone Joint Surg* 1971;53B:455–461.
12. Colson JM: An effective orthotic design for controlling the unstable subtalar joint. *Orthot Prosthet* 1979;33:39–49.
13. Drennan JC: *Orthopaedic Management of Neuromuscular Disorders*. Philadelphia, JB Lippincott, 1983.
14. Mitchell GP: Posterior displacement osteotomy of the calcaneus. *J Bone Joint Surg* 1977;59B:233–235.
15. Dias LS: Ankle valgus in children with myelomeningocele. *Dev Med Child Neurol* 1978;20:627–633.
16. Burkus JK, Moore DW, Raycroft JF: Valgus deformity of the ankle in myelodysplastic patients: Correction by stapling of the medial part of the distal tibial physis. *J Bone Joint Surg* 1983; 65A:1157–1162.
17. McNicol D, Leong JC, Hsu LC: Supramalleolar derotation osteotomy for lateral tibial torsion and associated equinovarus deformity of the foot. *J Bone Joint Surg* 1983;65B:166–170.

Index

Cumulative Index
Volumes 26 through 40

Volumes 36 through 40 of the Instructional
Course Lectures were published by the
American Academy of Orthopaedic
Surgeons, Park Ridge, Illinois. Volumes 26
through 35 were published by the C.V.
Mosby Company, St. Louis, Missouri.

Instructional Course Lectures

Volume number	Year published	Editor
XXVI	1977	H. Andrew Wissinger, MD
XXVII	1978	H. Andrew Wissinger, MD
XXVIII	1979	Reginald R. Cooper, MD
XXIX	1980	Hanes H. Brindley, MD
XXX	1981	David G. Murray, MD
XXXI	1982	Victor H. Frankel, MD
XXXII	1983	C. McCollister Evarts, MD
XXXIII	1984	John A. Murray, MD
XXXIV	1985	E. Shannon Stauffer, MD
XXXV	1986	Lewis D. Anderson, MD
XXXVI	1987	Paul P. Griffin, MD
XXXVII	1988	Frank H. Bassett III, MD
XXXVIII	1989	Joseph S. Barr, Jr., MD
XXXIX	1990	Walter B. Greene, MD
XL	1991	Hugh S. Tullos, MD

Author Index

A

ADELAAR RS: Fractures of the talus, 39:147

ADELAAR RS: The treatment of tarsometatarsal fracture-dislocation, 39:141

AGUILAR EA, SWOOP TF, DABEZIES EJ, D'AMBROSIA RD: Clinical research database system for orthopaedic surgery, 38:429

ALKER G: Radiographic evaluation of patients with cervical spine injury, 36:473

ALLEN BL Jr: Spinal instrumentation: Part II. Segmental spinal instrumentation with L-rods, 32:202

ALLMAN FL Jr: Rehabilitative exercises in sports medicine, 34:389

ALONSO JE, HUGHES JL: External fixation of the femur, 39:199

ALTCHEK DW, SKYHAR MJ, WARREN RF: Shoulder arthroscopy for shoulder instability, 38:187

AMSTUTZ HC: Fixation failure and techniques of revision surgery in total hip replacement, 30:414

AMSTUTZ HC, GRAFF-RADFORD A: THARIES approach to surface replacement of hip, 30:422

ANDERSON LD, MEYER FN: Nonunion of the diaphysis of the radius and ulna, 37:157

ANDERSON TE, CIOLEK J: Specific rehabilitation programs for the throwing athlete, 38:487

ANDREWS JR: Bony injuries about the elbow in the throwing athlete, 34:323

ANDREWS JR: See HUNTER LY, 31:126

ANDREWS JR: See McCUE FC III, 26:103

ANDRIACCHI TP: Evaluation of surgical procedures and/or joint implants with gait analysis, 39:343

ANSPACH WE Jr: Barrier materials and special air-handling systems for bacteriologic control in the operating room, 26:47

ARNOCZKY SP: Basic science of anterior cruciate ligament repair and reconstruction, 40:201

ARONSON J: Osteoarthritis of the young adult hip: Etiology and treatment, 35:119

ARONSON J, HARP JH Jr: Factors influencing the choice of external fixation for distraction osteogenesis, 39:175

B

BAILEY RW: Instability of the cervical spine, 27:159

BAILEY RW: Rheumatoid arthritis and spondylitis rhizomélique, 27:173

BAILEY RW: See SMITH WS, 27:179

BASSETT CAL: Un-united fractures: Part I. Pulsing electromagnetic fields. A nonoperative method to produce bony union, 31:88

BASSETT GS: Lower-extremity abnormalities in dwarfing conditions, 39:389

BASSETT GS: Orthopaedic aspects of skeletal dysplasias, 39:381

BAUER GCH: Treatment of gonarthrosis, 31:152

BEATY JH: Legg-Calvé-Perthes disease: Diagnostic and prognostic techniques, 38:291

BEHRENS F: External fixation in children: Lower extremity, 39:205

BEHRENS F: External fixation: Special indications and techniques, 39:173

BEHRENS F: External skeletal fixation: Part A. Introduction to external skeletal fixation, 30:112

BEHRENS F: External skeletal fixation: Part B. Basic concepts, 30:118

BEHRENS F: External skeletal fixation: Part E. Bone grafting. General principles and use in open fractures, 30:152

BEHRENS F: External skeletal fixation: Part H. Complications of external skeletal fixation, 30:179

BEHRENS F: External skeletal fixation: Part I. Basic concepts and applications in open tibial fractures, 33:124

BEHRENS F, JONES RE III, FISCHER DA: External skeletal fixation: Part C. External fixator application, 30:125

BEHRENS F, MEARS DC, JONES RE III: External skeletal fixation: Part F. External fixation in open fractures, 30:156

BEISAW NE: See PAIEMENT GD, 39:413

BELL T: The art of being understood: Part I. The art of being understood, 32:1

BELLE RM: See HAWKINS RJ, 38:211

BEN-MENACHEM Y: Massive blunt trauma: Radiologic diagnosis and intervention, 35:31

BEN-MENACHEM Y: Pelvic fractures: Diagnostic and therapeutic angiography, 37:139

BENNETT J: See TULLOS HS, 35:69

BENNETT JB: See TULLOS HS, 30:185

BENNETT JB: See TULLOS HS, 33:364

BENSON DR, KEENEN TL: Evaluation and treatment of trauma to the vertebral column, 39:577

BERNREUTER WK: See DUNHAM WK, 38:419

BIGLIANI LU: Treatment of two- and three-part fractures of the proximal humerus, 38:231

BLACK JD: See GREENWALD AS, 30:301

BLAHA JD, NELSON CL, FREVERT LF, HENRY SL, SELIGSON D, ESTERHAI JL Jr, HEPPENSTAL RB, CALHOUN J, COBOS J, MADER J: The use of Septopal (polymethylmethacrylate beads with gentamicin) in the treatment of chronic osteomyelitis, 39:509

BLAIR SJ: Evaluation of impairment of hand and upper extremity function: Part A. Foreword, 38:73

E

F

N

Subject Index

For each entry, the number preceding the colon is the volume number and the number following the colon is the first page of the chapter in which the key word is discussed.

A

Acetabulum

Abnormal growth and development of the pediatric hip, 34:423

Bone grafting in revision total hip arthroplasty, 40:177

Congenital hip dislocation: Techniques for primary open reduction including femoral shortening, 38:343

Fracture treatment for the multiply injured patient, 35:13

Fractures of the pelvic ring and acetabulum in patients with severe polytrauma, 39:591

Management of unstable pathologic fractures—dislocations of the spine and acetabulum, secondary to metastatic malignancy, 29:51

Principles, techniques, results, and complications with a porous-coated sintered metal system, 35:169

Revision total hip arthroplasty for aseptic component loosening, tilting, and/or migration: Part D. Revision of total hip arthroplasty for aseptic loosening. The acetabulum, 35:157

Surgical management of acetabular fractures, 35:382

Achondroplasia

Lower-extremity abnormalities in dwarfing conditions, 39:389

Orthopaedic aspects of skeletal dysplasias, 39:381

Spinal deformity in short-stature syndromes, 39:399

Acquired immune deficiency syndrome

Acquired immune deficiency syndrome associated with hemophilia in the United States, 38:357

Blood conservation techniques in orthopaedic surgery, 39:425

Blood products: Optimal use, conservation, and safety, 39:431

Allen test

Current status of noninvasive techniques in the diagnosis of upper extremity disorders: Part I. Evaluation of vascular competency, 32:61

Allergy

Antimicrobial treatment of orthopaedic sepsis, 26:24

Amputation

Current concepts in above-knee socket design, 39:373

Evaluation of impairment of hand and upper extremity: Part B. Evaluation of impairment, 38:73

Management of open fractures and complications: Part II. Management of open fractures and complications, 31:64

Management of the diabetic-neurotrophic foot: Part I. Diabetic-neurotrophic foot. Diagnosis and treatment, 28:118

Management of the diabetic-neurotrophic foot: Part II. A classification and treatment program for diabetic, neuropathic, and dysvascular foot problems, 28:143

Microsurgical techniques in vessel and nerve repair: Part II. Replantation of amputated hands and digits, 27:15

New concepts in lower-limb amputation and prosthetic management, 39:361

Overview of prosthetic feet, 39:367

Surgical techniques for conserving tissue and function in lower-limb amputation for trauma, infection, and vascular disease, 39:355

The orthopaedist as prosthetic team leader: Getting the best for your patient from the team, 39:353

Anatomy and physiology

Acute shoulder dislocations: Factors influencing diagnosis and treatment, 33:364

Adult forefoot: Part III. Rupture of the tibialis posterior tendon, 33:302

Advances in our understanding of the implant-bone interface: Factors affecting formation and degeneration, 40:101

Anatomy and kinematics of the elbow, 40:11

Ankle fractures with diastasis, 39:95

Arthroscopic anatomy and how to see it, 27:127

Articular cartilage, 32:349

Assessment of pelvic stability, 37:119

Basic science of anterior cruciate ligament repair and reconstruction, 40:201

Blood supply to bone and proximal femur: A synopsis, 37:27

Bone grafting in revision total hip arthroplasty, 40:177

Bone structure and function, 36:27

Comminuted fractures of the distal radius, 39:255

Compartment syndromes of the foot, 39:127

Compartment syndromes: Part A. Pathophysiology of compartment syndromes, 38:463

Compartment syndromes: Part B. The diagnosis and management of chronic compartment syndrome, 38:466

Computerized tomography of spinal trauma and degenerative disease, 34:85

Condylocephalic nailing of intertrochanteric and subtrochanteric fractures of the femur: Part II. Condylocephalic nailing of intertrochanteric fractures, 29:29

Congenital clubfoot: Pathoanatomy and treatment, 36:117

Congenital hip dislocation: Techniques for primary open reduction including femoral shortening, 38:343

Congenital malformations and deformities of the hand: Part A. General concepts, 38:31

Current concepts in snap-fit, sloppy-hinge total elbow arthroplasty, 40:61

Current management of clubfoot, 31:218

Current status of noninvasive techniques in the diagnosis

E

Fracture-dislocation

G

Histiocytoma

History of medicine

Humerus

Hyperemia

Hypertrophy

I

J

K

M

O

P

R

T

W